PUBLIC POLICY AND CANADIAN NURSING

PUBLIC POLICY AND CANADIAN NURSING

LESSONS FROM THE FIELD

MICHAEL J. VILLENEUVE

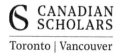

CANADIAN
SCHOLARS

Toronto | Vancouver

Public Policy and Canadian Nursing: Lessons from the Field
By Michael J. Villeneuve

First published in 2017 by
Canadian Scholars
425 Adelaide Street West, Suite 200
Toronto, Ontario
M5V 3C1

www.canadianscholars.ca

Library and Archives Canada Cataloguing in Publication

Villeneuve, Michael J. (Michael Jon), 1959-, author
        Public policy and Canadian nursing : lessons from the field / Michael J. Villeneuve.

Includes bibliographical references and index.
Issued in print and electronic formats.
ISBN 978-1-55130-970-5 (softcover).--ISBN 978-1-55130-972-9 (EPUB).--ISBN 978-1-55130-971-2 (PDF)

1. Medical policy--Canada. 2. Nursing--Canada. I. Title.

RA395.C3V55 2017   362.10971   C2017-902095-1
                                             C2017-902096-X

Cover and interior design by Elisabeth Springate

Printed and bound in Canada by Webcom

Canadä

MIX
Paper from
responsible sources
FSC® C004071

TABLE OF CONTENTS

LIST OF COMMON ABBREVIATIONS

Some of the following common abbreviations used in this text.

ACEN	Academy of Canadian Executive Nurses
ANA	American Nurses Association
ARNBC	Association of Registered Nurses of British Columbia
ARNM	Association of Registered Nurses of Manitoba
ARNNL	Association of Registered Nurses of Newfoundland and Labrador
ARNPEI	Association of Registered Nurses of Prince Edward Island
CAAPN	Canadian Association of Advanced Practice Nurses
CANR	Canadian Association for Nursing Research
CARNA	College and Association of Registered Nurses of Manitoba
CASN	Canadian Association of Schools of Nursing
CASW	Canadian Association of Social Workers
CCPNR	Canadian Council of Practical Nurse Regulators
CCRNR	Canadian Council of Registered Nurse Regulators
CDA	Canadian Dental Association
CFHI	Canadian Foundation for Healthcare Improvement
CFNU	Canadian Federation of Nurses Unions
CHI	Canada Health Infoway
CIHI	Canadian Institute for Health Information
CMA	Canadian Medical Association
CNA	Canadian Nurses Association
CNAC	Canadian Nursing Advisory Committee
CNF	Canadian Nurses Foundation
CNO	College of Nurses of Ontario
CNPI	Canadian Nurse Practitioner Initiative
CNPS	Canadian Nurses Protective Society
CNSA	Canadian Nursing Students' Association
COF	Council of the Federation
CPhA	Canadian Pharmacists Association
CPHA	Canadian Public Health Association
CPSI	Canadian Patient Safety Institute
CRNBC	College of Registered Nurses of British Columbia
CRNE	Canadian Registered Nurse Examination
CRNM	College of Registered Nurses of Manitoba
CRNNS	College of Registered Nurses of Nova Scotia
HHR	Health Human Resources
ICN	International Council of Nurses
IHI	Institute for Healthcare Improvement
MDGs	Millennium Development Goals
MHCC	Mental Health Commission of Canada
NANB	Nurses Association of New Brunswick
NCLEX–RN	National Council Licensure Examination for Registered Nurses
OECD	Organisation for Economic Co–operation and Development
OIIQ	Ordre des infirmières et des infirmiers du Québec
ONP	Office of Nursing Policy (Health Canada)
RCPSC	Royal College of Physicians and Surgeons of Canada
RNAO	Registered Nurses Association of Ontario
RNANTNU	Registered Nurses Association of the Northwest Territories and Nunavut
RPNAO	Registered Practical Nurses Association of Ontario
RPNRC	Registered Psychiatric Nurse Regulators of Canada
SDGs	Sustainable Development Goals
SRNA	Saskatchewan Registered Nurses Association
TRCC	Truth and Reconciliation Commission of Canada
UN	United Nations
WHA	World Health Assembly
WHO	World Health Organization
YRNA	Yukon Registered Nurses Association

ACKNOWLEDGEMENTS

One of the greatest supports in my life and career has been the gift of great teachers. From kindergarten to graduate school, I had the good fortune to run into a steady stream of superb educators—women and men of very high standards who were caring, smart, and tough. They opened my mind to the whole world. I cannot say enough about the value of great teachers and a rigorous education. I owe much of my success to their hard, loving work in helping me start life with a solid foundation.

I am deeply grateful for the people throughout my career who coached me, disciplined me a time or two, and helped me learn life lessons along the way. I especially had a lot of guidance after landing in Ottawa, in the year 2000, in my first formal policy role, and I learned so much from the amazingly bright, generous team of people who make up the elected officials and public service at Health Canada. Their impact is with me every day, and I want to thank them all.

In the preparation of this book, I was blessed to have the generous input of the four, anonymous, external reviewers, who each gave so much time and thoughtful attention to the feedback they provided. And I was well supported by the entire team at Canadian Scholars. I offer a deep nod of gratitude to each of them, and any errors and inconsistencies in the final narrative are mine entirely. I am also sincerely thankful to Gail Donner and Kathleen MacMillan for making time to review the book and for their very kind words of support.

Finally, like my teachers, my parents—Ron and Vivian Villeneuve—were fully behind me from day one. Unapologetic in their tough-love approach to life, they surrounded their three children with aunts, uncles, and godparents who held the same kinds of values. None of them were wealthy people; my mother started her adult life as a rural, one-room-schoolhouse teacher and my father sold insurance. They set high expectations of their kids and put in place whatever supports they could afford to help us achieve whatever we wanted in life. The goals were ours. But whatever they were, failure was not an option. I know they would be proud of this book, and I dedicate it with a lot of love in their memory.

PREFACE

"If nurses mobilize, change could happen overnight. We do not have the right to be uninvolved."
— *Marion Dewar, CM, former mayor of Ottawa and former public health nurse*

The notions that *every nurse is a leader* and *every nurse is an advocate* have become entrenched across Canadian nursing over the past quarter century. While these are laudable ideas, evidence that the great body of nurses is equipped to take on either role comfortably and effectively is much less certain.

The public image of nursing in Canada is strong; Canadians accord registered nurses in Canada and the United States tremendous levels of trust—in many polls higher than any other occupational group. But the lack of comfort many nurses feel in tackling the politics of leadership, administration, and policy development reveals that something is missing in their education and socialization, the translation of learning to practice, structures for support and opportunity, or perhaps elements of all of these.

Canada's Margaret Hilson was honoured with the first International Achievement Award of the Florence Nightingale International Foundation at the centennial meeting of the International Council of Nurses in 1999. When accepting the award she implored, "To really improve the health of a people, as nurses we must be more than health service providers; we must be political activists and agents of change."[1] A year later, leaders of the Canadian Nurses Association (CNA) said: "If we think of health as something broadly defined and influenced, we begin to arrive at the inescapable conclusion that to be concerned with health is to be concerned with the social context, and that nursing is, indeed, a political act."[2] So while effective nurses have always been smart political actors, the gauntlet was laid down explicitly coming into the 21st century, and most leading nursing organizations are well aligned with that position today.

What does this mean for nursing students and for nurses in practice today? Things are slowly changing, in that a growing number of undergraduate programs now include more education in the area of health systems and health policy. Many nursing graduate programs now offer similar courses that may be optional or even required—especially programs focused in the leadership and administration sector. Students in the Master of Science in Nursing program at Trinity Western University in British Columbia, for example, take part in a one-week residency in Ottawa focused on policy and politics as a mandatory component of their education. The Master of Nursing program in Health Systems Leadership and Administration at the University of Toronto now requires all students to complete a course in health systems and health policy development, and graduate students in the clinical programs can choose the course as an elective. Undergraduate students in the faculty also study health systems and public policy.

There are other examples, of course, but the reality is that most newly graduated registered nurses still say they have limited exposure during their undergraduate education to understanding the structure, governance, economics, and politics of the health care systems in which it is hoped they will spend a career. If they do study content in this area, it competes with the immediate pressures of clinical learning and impending registration examinations—all of which might sideline the political advocacy and policy side of nursing in the long list of priorities for the majority of students. The problem is that for most nurses, such learning is never formally picked up again; as they move into professional roles, nurses are pulled, quite understandably, into advanced learning within specialty streams like mental health, critical care, or public health nursing. And here too the policy side of the work may take a back seat to pressing clinical and care issues.

The result is both clear and worrying: in a blunt 2010 commentary, Steven Lewis—who has emerged as one of Canada's most astute health policy experts and commentators—summarized the problem by observing that "nursing's combination of numbers, reputation and reach should translate into power and influence over how health care is financed, organized and delivered. Yet politically, the profession punches below its weight. The country is the worse for it."[3]

Lewis's assertion finds uneasy company in the reality that the world's 18 million-plus nurses—typically the largest sector of health professionals and the largest group of educated women in most countries—can sometimes seem nearly invisible in the arenas of public policy deliberation and legislation in their nations. Speaking to the debate over health care reform that began in the late 1990s, health journalist André Picard said that "the collective voice of Canada's ... nurses has largely been ignored, often with devastating results."[4] Commonly in most countries, nurses hold the burden of delivering on (or responding to the consequences of) many of the health and social policy choices made by politicians and other senior decision makers—more than likely men who rarely have education or experience in health sciences, and who are almost never a nurse.

In a poll of Canadians leading up to the October 2015 federal election, two-thirds of respondents said they believed nurses should exert a greater role in improving the health care system.[5] (Only 37 per cent of Canadians said politicians should do so.) Nurses should expect to have a seat at every table where public policy decisions are being made that will impact their everyday practice. But they must be prepared and willing to act effectively in that seat, not just keep it warm. Policy is a tough game and nurses have fierce competitors at those decision-making tables that are only too happy to speak up. Liaschenko and Peter[6] urged nurses to "exercise power more deliberately," not through domination but by taking their places appropriately in the discourse, being able to speak and command respect, and holding themselves and others accountable. The challenge can be daunting, but as Maggie Kuhn—who founded the Gray Panthers movement in the United States—famously said, "Stand before the people you fear and speak your mind, even if your voice shakes."[7] Understanding more about public policy, especially about evidence-informed policy, can bolster a skill set to embolden the soul and perhaps help steady the shaky voice at least a little.

Nurses and their associations can play an important role in amplifying individual and disparate voices; it was at the 1998 CNA convention in Ottawa that the former federal health minister, the Honourable Monique Bégin, encouraged nurses to "think big and say it loud."[8] She implied then that nurses had not fully mined or exploited their significant political power. In the presence of the sitting federal minister of health, the Honourable Allan Rock, she publicly pushed CNA to ramp up nursing activity around lobbying and advocacy.[9]

In its final report in 2012, the National Expert Commission concluded with enthusiasm that, through their numbers and collective knowledge, nurses "are a mighty force for change."[10] But given Lewis's pointed observation cited earlier, a note of caution about that cheer is warranted. As former CNA executive director (1981–1989) and later president (2000–2002) Ginette Lemire Rodger said, "We are so potentially powerful and influential.… If we can focus and hone that energy … we will truly be a political force to be reckoned with in Canada."[11] So perhaps it might more accurately be said that, with the right knowledge, supports, and coalitions, nurses have the *potential* to be "a mighty force for change." It is the gap between those two ideas that this book hopes to help narrow.

WHAT IS THIS BOOK ALL ABOUT?

Myriad excellent publications already exist in the public policy, governance, and politics canon—some from this same publishing house—and many of them are cited in this book. So while pieces of the same material will necessarily be covered, it is not the intention of this book simply to restate what others have already so ably written. Indeed, many of the topics merit and already are explored in entire books on their own. For example, the areas of First Nations, Inuit, and Métis history, colonization, and governance, and how they interlink to health and social outcomes today merit a depth of expertise and volumes of work that are beyond the parameters of this text.

The same can be said of the complex and complicated issue of gender in nursing. This new resource hopes to introduce and frame some of the important pieces of theory, evidence, and opinion from and about the world of public policy in a context that applies to the thinking, practice, and experiences of Canadian nursing—offering nurses a taste of the most salient issues. From there, nurses may look more deeply into various topic areas using the many references and additional policy resources suggested.

Nursing has had a long-standing influence on health system programs and policy, but there is a need to extend our collective reach and become more purposeful and strategic in our actions. That is no small task to take on. When she was new to her role as executive director of the federal Office of Nursing Policy,

A Few Words About Evidence

A great deal of evidence is presented in this text, but it is important to acknowledge from the outset that while credible evidence is important to policy development, it is only one force informing policy. Furthermore, evidence is not (or not always) neutral; like other inputs, it may be laden with values and biases, and interpreting it may be similarly affected. Commenting in 2012 on evidence and policy, Humphreys and Piot argued that "there is no such thing as evidence based policy, only 'evidence informed' policy."[12] They reminded policy students and decision makers that scientists make mistakes too—and even if no errors are made, we see old "facts" overtaken by new evidence all the time. Moreover, they suggested, "Conflating facts and values allows scientists to use their authority inappropriately—that is, to cloak their effort to make society live by their values as a disinterested, objective, and unassailable stance."

Historically, health policy has sometimes been accused of being an entirely political—or sometimes entirely fiscal—affair where evidence has no role. But over the past decade it has become de rigueur to preface the word policy with the phrase evidence based, signalling the growing prominence of evidence as being essential to policy. Humphreys and Piot pull the evidence pendulum back a little, offering up the idea that "failure to value the influence of forces other than science in forming health policy can have dangerous consequences for the accountability of politicians and scientists, and for the justification of policies that violate fundamental principles in a democratic society."[13] More on all these forces is introduced throughout Module III and particularly in Chapter 11.

Judith Shamian commented that any of the nurses on the team could walk into any hospital around the world and in very short order figure out the important rules and routines. But walking into a government policy office "is like landing on Mars," she said, adding, "None of the rules are clear and nothing we do out there in clinical care applies to what we do in here."

To be clinically safe, effective, and confident "out there," nurses typically build up a complex knowledge of human anatomy, physiology, and pathophysiology. They then take part in long periods of practice related to each successive skill set. But for too long, nurses have been expected to somehow intuit the knowledge and skills required to operate within and across complex financial, policy, and political systems. Like the care of sick babies or of frail seniors, policy skills have to be taught, studied, and practiced. To extend the clinical metaphor, this book lays out some of the landscape of this field of knowledge (the anatomy), talks about how the basic systems function and relate to one another (the physiology), points to examples of problems amenable to policy solutions (the pathophysiology), and, finally, lays out some of the basic tools of policy analysis and development to help in decision-making (the diagnosis and treatment plan). The intention is to help nurses strengthen their policy competency.

At the Canadian Association for Health Services and Policy Research conference in 2004, health economist Robert Evans responded to a question about causes of the apparent nursing shortage by saying simply, "because policy is possible."[14] What he meant was that there was an apparent shortage of nurses in 2004 because policy had been designed starting in the mid-1990s to reduce the number of nursing students and nurses; a decade later, the policy had worked. If policy is possible, then so is learning about it. The evolution of a nursing professional from student to novice practitioner to competent leader and successful advocate rests first in understanding the structure and context in which one is operating—in the case of policy, this means the governance of Canada and its health systems; knowledge of the people, economic factors, and politics that influence policy; and insights into the ways policy is developed, legislated, and evaluated.

To address those concepts, the content in this book is divided into three modules:

- Module I focuses on the basics and background, including terminology, governance, and structures—in essence, where, how, and why things happen the way they do.

- Module II turns to an examination of the development of Canadian health care and our history of reform, what we are spending, and key population health and system performance measures. What is health care supposed to be for, what does it cost, and what is it achieving?

- Module III introduces models and tools to help understand how to undertake the work of policy, and how different forces might shape the ways tough decisions are made. The book concludes by looking forward to consider some of the important, looming system challenges for which policy interventions by nurses might make a valuable difference.

Throughout the text, the focus of the content is on nurses, the nursing profession as a whole, and the people and other forces surrounding both. Examples of nursing action in public policy are cited throughout this text. Like leadership, advocacy and policy expertise are not tied to titles or positions, and of course, one need not occupy a visible public role to take on valuable policy work. Policy advocacy—defined by Spenceley and colleagues as "knowledge-based action intended to improve health by influencing system-level decisions"[15]—is required in many roles. However, since some examples of nursing policy leadership have been more publicly documented than others, some of these more visible leaders and examples are cited throughout the text. This includes, in particular, examples from Health Canada's Office of Nursing Policy, the CNA, the Canadian Federation of Nurses Unions (CFNU), and all their provincial and territorial counterparts, since so many of them were well documented. The intent is not to diminish less visible (but equally important) policy work or to imply that nurses must have formal titles or senior roles to become involved in policy analysis and development.

To introduce nurses to a variety of historical, current, and emerging policy influencers, brief sketches of these leaders are introduced throughout the book. Finally, while there are scientific references and resources cited throughout the text, additional resources and applications are brought to the attention of the reader using call-out boxes, and each chapter concludes with a list of discussion questions and additional policy resources. For instructors, accompanying PowerPoint slides are available for each chapter.

ABOUT THE AUTHOR

Along with the evidence presented, this text is informed by my own work and observations over a long career in health care. Since 1978, I have had the privilege of holding a variety of roles in nursing clinical practice, education, research, administration, and policy. I began my career in the late 1970s with my first tentative and excited steps into health care by working as an orderly at l'Hôpital Montfort in Ottawa. I continued that work—some elements of it being not unlike what we would now call a personal support worker—in medical/surgical settings, and for three years in an emergency department, where I gained clinical confidence, competency in skills, and insight into human behaviour. After completing my BScN at the University of Toronto in 1983, I went on to work as a staff nurse, and later a clinical instructor, nurse clinician, and manager in the Neurosurgical Intensive Care and Neurosurgery/Trauma units at Sunnybrook Health Sciences Centre in Toronto. Along the way I spent a year working at the God's Lake Narrows First Nation nursing station in northern Manitoba, spent three years coordinating the Quality of Nursing Worklife Research Unit at the University of Toronto, and completed my MSc at the University of Toronto.

After accepting an offer early in 2000 to serve as senior nursing consultant in the federal Office of Nursing Policy in Ottawa, my interest in public policy deepened quickly and significantly—and I have worked in a variety of policy roles since then. It has been an interesting exercise during the writing of this text to stand back and think about that journey and the lessons along the way that inform my policy work today. Those roles gave me the opportunity to see nearly every corner of Canada and to visit many other countries—a very special privilege. And they allowed me to lead or participate in numerous national and international health system and nursing initiatives, including serving as the staff lead for the Canadian Nursing Advisory Committee, visiting consultant with the Organisation for Economic Co-operation and Development (OECD) in Paris, scholar-in-residence at CNA, and executive lead for CNA's National Expert Commission.

In 2012, I was offered the special opportunity to join the design team developing the Master of Nursing program in Health Systems Leadership and Administration at the Lawrence S. Bloomberg Faculty of Nursing, University of Toronto. I remain on the faculty, currently as a lecturer in public policy, leadership, and administration courses, and I was the program lead from 2015 to 2016. I also operate an independent health policy consultancy in the National Capital Region, which has allowed me to maintain strong, ongoing consulting relationships with organizations like Health Canada, CNA, and the CFNU, as well as organizations across the country and beyond. I am pleased to serve as vice chair for the Winchester District Memorial Hospital Board of Directors in eastern Ontario near my home, and am honoured to have the opportunity to spend some time in Halifax in 2017–2018 as the virtual visiting scholar at the Dalhousie University School of Nursing.

Just as this book was going to print, I was offered the exciting and daunting challenge of serving as the twelfth chief executive officer of CNA. The role brought me back to an organization I care deeply about, and one that I believe is an essential force in a large and complex nation like Canada. If we believe in the value and power of a strongly unified federation of provinces and territories, as I do, then the centre has to hold; it must be strong and effective. The same holds true for nursing and its structures. I am humbled to take the reins and I am keen to build on the foundations laid down so ably by Anne Sutherland Boal, her preceding 10 executive leaders, and the four-dozen elected presidents who have shaped CNA over the past century.

NURSING TERMINOLOGY

The family of nursing in Canada includes nurses in four regulated categories: (1) registered nurses; (2) nurse practitioners (registered nurses separately regulated for advanced nursing practice); (3) licensed practical nurses (titled as registered practical nurses in Ontario); and (4) registered psychiatric nurses. In addition, there are tens of thousands of unregulated care providers holding a variety of titles who carry out aspects of nursing care, either under the supervision of a regulated nurse or independently. In this text, unless stated otherwise, *nurse* and *nursing* are intended to refer to the regulated categories collectively; the *nursing family* includes the regulated and unregulated categories. The titles used for the five groups in this text are:

1. Registered nurse
2. Nurse practitioner
3. Licensed practical nurse
4. Registered psychiatric nurse
5. Personal support worker (unregulated care providers)

A FEW WORDS ABOUT NURSING ASSOCIATIONS CITED IN THIS TEXT

The Canadian Association of Schools of Nursing (CASN), CFNU, CNA, and other nursing organizations are cited in examples throughout this text. Readers are reminded that while these associations have headquarters and physical spaces, they are, of course, made up of members from across the country. A reference to CNA, for example, points to work done by and for 139,000 members across all 13 provincial and territorial jurisdictions, as well as its affiliation with the 45 national associations making up the Canadian Network of Nursing Specialties. The CFNU represents 136,000 nurses belonging to eight provincial unions. The direct members of both organizations are provincial and territorial jurisdictional associations and, in the case of CNA, also include individual direct members. In addition to the membership numbers cited here, both organizations welcome roughly 25,000 nursing students as additional members. The CASN members include the schools of nursing in every region of the country. It is important to remember that when these sorts of organizations are cited in examples of policy work, they should be interpreted in the context of collective views and work on behalf of thousands of members, approved by boards of directors, and not narrowed just to the work of operational teams or individuals within these organizations.

MODULE I

Introduction to Canadian Health Policy, Politics, and Governance

This book begins by identifying and defining some of the terms and concepts of the policy business, and thinking about why nurses should care about and be involved in this domain of practice. Similar to the process for developing expertise in complex clinical topics, it is vital to start by understanding core concepts in the policy arena, and to have some idea of the underlying theoretical models that may guide policy work or at least explain outcomes.

Building on that base, it helps to understand the structure of the country before exploring the complexities of health systems or the place of nursing within them. The word *governance* may threaten to cause eyes to glaze over. However, like the construction of a solid house, it is prudent to build a strong foundation before thinking about constructing the walls, ceilings, and roof. Governance in this context really speaks to who does what (or who should be doing what), which people and roles are involved, their areas of authority and responsibility, and how decisions are made.

All of this is true whether we are talking about our country, our province or territory, our employer, our community, or even our friends and family. Every system, even the simplest one, has rules, explicit or otherwise, that help us understand how decisions are made, who makes them, and how things get done. What does it mean when we say that Canada is a federation and a constitutional monarchy? What exactly are the Constitution and the Charter of Rights and Freedoms, and how do they affect nurses and those they serve? What are the differences among the roles and responsibilities of the federal government and the governance of the provinces, territories, and lands of Aboriginal Peoples? These institutions and structures all underpin and drive the directions of Canadian public policy. Nurses need to understand them to have a grasp of the ways health and nursing policy develop, and how ideas move from conversation to legislation.

In this context, governance is at the base of everything else discussed in this book. After starting the story in Chapter 1 by defining terms and introducing theoretical perspectives, Chapter 2 explores the governance of Canada and its evolution. Chapter 3 focuses on the governance of Canada's health systems, defining *medicare* as the term is used in Canada, and exploring the ways different services are delivered in the public and private spheres of our health systems. The structures, chains of authority and responsibility, and regulations and important pieces of legislation that have built today's health care systems in Canada are identified. Looking at this complex mix of variables, links to public policy, health policy, and implications for nurses and nursing are examined. Finally, in Chapter 4, health human resources are introduced. The focus is on nursing, where the governance and structures of the profession are examined along with a high-level introductory look at some of the policy challenges that have arisen in its regulatory, professional, union, and other structures.

CHAPTER 1

Politics, Policy, and Health Systems: What Are We Talking About and Why Does All This Matter to Nurses?

CHAPTER HIGHLIGHTS

- Why Should Nurses Study the Theory and Practice of Public Policy?
- Historical Examples of Public Policy, Health Policy, and Nursing Influence
- Terminology and Key Concepts
- Policy Development: Theories and Frameworks/Models
- Nursing Engagement with Canadian Policy: Political Realities
- Summary and Implications
- Discussion Questions
- Additional Policy Resources

LEARNING OUTCOMES

1. Discuss why it is important for nurses to study and engage in health policy.
2. Define the key terms and concepts of public policy development.
3. Differentiate among policies, procedures, guidelines, rules, and legislation.
4. Describe three policy theory paradigms or frameworks.

Policy Influencer: Anne Marie Rafferty

Dr. Anne Marie Rafferty, CBE, RN, PhD, FRCN, FAAN, is past dean of the Florence Nightingale Faculty of Nursing and Midwifery at King's College in London and is now the first chair of nursing policy in the United Kingdom. From 2013 to 2014, she was the Frances Bloomberg International Distinguished Visiting Professor at the Lawrence S. Bloomberg Faculty of Nursing, University of Toronto. She served on the Prime Minister's Commission on the Future of Nursing and Midwifery in England and is sought out as one of the world's foremost health policy thinkers and experts in areas of history, health policy, and health services. Her science focus has included "research linking staffing numbers to patient outcomes [showing] how nurses make a profound difference to patients and the chances of their survival."[1] With Rafferty's input, the Prime Minister's Commission in England called on nurses "to swear an oath that we cannot live with anything less than the best. We need to join with the other professions and patients themselves to develop a coalition for quality which is committed to 100% achievement of quality benchmarks."[2]

"When the opportunity presents itself, always sit at the table. No one listens to the people sitting at the side of the room."

—*Sheryl Sandberg, Chief Operating Officer, Facebook*

WHY SHOULD NURSES STUDY THE THEORY AND PRACTICE OF PUBLIC POLICY?

When he was deputy director of the Government Social Research Unit in the United Kingdom under Prime Minister Tony Blair, Philip Davies observed that "most professions build themselves around good solid evidence. It's only policy making that in many spheres thinks of itself as an amateur enterprise—dilettantes doing their best, so to speak. And that's not sustainable in the 21st century."[3] As a solution he argued that "policy making should be a profession."

Over the years since Davies made those comments to his Canadian audience, policy has emerged as a much more prominent theme in nursing discussions and debate. Certainly some of that evolution was fuelled by the presence of nurses working in policy roles in federal, provincial, and territorial governments, becoming more visible in the late 1990s. But over the past 20 years, nursing's professional, administrative, union, and specialty organizations and associations

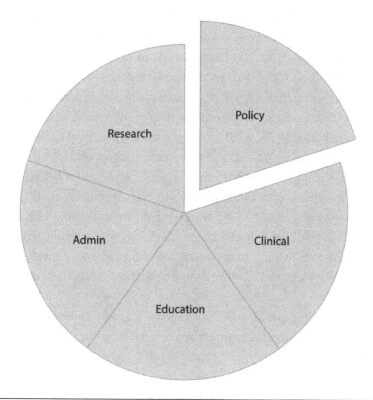

Figure 1.1: Domains of Nursing Practice

all have recognized the need to be more savvy and strategic in understanding and framing their positions in a policy context—especially paying attention to the link between evidence and policy decision-making.

The momentum continues to grow as courses focused on health policy and health systems have emerged in graduate and even undergraduate nursing programs over the last decade. Policy has become so important to the profession that the four practice domains of nursing—traditionally described as clinical (referring to the whole area of direct service delivery to patients, residents, and clients across the continuum of care), education, administration, and research—have been expanded in most contemporary models to include policy as a fifth pillar, as shown in Figure 1.1.

But why should any of this matter to the great body of Canadian nurses, the vast majority of whom are working at an exhausting pace delivering the care services that are the core of nursing? The answer is both simple and complex: because if nurses don't carry out this work, others surely will—and they already are. Consider just a few facts that are explored further in this text:

- Canadians spent more than $219 billion on health care in 2015—just shy of 11 per cent of the gross domestic product (GDP).
- There are roughly 73,000 hospital beds in operation across Canada[4] and about 1 million Canadians receiving home care at any given time.[5]
- There are more than 77,000 physicians practicing in Canada[6] and in 2015 the regulated nursing workforce numbered more than 415,000, including registered nurses (292,378), licensed practical nurses (113,367), registered psychiatric nurses (5,766), and nurse practitioners (4,353).[7]
- The CFNU reported in 2015 that "21,000 public sector health care nurses are absent due to own illness or disability on a weekly basis. This represents an absenteeism rate of 7.9%," triggering an annual cost to Canadians conservatively estimated at $846.1 million.[8] Partly as a result, nurses worked more than 19 million hours of aggregated paid and unpaid overtime in 2014, equivalent to 10,700 full-time positions, at a further cost of $871.8 million.
- In its 2016 report, the OECD reports Canada as having 95,530 beds in all general, specialty, psychiatric, rehabilitation, and long-term care hospitals.[9]

Is that the right number of beds to meet population needs? The right mix? What is the right number and mix of regulated nurses and physicians? What outcomes do we want them to achieve? Why are there 292,000 registered nurses and not 200,000 or 400,000? And why are their absenteeism and overtime rates so high? Who makes the decisions that lead to these outcomes?

Of course, none of these results happened magically. They are each the product of a series of deliberate public policy choices—for better or worse. Indeed, many are the result of years of debate and agonizing decisions within and among elected government officials, their bureaucrats, and, sometimes, professional groups and the public. And the choices made by those governments about how much Canadians will spend on health care, how that funding is allocated, and who will deliver the care all impact the practice and work settings of nurses every day of their careers.

In her 2015 Nursing Week blog for rabble.ca, prominent Toronto-based nurse advocate Cathy Crowe cited Florence Nightingale's words from an 1892 letter to the editor in which she said, "We must create a public opinion which must drive the government, instead of the government having to drive us—an enlightened public, wise in principles, wise in details."[10] Crowe noted that "Naomi Klein essentially says the same thing today. She puts it this way—that in order to create policy change, we the public, and I would add 'we the nurses,' need to build 'movement muscle.' Then we can walk the talk."[11] Crowe is one of Canada's most well-known nurses in this area of practice and serves as Distinguished Visiting Practitioner in the Politics and Public Administration Department at Ryerson University in Toronto.

Nurses and physicians, who make up the largest proportion of health care providers in Canada, have a deep and vested interest in being aware of, engaging in, and, where feasible, taking part in making the health policy decisions that will govern and shape every aspect of the scope, quality, and outcomes of care they will spend their careers delivering. At the very least, nurses need to exercise that "movement muscle" by understanding what policy decisions are being made in their name, how they are being made, and by whom.

HISTORICAL EXAMPLES OF PUBLIC POLICY, HEALTH POLICY, AND NURSING INFLUENCE

Policy may be as simple as a family decision to make an effort to reduce waste and use energy more mindfully. On the other end of the spectrum, it may be as broad and complex as the challenge Canadian governments faced in their struggle to respond to the Supreme Court of Canada's February 2015 decision to strike down the ban on physician-assisted death for mentally competent individuals.

As examples throughout this book explore in more detail, public health policies that may be developed and delivered by and with nurses change the course of history and society every day:

- In 2015, a vaccine effective in preventing Ebola was discovered by Canadian scientists. A policy requiring its use in high-risk areas could dramatically reduce deaths from the disease—and not just reduce the deaths of patients, but the deaths of nurses and doctors providing their care.
- During the early 1980s, infection with the human immunodeficiency virus (HIV) and its common sequel, acquired immune deficiency syndrome (AIDS), was a virtual death sentence. But public policy choices to fund research resulted in treatments that have led to plummeting death rates. The reversal is so great that in April 2016, Canada's Manulife Financial reached a landmark decision to offer its life insurance products to HIV-positive individuals after concluding that the disease is now akin to a chronic illness that can be managed well with medications. The search for a vaccine—again with the benefit of some public funds—continues. In 2014, in a sign of the times, for the first time in a generation only one baby in Canada was born carrying HIV.

- Over the past 50 years in North America, public safety policy has evolved from the point where seat belts were a luxury option available in the front seats of cars to the requirement today that seat belts (and, in some cases, more sophisticated passive restraints such as air bags) be standard equipment in even the cheapest vehicles—and there are serious penalties for failure to use them. The result? Death and injury rates from motor vehicle collisions have dropped dramatically.

- In conjunction with health professionals and the private sector, governments at every level and in most jurisdictions have taken on the issue of tobacco smoking over the past 40 years through multi-pronged public policy efforts—taxes, advertising, access, employer policies, and municipal bylaws. Despite the vigorous resistance of the tobacco lobby, there has been a steady and significant decline in the number of men smoking and a concomitant drop in lung cancer rates (the curve for women seems to mirror the pattern for men but is delayed because in Canada more women started smoking later than most men). Policy developed to tackle smoking has been contentious to say the least—but it is working, and Canada's success is commended around the world. Examples in Ontario include the Smoke-Free Ontario Act (2006) "prohibiting smoking in enclosed public spaces ... and restricting the public display of tobacco products," and, in a 2009 amendment, prohibiting smoking in motor vehicles carrying children under the age of 16.[12]

The preceding examples of policy were all intended to maintain or improve health, quality of life, and safety. But history teaches us that public and health policy may have unintended adverse effects, and while it may seem unnecessary to say so, the University College London Lancet Commission report linking health outcomes to urban planning reminded readers that "policy makers should be alert to the unintended consequences of their policies."[13] For example, despite the refusal of officials to authorize its use in the United States, the drug thalidomide was approved by the federal government for use in Canada in 1961 as an effective antidote to morning sickness in pregnant women. Less than a year later, it was withdrawn from the Canadian market in the wake of overwhelming global evidence about infant deaths as well as blindness, deafness, and catastrophic limb and organ malformations in babies born to mothers who had used the drug. The drug also injured women who took it, with side effects such as peripheral neuritis. In 2015, according to the then federal minister of health, the Honourable Rona Ambrose, there were 92 survivors in Canada, then reaching their mid-50s. Governments are still providing them with compensation in the form of lump-sum payments and pensions as part of the fallout of the decision to approve the drug.

Choosing to act indecisively in any given area of public policy—or to act in a way that minimizes political risk—may also shape legislation. For example, in the United States in 1993, newly elected President Bill Clinton had promised during his election campaign to repeal the ban on homosexuals serving in the military if he was elected. Once in office, however, he encountered immediate and tremendous resistance from members of Congress. In the end, Clinton compromised heavily with the now infamous "Don't Ask, Don't Tell" policy, which permitted homosexual men and women to serve in the military provided they not disclose their sexual orientation; the law also directed leaders in the armed forces not to question or harass service members whom they thought might be homosexual. The controversial compromise remained federal policy for 18 years until President Barack Obama repealed it in 2011, striking down any conditions related to sexual orientation for those serving in the United States military.

Finally, public policy may be deliberately malevolent. A glance at any news report makes plain that official public policy around the world continues to have devastating impacts on people, basic human rights, social and economic systems, and the physical environment. Think of the government of Adolph Hitler, the apartheid system of racial segregation in South Africa, or the failure to grant basic civil rights to African Americans in the United States until the 1960s. In our own time, it was official Canadian government policy to remove children from Aboriginal families and place them in residential schools in an effort to assimilate them into the majority culture of people who had settled on Aboriginal lands. Much of the treatment of those children, we now know, was cruel to the point of being inhuman, and if that was not an explicit part of the policy, it was at least condoned. Residential schools are not the only issue: as a signatory to the United Nations Convention on the Elimination of All Forms of Discrimination against Women,[14] Canada was admonished in 2015 for its "grave violation" of human rights by failing to take on the issue of disproportionate levels of violence toward Aboriginal women.

The catastrophic socio-cultural damage of colonization to Aboriginal Peoples and now, in its wake, to the reputation and integrity of Canada are incalculable. Canadians have learned through the Truth and Reconciliation Commission that efforts to understand and confront the weight and meaning of this area of public policy are only in their infancy.[15] As discussed later in this text, most policy decisions will benefit some and disadvantage others; there is perhaps no starker example in Canada's history than the one executed through the past century to extinguish the cultures of the First Peoples of the land we now all share.

Nursing Influences on Policy

Although it would not have been expressed as such at the time, among the earliest records of health policy development in Canada was the work of Jeanne Mance (1606–1673), a French woman who settled in New France—now the province of Quebec. She would be described now as a lay nurse because she had no formal training, as we understand it today. But Mance used her basic training and practical experience from France to establish the original Hotel-Dieu de Montréal hospital inside the fort at Ville Marie in the fall of 1642, and a separate hospital outside the fort in 1645.[16] Apart from treating diseases among the settlers, records from the time indicate that she and her team provided care for Huron people injured in attacks by the Iroquois Nation, and later for French settlers who were similarly afflicted. Mance provided direct care but also travelled between Montreal and France, proving to be a highly effective policy advocate, using her personal connections to recruit staff, raise funds, and improve standards of care. In short, she identified problems, discussed options, secured funding, implemented solutions, evaluated outcomes, and so on—a perfect example of the policy cycle model that is explored in Module III.

Jeanne Mance is the earliest recorded nurse in North America, and she set down a challenging model for the nursing role by dividing her time amongst direct care, administration, and policy/advocacy functions—including advocating for the provision of free care for the poor and actually delivering it. Beyond her immediate health care duties it was noted that "with remarkable zeal, she directed her energy towards laying the colony's very foundations."[17] With Paul de Chomedey de Maisonneuve, Mance is credited as co-founder of the city of Montreal (May 17, 1642), and the Hotel-Dieu de Montréal she founded is still in operation today as part of the Université de Montréal hospital system.

Despite Mance's historic contributions to Canada's early social and nursing history, Florence Nightingale (1820–1910) is more familiar to most nurses in Canada and globally. It is certainly a well-earned legacy, overshadowing Mance's story not just because it occurred so much more recently and was so extensively documented, but because Nightingale's reach was as vast as the scope and complexity of the work she took on. Looking back now on her life, Nightingale emerges as one of the most prominent and transformative figures of the 19th century—so much more than the sentimental images of the lady with the lamp. In its entry on Nightingale, Encyclopædia Britannica opens by describing her as the "foundational philosopher of modern nursing, statistician, and social reformer."[18]

Nightingale's success in dramatically reforming sanitation and health care for members of the military in the Crimean War quickly expanded her already considerable social network in England. Her work led to "marked reform in the military medical and purveyance systems."[19] And Nightingale's statistical proficiency gained such notoriety that she became the first woman admitted to the Royal Statistical Society.

Despite her association with hospitals and her influence on institutional care, Nightingale wrote extensively about home care and sanitation, and she was a prominent policy advocate for health care for the most vulnerable citizens. Her *Notes on Nursing* was a landmark publication used around the world to help ordinary people who were charged with providing care to the sick or injured, usually in home settings but also in the emerging hospital sector. Nightingale's model of nursing underpinned much of modern nursing education for the next century. The original school in her name, now the Florence Nightingale Faculty of Nursing and Midwifery at King's College in London, continues as a world leader in education today.

While not segregated into two discrete streams or models, the work of Mance and Nightingale, respectively, gave rise to what are sometimes described as the Franco/Catholic and Anglo/Protestant traditions that have shaped health care in Canada and beyond. Jeanne Mance was not a nun, but she worked closely with a priest and with the Augustinian nuns who delivered care. That branch of the nursing tree in Canada was grounded in religious faith, tying nursing fairly narrowly in the earliest years to Roman Catholic nurses who were likely to be nuns. Others followed and built on the tradition, perhaps most famously in Canada Sister (and later Saint) Marie-Marguerite d'Youville, founder of the Sisters of Charity—*les sœurs grises*, or the Grey Nuns of Montreal, as they came to be known. That order grew and established many

Florence Nightingale

Lynn McDonald, former Member of Parliament (New Democratic Party) in Toronto and former president of the National Action Committee on the Status of Women, is the director and editor of the 16 volumes of *The Collected Works of Florence Nightingale*—the most definitive collection of all of Nightingale's writing. To learn more, go to http://www.uoguelph.ca/~cwfn.

For an introduction to the life and world of Florence Nightingale, download the free iTunes app, *Navigating Nightingale*.[20]

other health care settings across the continent, some still in operation more than 250 years later. Later, nuns from other faiths—Anglicans (Church of England), for example—and other Christian women continued to tie nursing to faith, charity, self-sacrifice, and human caring. In this tradition, the act of nursing is aligned with love and mercy, and some maintain that tradition today even though most historically faith-based hospitals have become part of public systems in Canada.

Nightingale's Anglo tradition deliberately positioned nursing away from a religious calling and established it as paid, respectable, secular work for women. As Richards put it in 1902, "It was Florence Nightingale who introduced the spirit of reformation and teaching into the work of nursing. She ... overthrew the old systems and replaced them with a mission for the nurse, to teach and practice sanitation and hygiene with authority. With her began a new era of nursing."[21] While faith-based nurses certainly used evidence and were known to provide care in a well-organized network of health care organizations, the religious tradition was sometimes cast as being grounded in faith, love, and intuition rather than science. With that said, secular nurses would work until they were married and then leave their jobs, whereas nuns mostly spent a lifetime in service,[22] which could have boosted the career expertise of the latter. The two traditions borrowed from one another, but the Nightingale tradition situated nursing as a career option for women based in a model of education and practice beyond personal religious beliefs. As Nelson and Rafferty said in 2010,

> Nightingale's endeavours to build a respectable secular profession for women through the development of training programs for nurses, who would then lead the reform of the hospital, was a breakthrough moment for nursing as it evolved from its previous confines as either religiously motivated or stigmatized as domestic work.[23]

Significantly, both traditions entrenched the link between the work and women, creating a space that, in the early years in Canada and the United States, was respectable and indeed offered a range of opportunities for advancement into interesting and progressive career tracks beyond the bedside (e.g., education, administration). While most institutions were dominated by men (often physicians, in the case of health care), within the ranks of nursing women had at least some measure of autonomy, choice, control, and influence nearly unparalleled in other areas of work. Liaschenko and Peter liken the situation to upper-class Victorian households, "organized by hierarchies of power and status marked by gender and social position. The physician was the head of the household and the final authority; the sister or matron of the hospital was the wife with significant authority over her charges, which included the nurses and the patients."[24] They point to this model as a source of nursing's "long history of embeddedness in hierarchical, bureaucratic institutions where everyone knew and kept their place."[25]

In the wake of Mance and Nightingale, the 20th and 21st centuries are replete with examples of Canadian nurses who helped shape health and social policy, not just through nursing or traditional health care roles. Georgina Fane Pope (1862–1938), for example, left what could have been a life of relative leisure on Prince Edward Island to study nursing at Bellevue in New York, going on to become the first matron commander of the Canadian Army Medical Corps. In honour of her impact on health care in the military during the Boer War and World War I, Pope was the first woman to receive the Royal Red Cross.

A generation later, Nova Scotia's Lyle Morrison Creelman (1908–2007) was recruited to be chief nurse in the British Zone of occupied Germany after World War II. She had a broad impact on population health, organizing nursing services "to help care for millions of people of many nationalities who had been displaced during the war."[26] In 1950 she became the first Canadian nurse to work for the World Health Organization (WHO), eventually rising to the role of chief nursing officer of the organization, 1954–1968, where the International Council of Nurses concluded she "probably achieved more for nursing throughout the world than any other nurse of her time."[27] So significant was Creelman's impact on global public health policy that in a 2012 book exploring unsung Canadian heroes, she was chosen as one of the 50 people whose lives changed Canada.[28]

Later in the 20th century, nurses acted en masse to shift their own education, making it tougher and more expensive, in an effort to better serve the public. At the same time, nurses did battle to force changes in what became the Canada Health Act (1984), again in the interest of the Canadian public. Early in this century, Office of Nursing Policy team members at Health Canada—including nurses— were awarded for their instrumental role in shaping the 2003 First Ministers' Accord on Health Care Renewal. That accord included $90 million in funding that was distributed across Canada and across professions "to strengthen the evidence base for national planning, promote interdisciplinary provider education, improve recruitment and retention, and ensure the supply of needed health providers (including nurse practitioners, pharmacists and diagnostic technologists)."[29]

And at the time this book is being written, Leigh Chapman, a young doctoral candidate in nursing at the University of Toronto, has made repeated appearances in municipal government settings in Toronto advocating for better shelters and housing for homeless people and for the establishment of safe injection sites. This action signals a new generation of nurses taking up the mantle of what often has been called "street nursing," carried out so ably by generations of nurse leaders, such as Lillian Wald in the early 1900s, Liz James in Vancouver in the 1970s, and Cathy Crowe and her contemporaries in Toronto today. Also, from the early 20th century, the Victorian Order of Nurses (now VON Canada) employed nurses who were skilled in making the links "between the broader social determinants of health, such as housing conditions and income, and the need to reform policies that would improve the health of individuals."[30]

These are but a handful of examples of nursing impacts on policy and population health, in very different sectors and led by nurses in very different roles. Indeed, the presence and influence of nurses can be found everywhere in the worlds of social and health policy. Policy change requires strategic inputs from the national level to provincial and territorial, and on to regional, municipal, and organizational. Many examples of this work are discussed throughout this text.

TERMINOLOGY AND KEY CONCEPTS

The Politics of Policy

The focus of this book is policy, but policy debate, development, legislation, and revision are virtually inseparable from politics, whether that refers to the relationships within a small workplace team or the formal positions of elected premiers sitting at the Council of the Federation table. In its formal definition, *politics* may be used as either a singular or plural noun referring collectively to the "activities that relate to influencing the actions and policies of a government or getting and keeping power in a government."[31] The term also is used commonly to refer to a profession—the work of people elected or appointed to governments is often simply called politics.

Politics has gained a rather sullied reputation in some quarters, or at least often carries negative associations. Nurses are not the only professionals who shy away from policy work because "it's all politics" or because they're "not interested in politics." Inferred is a disdain for public mudslinging by politicians or the power games that may surround public policy development, and not for the idea of policy development more narrowly. This view of politics refers more directly to yet another definition of politics, that is, "opinions ... about what should be done by governments: a person's political thoughts and opinions."[32]

In her treatise on public policy, Miljan describes the related topic of the *political agenda*—another potentially loaded term. When we speak of an administrator, for example, having a political agenda, it is not likely meant as a compliment; at best it may arouse suspicion of motives. But Miljan notes that the term is meant to represent "what is relevant in political life, how issues are understood, whose views should be taken seriously, and what sort of 'solutions' are tenable."[33] Identifying and understanding political agendas is key to success in the policy game, to say nothing of surviving a long career in health care, where politics and policy are a constant force.

Public Policy

For many nurses, policy historically meant dusty binders full of paper sitting on hospital nursing station shelves. Today it may mean rarely read policies within digital folders on an employer's computer network. It is important to differentiate between workplace policies and procedures and the much broader concept of public policy.

In its purest form, a *policy* may be defined as "a statement of direction resulting from a decision-making process that applies reason, evidence and values in public or private settings."[34] It implies some sort of action (including the choice to not act in a given situation) that is driven by thoughtful decision-making and supported with data if possible; a purposeful choice is made with the intention to meet a defined goal, objective, or outcome. The National Collaborating Centre on Healthy Public Policy defines a public policy as "a statement produced by a public authority that defines one or more problems affecting the population or one or more groups within it, and that also furnishes (to varying degrees) a response to that problem in terms of objectives, actions and actors."[35]

Taken to the population and government levels, Brooks defines the larger landscape of *public policy* as "the broad framework of ideas and values within which decisions are taken and action, or inaction, is pursued by governments in relation to some issue or problem."[36] Health policy is one subset of public policy that may sit alongside education policy, housing policy, transportation policy, and so on. The rest of this book centres around this larger view of public policy—focused on population health and health care policy—as defined by Brooks. But it also looks more narrowly at the development of public policies by examining the various steps and dynamics implied in the National Collaborating Centre's definition.

The formal study of this field—health policy research—is defined by the Canadian Association for Health Services and Policy Research as "a multidisciplinary field involving instrumental analyses of policy alternatives that affect the health care system or the health of the general public, and scholarly inquiries into the process of health policy making and how it is shaped by ideas, interests, and institutional arrangements."[37] Much of the evidence used in policy development has emerged from the field of health services and policy science; there is a large sector of this research across Canada. Nurse scientists and non-nurse scientists studying nursing have made significant contributions to the body of health systems evidence within Canada and globally—among them now-famous names like Baumann, Birch, Bourgeault, Browne, Cummings, Deber, Doran, Edwards, Estabrooks, Evans, Flood, Giovannetti, McGillis Hall, McGrail, O'Brien-Pallas, Pringle, Roos, Spence-Laschinger, Tamblyn, Tomblin Murphy, Tourangeau, and many more. Their names are renowned in the global world of health services research, and their body of work—examining the interacting effects of nurse, nursing team, and organizational characteristics on individual, organizational, and system outcomes—is vast and increasingly well documented.

These definitions of policy differ significantly from the policy manuals mentioned earlier, from that with which nurses typically may be most familiar from their roles in service settings. While often labelled as such, many of the organizational policies nurses and other providers encounter in health care settings are really procedures, guidelines, and/or rules. These terms may be differentiated from one another as follows:

- *Procedures* are the "established or official ways of doing something"[38]—for example, endotracheal suctioning in an intensive care unit, administration of a vaccine in a school clinic, or the method for ordering supplies in a home care setting.
- *Guidelines* are suggested courses of action or advice, typically based in evidence, seen in examples such as Canada's Food Guide[39]; in the approaches to treatment, support, and follow-up outlined in Alberta Health Services' *Cancer Guidelines*[40]; and in the wide range of nursing best practice guidelines developed by the Registered Nurses' Association of Ontario (RNAO).[41]
- *Rules* represent "explicit or understood regulations or principles governing conduct or procedure within a particular area of activity."[42] Examples could include clauses contained in a collective union agreement (such as how many minutes of break time are allowed on each tour of duty in a hospital), the established visiting hours in a nursing home, or expectations regarding the timing of submission of staff schedules by patient care managers in an organization.

Public policy is, of course, highly contextual, and for better or worse mirrors the world in which it is developed. Any one policy may affect different settings, jurisdictions, and/or population groups in different ways, and in reality most policies can't help but be seen as a benefit to some and a detriment to others. More on that conundrum follows in Chapter 11. As Miljan said of political agendas, "Political issues and policy problems are not inevitable and inherent; rather they are constructed out of the conflicting values and terminologies that different groups put forward when they are competing for something that cannot be shared to satisfy all of them fully."[43] Few policies will please (or benefit) all sides of any issue.

The range and complexity of public policy issues are vast. For example, in a 2005 survey of its member countries' main policy concerns, the United Nations found that HIV/AIDS was the leading concern among both developing and developed countries (essentially less-wealthy and more-wealthy nations, respectively). But there the similarities ended. Developing countries, for example, identified concerns around high fertility (and especially high adolescent fertility), high population growth, and large, young, working-age populations—precisely the opposite of wealthy nations like Canada, which has low fertility, an aging population, and a smaller working-age population. Of course, those opposing dynamics can lead to tremendous tensions around issues such as international migration—with some countries bursting with young, unemployed (or under-employed) citizens looking for a better life, set against others with much older populations who need an influx of young workers but have not developed effective mechanisms to attract or integrate them. Global conflicts and the refugee issue only complicate the migration challenge.

Nurses may not see these high-level policy issues as their business, but there are urgent implications. Nursing has been entangled in international migration policy for the past generation as some employers and even governments have sought to attract nurses from other countries to shore up domestic shortages. The ethics of nursing recruitment have been called into question in cases—in Africa, for example—where countries cannot afford to lose any of their precious health human resources. The CNA issued its first public position statement on the issue, *Immigration and Employment of Nurses from Abroad* (1969), responding to the growing number of nurses migrating to Canada. Policies within governments and professional associations around internationally educated nurses have been developed in response to criticism, but the tremendous pressure from over-crowded and economically disadvantaged regions in Africa, India, and Asia to move to places like Canada is not likely to go away as populations in those areas continue to grow. In a medium-fertility scenario, global population is set to grow by about 3 billion between now and 2050, and nearly all of it in the southern hemisphere. Canada and its nurses must tackle this issue to have any hope of a sufficient tax base to provide care to the rapidly growing sector of seniors leaving the workforce, and whose numbers are overwhelming the number of younger workers still in it.

To say nothing of a staggering payment problem, Canada faces a looming mismatch in human resources supply and demand: the Canadian Institute for Health Information reported that in 2014, after a decade of growth, the number of regulated nurses who did not renew their annual registration exceeded the number of new graduates.[44] The numbers are up again in 2015, but as baby boomers retire from nursing and eventually need more care themselves, Canada will need a lot more nurses entering its workforce over the coming 10 to 20 years.

Across the world in 2005 were common issues related to population size and growth, urbanization and the growth of cities, population aging, fertility and contraception, mortality (including the prominent issue of HIV/AIDS), international migration, and population policies.[45] Note that while that list touches on the determinants of health, health care is not even mentioned explicitly beyond HIV/AIDS. And other than HIV/AIDS, which has at least been tamed, those issues are all still prominent in Canada today. Despite the span and complexity of these public policy issues, they do not touch on the environment, natural resources, the economy, relationships with Aboriginal Peoples, or global conflicts—all of which confront governments every day.

Healthy Public Policy

According to the WHO, *healthy public policy* is "characterized by explicit concerns for health and equity in all areas of policy and by an accountability for health impact."[46] Canada's National Collaborating Centre for Healthy Public Policy describes the term as "public policy that potentially enhances populations' health by having a positive impact on the social, economic, and environmental determinants of health."[47] Certainly governments focus on the economic impacts of public policy as it is developed; media stories every day report on debates surrounding the impact of different policy options on jobs and the economy. Healthy public policy would put accountability for the health consequences of public policy decisions on an equal footing with the economic ones. Put most simply, "government sectors concerned with agriculture, trade, education, industry, and communications need to take into account health as an essential factor" in the formulation of public policy.[48]

That approach often is described as "Health in All Policies." It requires the use of some sort of lens by which proposed legislation can be screened for its impact on population health, and then adjusted as necessary, depending on the findings. When Finland took on the presidency of the European Union in 2006 (the role rotates among the member nations), it adopted Health in All Policies as the health theme for its leadership tenure[49] in order to focus attention and advance action on the issue. Closer to home, the National Expert Commission made a recommendation about Health in All Policies in its 2012 report (see Chapter 6 for further discussion). Change in this area may be emerging: for example, in his comments to the Ontario Hospital Association in November 2015, Ontario minister of health and long-term care Eric Hoskins commented that "delivering on a promise of health equity isn't something the health care system can do alone. True health equity requires a 'Health in All Policies' approach. It requires breaking down the silos between health policy and social policy. It requires better integration not just within a system, but across government."[50] Minister Hoskins committed to working across government to implement this approach and to address broad determinants of health.

Legislation and Regulation

The ultimate intent of health policy development is often to support new or revised legislation and/or regulations—and legislative policies that are "laws or ordinances created by elected representatives."[51] The first definition of the word *legislation* really means the act of legislating, that is, "the exercise of the power and function of making rules (as laws) that have the force of authority by virtue of their promulgation by an official organ of a state or other organization."[52] As a mass noun, *legislation* refers to individual laws or sets of laws considered collectively, and *legislative power* means "the power to make law or policy."[53]

Regulation(s) may flow from legislation or stand alone as the result of policy development. Regulatory policies may include "rules, guidelines, principles, or methods created by government agencies with regulatory authority for products or services."[54] In the context of this book, *regulations* are assumed to refer to laws, rules, or other orders "prescribed by authority, especially to regulate conduct."[55] Canadian nurses will be familiar with the concept of legislation regarding health professionals in each province and territory—the Health Professions Act in British Columbia and Regulated Health Professions Act in Prince Edward Island, for example. Regulations regarding their professional conduct flow from that legislation and typically are enforced by a licensing or similar regulatory body—for example, the College of Registered Nurses of Manitoba and the regulatory arm of the Yukon Registered Nurses Association. More on nursing regulation follows in Chapter 4.

Medicare

Because medicare is mentioned repeatedly throughout this text, it is important to clarify its meaning. In Canada, *medicare* is not an official term. However, as Health Canada has noted, it is the term by which Canadians have often come to refer to their national health insurance program, the interlocking system of 13 provincial and territorial health insurance plans "designed to ensure that all residents have reasonable access to medically necessary hospital and physician services, on a prepaid basis."[56] Students of health policy should be clear not to confuse Canada's public medicare system with the formal titles of the Medicare[57] and Medicaid[58] insurance programs in the United States.

For Canadians, medicare has, of course, come to mean so much more than a set of insurance systems. The health care system it represents is emblematic of Canadian values—in fact, to many Canadians universal health care is the single most important reflection of what it means to be Canadian. As such, any discussion of medicare, especially of reforming it, can quickly rouse prickly emotions on all sides; it is seen—and perhaps purposefully framed by some interest groups— not as a critique of a business model, but rather as an attack on core values. Few programs in Canada prompt more impassioned, often enraged, responses. Elected officials seem either stymied by or terrified of the notion of decisive intervention. In a 2013 report for the Health Action Lobby, Tholl, Bujold, and Grimes noted that health care consistently ranks as one of the top concerns of Canadians, and observed that successive governments seem to lack either the will or the ability (or both) to deal with its problems; they called it "medicare malaise."[59] But in his 2012 analysis of Canadian health policy and health care, Jeffrey Simpson was more pointed, saying, "Medicare is the third rail of Canadian politics. Touch it and you die. Every politician knows this truth."[60]

POLICY DEVELOPMENT: THEORIES AND FRAMEWORKS/MODELS

> "Health policy-making involves a careful balance of trade-offs, reflecting the weights assigned to a range of important goals and a great deal of uncertainty. Even when the tough choices are made, changing systems so as to improve performance is never easy ..."
>
> —*Organisation for Economic Co-operation and Development, 2004*[61]

Oxford Dictionaries defines *theory* as a "supposition or a system of ideas intended to explain something," and theories include principles or ideas to ground and justify courses of action or to account for a given situation.[62] Theories should reliably and systematically help to explain and predict outcomes in the presence of certain variables and courses of action. *Frameworks* lay out sets of facts that support any given idea and put a structure around sets of ideas.[63] Similar to frameworks, *conceptual models* show factors and relationships that may be concrete or abstract, and that when acting together may lead to a certain outcome. Myriad theories and frameworks or models have been published to explain the elements and process of what Brownson and colleagues called the "science and art"[65] of policy development and change.

Policy design and implementation have been described as "a complex, multi-directional, fragmented and unpredictable process."[66] As a result, theory in this sector is more fluid and less predictable than common mathematical or physics theories like the theory of gravity. But there are fundamental process steps, including a set of variables, phases, a trajectory, and an outcome. At its most basic level, policy development generally includes four basic stages,[67] as shown in Figure 1.2, which are useful in organizing issues, research, and phases of policy development. Walt and colleagues cited analysts, however, who have been critical of this model "for presuming a linearity to the public policy process that does not exist in reality, for postulating neat demarcations between stages that are blurred in practice, and for offering no propositions on causality."[68] Walt and Gilson's policy triangle framework, and later network frameworks, build on the basic linear process shown here to include multiple factors and policy actors. Cairney, too, observed that "policymaking does not operate in discrete stages," adding that it is a messy affair in which it is "difficult to link policy outcomes to particular individuals or organisations."[69] He went on to note that the uncertainty of messy policy making "is not an argument likely to be embraced in 'Westminster' systems where practitioners may feel obliged to uphold the idea of accountability to the public via ministers and Parliament"—and which, he added importantly, "is based on the idea that power is concentrated at the centre

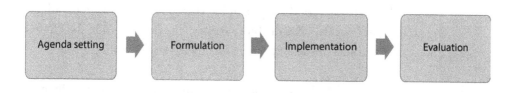

Figure 1.2: Basic Public Policy Process

of government."[70]

Cairney and others have offered some criticism of circular models often used to explain, plan, and predict policy development outcomes, but they remain popular nonetheless. Cairney noted, for example, that an internal review by the Scottish government of its own processes found that five models were used—all circular in nature.[71] There is no one right model; however, a model that takes into account a series of inputs and phases that may be useful to understanding policy development by nurses and others is described and explored extensively in Chapter 9.

As important as the stages and steps of policy frameworks are, the more complex issue of why policy unfolds as it does (or does not) also merits exploration by students of policy. Theories can be helpful because they lay out ideas that are intended to explain, understand, and sometimes predict facts or events—in short, to help shed light on why things happen the way they do. Numerous theories of public policy have been developed to explain and predict key concepts, variables, and relationships—and of course to enable testing of each. Given the extensive literature on policy theory and models, this text does not tackle the topic in detail here. However, it is useful for nurses to have some key ideas and concepts in mind while exploring other facets of public policy development.

Different analysts have divided policy theories into many categories. For example:

- Policy may be conceptualized as a top-down versus bottom-up exercise and/or as an inside versus outside government activity.
- In an OECD review of theoretical approaches in policy change, Cerna organized a number of theories according to outcomes categorized as "policy change" and "policy implementation."[72]
- In her book for this same publishing house, Bryant explores the public versus private financing model and the issue of societal values (health as a human right) versus the open market (health care as a commodity) as policy drivers.[73]
- Decter referred to some of these principles when he divided value sets affecting policy into the categories of ability-to-pay, like the system in the United States, versus ability-to-benefit, such as Canada's largely public system.[74]

Two taxonomies may be of help to nurses wanting to explore policy theories in greater depth. In the first of these, Bryant ultimately organized her discussion of theories into three categories, arguing that the third is the most useful for understanding policy making:[75]

1. *Pluralism*: Power is divided among interest groups across society that compete to dominate/control policy.
2. *New Institutionalism*: Decision-making is the result of the interplay of dynamics and rules among societal institutions (compared to "old institutionalism," in which decision-making was vested in the state and/or government).
3. *Political Economy*: This lens "broadens operational considerations beyond technical solutions to include an emphasis on stakeholders, institutions and processes by which policy reform is negotiated and played out in the policy arena."[76]

Miljan divided her discussion into the categories of structuralist and dynamic theories and models, including the examples shown in Table 1.1; she also positioned systems theory as a bridge between the two.[77] A fundamental divide between Miljan's two categories lies in the locus of influence. Understanding these may be helpful to nurses in understanding policy theory.

Structuralist theories posit that public policy ultimately is driven by politics, institutions, bureaucracies, and society (including class groups). Falling into this category, an institutionalist theory, for example, would position public policy as an output of institutions, derived by executive, legislative, and judicial branches of governments—a largely top-down exercise rigidly and authoritatively controlled and determined from the centre. In this theoretical view, nurses may see little room to influence policy, which is cast as government- or institution-driven (e.g., a regulator) and therefore not open to input from outside.

On the other hand, dynamic theories assume that public policy is driven in more fluid ways by competing groups and interests—theories in this stream would align with the pluralist category used by Bryant and cited above. Generally they are more individually focused than structural approaches. So here, nurses and nursing groups would assume they have a right to take part in and influence policy decision-making.

Table 1.1: Miljan's Categories of Theories and Models of Public Policy

STRUCTURALIST	SYSTEMS	DYNAMIC
Marxism	Political Systems Theory	Pluralism
Globalization		Public Choice
Institutionalism		
Incrementalism		
Environmental Determinism		

Finally, systems theory leaves room for some of the features of both. As Johnson defined it, systems theory "emphasizes the way in which organized systems (human and non-human) respond in an adaptive way to cope with significant changes in their external environments so as to maintain their basic structures intact."[78] This approach may have particular resonance for nursing, because it assumes that decision-making across groups and organizations emphasizes "their interaction with 'outside' actors and organizations and concentrates on identifying the particular elements in the environment of the group or organization that significantly affect the outcomes of its decision-making."[79] So in this sense nurses could bring nursing knowledge, science, and experience to bear on selected areas of policy with targeted outcomes that are amenable to nursing input.

NURSING ENGAGEMENT WITH CANADIAN POLICY: POLITICAL REALITIES

Two key issues may affect the nursing approach to policy—and also may explain some of the frustration nurses sometimes encounter when delving into policy work.

First, Canadian nurses generally are socialized through their education in a politically left-leaning model grounded in pluralist or systems theory. This is not to say that there is no influence of neoliberal political ideology in nursing;[80] the decision to move the Canadian registration examination to the United States has raised that issue for some observers. But for the most part, nursing seems set to be at loggerheads with the neoliberal values that have become so prominent across the governments and societies of many wealthy Western nations over the past quarter century, where policies often tend to favour market forces and privatization. Peter and Liaschenko were blunt in making the link to nursing, charging that "the ideals of neoliberalism are inconsistent with an understanding of persons as interdependent in need of care, and at varying times to varying degrees, vulnerable"—the very stuff of nursing.[81]

Second, political action and advocacy are built into the expectations of nurse behaviour and even into some regulatory standards of practice. The first nursing school in the country, the St. Catharines Training School and Nurses' Home (later the Mack Training School for Nurses), opened in June 1874, and its motto, *video et taceo* (I see and I am silent), is infamous in Canadian nursing.[82] But nursing education, socialization, and practice has since made a complete 180-degree flip; today they all are underpinned by a fundamental assumption that nursing interest groups, professional bodies, and coalitions not only can shape public policy, but that it is their duty to do so. Certainly these beliefs are fundamental to the existence and operation of professional associations. Consider the expectations inherent in the language of three professional nursing associations:

- Association of Registered Nurses of British Columbia: "As partners in progress, we help make sure the voices of Registered Nurses and Nurse Practitioners are heard by government, health authorities, media, and the public."[83]
- Registered Nurses' Association of Ontario: "Since 1925, RNAO has advocated for healthy public policy, promoted excellence in nursing practice, increased nurses' contribution to shaping the health care system, and influenced decisions that affect nurses and the public they serve."[84]
- American Nurses Association: Its mandate includes "lobbying the Congress and regulatory agencies on health care issues affecting nurses and the public."[85]

Neoliberalism

Despite its pervasive use, *neoliberalism* is a term that in some ways defies an easy or precise definition. Merriam-Webster, for example, defines a neoliberal as "a liberal who de-emphasizes traditional liberal doctrines in order to seek progress by more pragmatic methods"[86]—arguably not that helpful. Collins Dictionary goes further, describing neoliberalism as a "modern politico-economic theory favouring free trade, privatization, minimal government intervention in business, reduced public expenditure on social services, etc."[87] But in his criticism of the concept, Monbiot gets to the crux of what troubles so many in the health care sector, making the case that "neoliberalism sees competition as the defining characteristic of human relations. It redefines citizens as consumers, whose democratic choices are best exercised by buying and selling, a process that rewards merit and punishes inefficiency. It maintains that 'the market' delivers benefits that could never be achieved by planning."[88] Among the social changes associated with the movement over the past generation are "tax cuts for the rich, the crushing of trade unions, deregulation, privatisation, outsourcing and competition in public services."[89] Fears in Canada about the creeping commodification of public health care and the constant push in some sectors favouring for-profit care have fuelled a growing backlash against the doctrine by many nurses and other health and social care providers.

Challenges in the Federal Policy Landscape

Aligning with Miljan's category of dynamic theories, this book assumes that nurses have a right and duty to lobby to influence policy and an expectation that their efforts, if well informed and executed, may make a difference to the outcomes. That stance can be harshly tested when pluralist beliefs come up against the rigid institutions, ideologies, and/or incrementalist stances of governments that see public policy development differently. This is especially so if one believes philosophically that pluralism "dismisses the monopoly of the ruling class."[90] Canadians witnessed a long-standing, public political battle of wills over health care reform between the Conservative government of the Right Honourable Stephen Harper and professional associations representing nurses and doctors, unions, and coalitions such as the Health Action Lobby. Individual provincial and territorial governments added their voices to the constant calls for a less rigidly centralized and more dynamic approach.

Calls for a more collaborative approach grew stronger around the hope for a negotiated successor to the 2004–2014 Health Accord. Mr. Harper had given every possible signal that he would not enter into a new health accord with provinces and territories, and he stood firm. Still, many groups seemed shocked when he shut down the conversation in December 2011 with a unilateral announcement of an ongoing funding formula—and no new accord. Throughout its tenure, the federal Conservative government adhered to many of the more rigid tenets of neoliberal ideology and structuralist theory (e.g., a top-down system, rigidly controlled from the centre). Formed in 2003 from a range of right-wing conservatives, including the Reform Party (later the Canadian Alliance), the new Conservative Party of Canada distinguished itself clearly from the former Progressive Conservative Party, or what some called "Red Tories" in a nod to their fiscally conservative and socially progressive beliefs. Evolving from a coalition of "discontented Western interest groups,"[91] the Reform Party roots of the Conservative Party of Canada were in part grounded in a western Canadian rejection of the Progressive Conservative Party. Accusations of extremism had been levelled at the Reform Party before it folded into the Conservative Party of Canada, and its more socially conservative ideology was followed rigidly during Harper's tenure. Martin characterized that stance as one of "venomous partisanship" in a July 2016 *Globe and Mail* piece about the contrast in tone (and indeed in age) of the new Liberal government elected in October 2015.[92]

On the world stage, Harper pulled Canada away from some of its traditional roles, and was seen by some others as a barrier in thorny global policy debates such as climate change. Within Canada the government embraced some of the Marxist principles Miljan laid out around the division of society into classes, with resulting "antagonism between the classes as the central fact of politics."[93] Government-employed scientists were (and/or felt) muzzled, long-standing traditions such as the long-form census were abandoned, and the media was kept at a distance. The prime minister largely avoided the tradition of the first ministers' meetings (the prime minister and premiers)—some saying rightly so, as those meetings tended to be mostly a political show and less than substantive. Still, with topics on the table during the 2013 premiers meeting that included pan-Canadian infrastructure, federal Senate reform, and the Canada–European Union free trade agreement,[94] expectation of a federal role was not unreasonable.

In its view of health care and the role of the federal government, Harper's approach was so hands-off that the *Globe and Mail*'s national health reporter, André Picard, called out the government in October 2015 as "constitutional fundamentalists"[95]—a reference to the constitutional division of powers related to health care discussed in Chapter 3. Behind those sorts of comments was the sharp departure from the Conservative Party's progressive social roots, and concerns about a perceived drift toward an American value set—for example, individual rather than collective rights, a neoliberal mindset around markets and profits, and social conservatism around military, prisons, and religion. That was problematic for many Canadians, including many conservatives, because some of those values were set to be at loggerheads from the get-go.

Boucher argued that Canadians are "fundamentally different" from Americans in origin, constitution, governance, and values, observing that "life, liberty, and the pursuit of happiness are the centre of the American constitutional tradition, while peace, order, and good government were the principle elements of the constitutional framework in Canada."[96] Despite that history, some commentators and social activists have argued that North American economic integration would lead inexorably to more cultural integration. However, Poisson suggested in 2013 that "while fears of Americanization remain," economic integration in fact "has not led to the development of a continental identity or political integration in the European Union style."[97] Adams called Canadians "avant-garde progressives" and described Canada and the United States as "distinct cultures, with unique socio-cultural trajectories."[98]

Canadians continue to resist continental assimilation, and they continue to share social values that in some ways are more akin to those of western Europeans than Americans. And indeed, the Pew Research Center found that Americans "continue to differ considerably from ... Western Europeans when it comes to views of individualism and the role of the state."[99] Of particular note, Americans continue to be "more individualistic and are less supportive of a strong safety net";

just over a third of Americans (35 per cent) said they believed "it is more important for the state to play an active role in society so as to guarantee that nobody is in need," while 58 per cent believed individuals should pursue their lives without interference from governments.[100] The social consequences are clear: Wu and Keysar cited evidence suggesting that "members of collectivistic cultures tend to be interdependent and to have self-concepts that are defined in terms of relationships and social obligations" whereas "members of individualistic cultures tend to strive for independence and to have self-concepts that are defined in terms of their own aspirations and achievements."[101]

From this complex mix of values emerges the bristle of Canadians around some American values, and in turn, the roots of some of the concerns around Harper's approach to policy in social sectors like health care. The worry was especially acute that the federal withdrawal from dialogue and leadership would further fragment health care for Canadians, and might add fuel to calls from some quarters for a more market-driven model that would favour private, for-profit options and solutions. Harper's beliefs and style proved a frustrating opposition for health care leaders and groups who believed in the value of a strong federal hand at the health policy table, and who, since the 1990s, had grown used to being consulted. Perhaps revealing the depth of the culture/values schism Harper seemed bent on driving, even the majority of Canadian conservatives (58 per cent) preferred Obama over his conservative (Republican) opponent in the run for president in the United States in 2012.[102] The influence of politics on policy is discussed in examples throughout the book, and explicitly in Chapter 11, where forces and models that may influence policy development are introduced (see Table 11.4).

SUMMARY AND IMPLICATIONS

Koon, Hawkins, and Mayhew described health policy as "a highly contested policy domain in which policy change is often incremental and slow."[103] Knowing something about policy models and policy theory can at least help us understand why it is that way. In a 2013 analysis of factors supporting success in European health policy, Mackenbach and colleagues concluded that, "in general, health policies tend to follow national income and to align with the values of their populations."[104] In addition, they noted that "in some cases, governments seem to be in the lead, doing more than might be expected, while in others they lag behind, doing less."[105] The federal Liberal government of the Right Honourable Justin Trudeau, elected by Canadians in October 2015, seems intent on having at least a leadership role (if not being in the lead) in a number of areas, including health, that its predecessor had eschewed.

In theory, the philosophy and decision-making style of the Justin Trudeau government, like previous Liberal governments over the past 50 years, would seem to signal a pluralist approach to its policy making. Demonstrating the shift from the Harper government in mandate letters to his cabinet ministers, the new prime minister stated his expectations around "a different style of leadership" that would include "close collaboration with your colleagues; meaningful engagement with Opposition Members of Parliament, Parliamentary Committees and the public service; constructive dialogue with Canadians, civil society, and stakeholders, including business, organized labour, the broader public sector, and the not-for-profit and charitable sectors" and others.[106]

In the prime minister's language, nurses and other health care providers saw an opening—an expectation that they would be included in the process of policy making. Discussing public engagement in policy development, Lenihan asserted that "many issues can't be solved by governments working alone," arguing that in policy areas such as population health "stakeholders and the general public often have a critical role to play."[107] This chapter has made a case that nurses and nursing organizations should be engaged in policy development and has identified historical examples of health policy and nursing interventions. But this chapter really is just the beginning of the beginning. Key terms in this area of work have been identified and defined, and categories of theories that may help guide the policy work of nurses have been introduced. These are expanded in Module III in a discussion of a more fulsome Canadian model that has been tested and continues to evolve with the input of nurses. The remainder of Module I is focused on governance of the country and its health systems so that nurses may understand points of accountability and possible points of input to policy development.

DISCUSSION QUESTIONS

1. Define public policy and discuss examples of public policy affecting nursing.
2. What is healthy public policy and how does it relate to nursing practice?
3. Contrast the various paradigms of public policy theory; what frameworks fit with the ideology (or ideologies) of nursing? Which ones have worked to facilitate nursing influence on public policy? Why are some more effective than others?
4. Discuss the impacts of neoliberal ideology on public policy in Canada. How is this movement affecting government decision-making in public policy? In health policy? What are the implications for nurses working in the policy arena?

ADDITIONAL POLICY RESOURCES

PUBLIC POLICY AND NURSING POLICY BASICS

Bryant, T. (2009). *An introduction to health policy.* Toronto: Canadian Scholars' Press Inc.

Humphreys, K., & Piot, P. (2012). Scientific evidence alone is not sufficient basis for health policy. *British Medical Journal, 344,* e1316. Available from http://dx.doi.org/10.1136/bmj.e1316.

Miljan, L. (2012). *Public policy in Canada: An introduction* (6th ed.). New York: Oxford University Press.

Spenceley, S., Reutter, L., & Allen, M. (2006). The road less travelled: Nursing advocacy at the policy level. *Policy, Politics, & Nursing Practice, 7*(3), 180–194.

CHAPTER 2

Canadian Federal, Provincial, Territorial, Municipal, and Aboriginal Governance: Who Does What?

CHAPTER HIGHLIGHTS

- Canada 101: What Nurses Need to Know
- The Governance of Canada
- Provincial and Territorial Governance
- Aboriginal Governance: First Nations, Inuit, and Métis Peoples
- Summary and Implications
- Discussion Questions
- Additional Policy Resources

LEARNING OUTCOMES

1. Describe the basic demographics and population distribution of people in Canada.
2. Describe the governance structures and functions of the three branches of Canada's federal government.
3. Define *federation, parliamentary democracy,* and *constitutional monarchy.*
4. Describe Canada's provincial and territorial governance structures.
5. Describe Aboriginal governance structures in Canada.

Policy Influencer: The Honourable Lucie Pépin

The Honourable Lucie Pépin, Chevalier de l'Ordre du Québec, RN, LLD (*honoris causa*), had an illustrious career in nursing in Montreal before turning her public service talents to politics. After holding the head nurse role in gynecology at Hôpital Notre Dame in Montreal during the 1960s, she was a force in establishing the first outpatient birth planning clinic in Quebec and subsequently helped spread the model Canada-wide.[1] She would remain a prominent advocate for women's reproductive rights all her life. Pépin was elected to the House of Commons in 1984 and later appointed to the Senate by Prime Minister Chrétien, where she served from 1997 to 2011. Among her many roles of policy influence she served as member of the Appeal Division of the National Parole Board, the Royal Commission on Electoral Reform and Party Financing, and the Special House Committee on Child Care—and she was vice president, then president, of the Canadian Advisory Council on the Status of Women. In her senatorial role, she co-led with Dr. Wilbert Keon a landmark Senate review of the determinants of health in 2009.[2]

"We are a geographically huge and diverse country; but for all the ways that geography defines us, Canada was formed not by accidents of nature, but by acts of national will."

— *The Right Honourable Charles Joseph Clark, former prime minister of Canada*[3]

CANADA 101: WHAT NURSES NEED TO KNOW

Bounded by the Pacific, Arctic, and Atlantic Oceans—the world's longest coastline—and the United States, the geographic scale of Canada is vast (see Figure 2.1). Spanning more than 5,500 km from Cape Spear in the east to the Yukon-Alaska border, and more than 4,600 km from Middle Island, Ontario, in the south to Cape Columbia, Nunavut,[4] Canada is the world's second-largest country after Russia. But with a population just over 35.5 million, Canada is one of the least densely populated nations; by comparison of scale, for example, with its roughly 1.3 billion citizens, all of India would fit inside Nunavut and the Northwest Territories, which together were home to about 80,000 Canadian citizens in 2015.

Within that space, Canadians are spread across 10 provinces, 3 territories, more

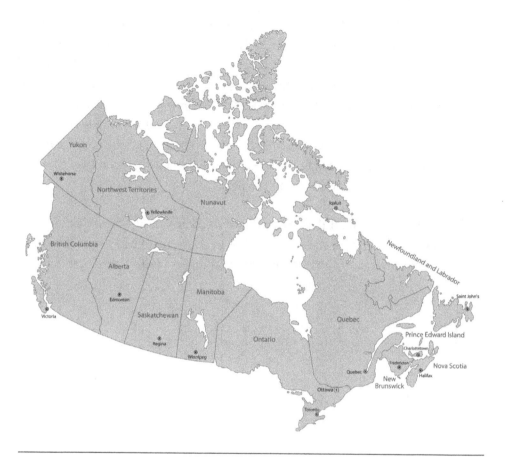

Figure 2.1: Map of Canada Showing Provinces, Territories, and Capital Cities

Source: Stockfresh.com

than 600 First Nations reserves, Crown land communities, and other Aboriginal territories, and 6 time zones in a highly skewed distribution (see Figure 2.2) that has given rise to some vexing governance and program challenges:

- Most Canadians live within about 200 km of the Canada–United States border. At nearly 9,000 km, it is the world's longest international border.[5]
- More than 60 per cent of Canadians live in Ontario (38 per cent) and Quebec (23 per cent) alone.[6]
- In one of the most ethnically diverse places on earth, more than 6 million Canadians live within an hour's drive of Toronto's iconic CN Tower—the Greater Toronto Area (Toronto, Durham, Halton, Peel, and York).[7] A million more Canadians live here than the populations of all of

Saskatchewan, Manitoba, the four Atlantic provinces, and all three territories combined. And if the trends continue in this region, foreign-born citizens will soon outnumber those born in Canada. To say nothing of the staggering infrastructure challenges posed by that volume and diversity of people and cultures, the resources both generated and required by this region and others like it—Vancouver and Montreal, for example—stand in stark contrast to those of most other areas of the country, which are much less densely populated but where citizens expect access to at least some of the same general services and privileges.

What the people in all these places have in common, of course, is that they all live in Canada. And so, whether they live in the heart of Montreal, on a farm outside Grand Prairie, or spend their lives working in God's Lake First Nation,

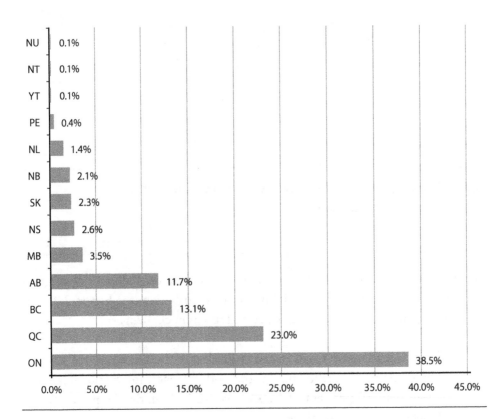

Figure 2.2: Proportion of Canadian Population by Province and Territory, 2015

Source: Statistics Canada. (2015). Estimates of population, Canada, provinces and territories: Second quarter 2015. Ottawa: Statistics Canada.

they share certain common rights, duties, and expectations related to their lives here. But Canada's geographic extremes and population distribution mean that delivering services like health care in relatively equitable ways can be a daunting challenge.

Canadians: A Population Snapshot

Canada's population growth leads the Group of Seven nations—usually simply called the G7. Population growth is highest in Nunavut, Alberta, Saskatchewan, and Manitoba, and has declined slightly in the Northwest Territories and in Newfoundland and Labrador.[8] Net international migration is responsible for two-thirds of Canada's population growth, with natural increase lowest in the Atlantic provinces and negative in Newfoundland and Labrador.

First Peoples

Evidence suggests that there were settlements in North America dating back to between 9,000 and 13,000 years before contact with Europeans—hence the use in Canada of the terms First Peoples, Indigenous, and Aboriginal, the latter referring to "the people and things that have been in a region from the earliest time."[9] In this text, the term Aboriginal is used to refer collectively to the First Peoples of this land. Certainly there is evidence of well-established, organized communities, trade, and agriculture across much of North America by 1,000 to 500 BC.

The Group of Seven (G7)

The G7 is a group of government leaders from wealthy nations that have advanced economies: Canada, France, Germany, Italy, Japan, the United Kingdom of Great Britain and Northern Ireland (hereafter the United Kingdom), and the United States of America (hereafter the United States). For various purposes other countries are sometimes included; for example, the G8 originally included the G7 countries plus Russia, but with Russia now suspended, the European Union is sometimes included as an eighth partner. There are also arrangements for meetings of a group of 10 countries and national banks called the G10, and a group of government and bank leaders from 20 nations called the G20, which describes itself broadly as "the premier forum for its members' international economic cooperation and decision-making."[10]

Some 1.4 million people in Canada (4.3 per cent of the population) claimed Aboriginal identity in the 2011 census, including First Nations (60.8 per cent), Métis (32.3 per cent), and Inuit (4.2 per cent) peoples. The Aboriginal population in 2011 had grown by 20.1 per cent since 2006—four times the rate of other Canadians, nearly all of that the result of natural increase. As a result, with a median age of 27 years, Aboriginal Peoples are much younger on average than other Canadians (median 40 years), with the youngest being Inuit (median 23 years), followed by First Nations (median 26 years) and Métis (median 31 years).[11]

Despite a history of attempts to eradicate their cultures, there is tremendous diversity among Canada's 618 First Nations,[12] who speak more than 60 languages in 12 distinct families.[13] The most common family of languages reported in the 2011 population census was Algonquian, including the Cree (e.g., Swampy Cree, Woods Cree, Moose Cree), Ojibway, Innu/Montagnais, Oji-Cree, Mi'kmaq, and Blackfoot languages.

The majority of First Nations are found in Ontario, the four western provinces, and in the Yukon and Northwest Territories. Métis nations can be found from Ontario to British Columbia. Most Inuit communities are in four areas together known as Inuit Nunangat: the autonomous area of Nunatsiavut (northern Labrador), Nunavik (northern Quebec), Nunavut, and the Inuvialuit Settlement Region (the western Arctic areas of Yukon and the Northwest Territories).

Aboriginal Peoples are spread across the country, living in urban, rural, and remote settings, with large concentrations of some groups in cities like Ottawa, Toronto, Winnipeg, Edmonton, and Vancouver. While many people with registered Indian status live on reserve lands, just over half now live off reserve, and a quarter of Inuit live outside the Inuit Nunangat. The largest concentration of First Nations people living off reserve (roughly 26,000 in 2014) is in Winnipeg.[14] A federal Urban Aboriginal Strategy was updated in 2014 to encourage partnerships and community planning and provide operational support to Aboriginal organizations.[15]

How Well Do You Know Canada's First Nations?

Check out this interactive map to learn more about Aboriginal territories, languages, and treaties: http://native-land.ca/full-map.html.

Look at the following interactive map to view profiles of individual First Nations and links to many of their websites: http://fnp-ppn.aandc-aadnc. gc.ca/fnp/Main/index.

Ethnicity of Non-Aboriginal Canadians

Historically, the vast majority of Canadian immigrants have come from a European background, the largest numbers being from Great Britain, Ireland, France, Germany, the Netherlands, Italy, and the Ukraine. But in reality, for much of its first half century, Canada was dominated heavily by citizens of British (51 per cent) and French (28 per cent) origin, and the country remained "strongly Eurocentric" at the end of World War II.[16]

Shifting social values through the 1960s, a more embracing public policy stance on multiculturalism by political leaders (whether genuine or, more cynically, Machiavellian[17]), amendments in 1978 and 1987 to the Immigration Act, and the new Multiculturalism Act (1988) all contributed to a dramatic shift in immigration patterns and in the present make-up and cultural integration of Canada's population. In 2011, 20.6 per cent of people in Canada identified themselves as having been born outside Canada (the highest among G7 nations), with most coming from East Asia, South Asia, and the Middle East. Among visible minorities—nearly a fifth of the Canadian population in 2011—South Asian, Chinese, and Black people made up 61.3 per cent of the sector. They are much younger on average than other Canadians and most immigrate to Ontario, British Columbia, Quebec, and Alberta—70 per cent settle in Toronto, Montreal, and Vancouver alone.[18] Some 95 per cent of all foreign-born Canadians live in these provinces, with half in Ontario. The largest group by far, South Asians, represent a quarter of all visible minorities and 4.8 per cent of the Canadian population.

In 2011, the largest self-identified ethnicity in Canada was Canadian (alone or with other ethnic origins), followed, in order of numbers, by English, French, Scottish, Irish, German, Italian, Chinese, First Nations, Ukrainian, East Indian, Dutch, and Polish—each group including more than 1 million people.

Language

Mirroring the ethnic diversity of the population, Canada is a place of many languages; more than 200 non-Aboriginal languages were reported in the 2011 population census. The numbers of English-only speakers (58 per cent) and French-only speakers (18.2 per cent) at home both dropped in 2011 from 2001, but the number reporting an ability to speak in either language rose slightly to 17.5 per cent. More than 6.5 million citizens reported speaking some other first language at home, with the highest growth being Tagalog, Mandarin, Arabic, Hindi, Creoles, Bengali, Persian, and Spanish. Matching the ethnic distribution, Toronto is home to the largest numbers of citizens speaking a language other than English or French, followed by Vancouver and Montreal.[19]

Religion

Roughly two-thirds of people in Canada identify as being affiliated with a Christian religion, the largest group being Roman Catholic (38.7 per cent), followed in number by affiliations with the United and Anglican churches. However, the second-largest group after Roman Catholic identified no religious affiliation (23.9 per cent), a sharp rise from 16.5 per cent a decade earlier. The next largest cluster of religions, at 7.2 per cent of all Canadians, includes Islam, Hinduism, Sikhism, and Buddhism—up from 4.9 per cent in 2001.[20] Muslims continue to be the fastest-growing group, just ahead of those having no religious affiliation.

Age

Like most of the wealthy Western world, with fertility gradually declining as longevity climbs, Canadians, on average, are aging. In 2014, for the first time in our history, the number of Canadians aged 55–64 exceeded those aged 15–24. On Canada Day in 2014, 15.7 per cent of Canadians were 65 or older—a marked rise from the mid-1960s when the number was just 10 per cent. By 2016, Canadians over the age of 64 are predicted to outnumber those under the age of 15, and seniors are set to represent 24–28 per cent of the population by 2063. Canadians in the Atlantic provinces are, on average, older than other Canadians, and in the territories they are younger.

Economy and Global Standing

Canada is a wealthy, modern democracy with a robust and fairly stable economy. Despite its small population (ranked 37th in size globally), the World Bank ranked Canada's economy as the world's eleventh largest in 2014 (in US dollars, see Figure 2.3),[21] and in thirteenth place as measured by gross domestic product (GDP) per capita.[22] The OECD defines GDP at market prices as "the expenditure on final goods and services minus imports: final consumption expenditures, gross capital formation, and exports less imports" with no deduction for depreciation.[23]

Canada's economy is heavily dominated by service industries (e.g., construction, education, health care, retail, tourism), where more than three-quarters of Canadians are employed.[24] More than 3.6 million people were employed by various levels of governments in public sector services alone in 2012—with their wages and salaries costing roughly $194.2 billion.[25] The two other leading industries are manufacturing (e.g., automobiles, food, paper, high-technology equipment) and natural resources (e.g., agriculture, fishing, forestry, mining). The United States is Canada's largest trading partner, and Canada takes part in a number of continental and other global trade agreements.

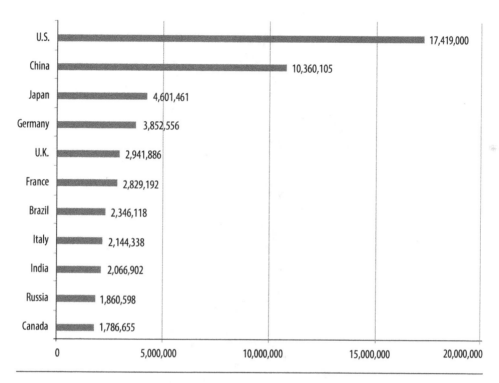

Figure 2.3: Gross Domestic Product of the Top 11 Economies, 2014 (USD Millions)

Source: The World Bank. (2015). *GDP ranking.* New York: The World Bank.

Among its many global affiliations, Canada is a member of the United Nations, the Commonwealth of Nations, the North Atlantic Treaty Organization (NATO), the World Trade Organization, the G7, and the OECD. The Washington-based Heritage Foundation—a conservative research think tank—describes Canada's "robust economic freedom" as resting on "a judicial system with an impeccable record of independence and transparency" and where corruption is vigorously prosecuted by governments.[26] The foundation ranks Canada in sixth place globally in its measures of economic freedom.

THE GOVERNANCE OF CANADA

"Governments in democracies are elected by the passengers to steer the ship of the nation. They are expected to hold it on course, to arrange for a prosperous voyage, and to be prepared to be thrown overboard if they fail in either duty."

—*The Honourable Eugene Forsey, former Senator, Canada*[27]

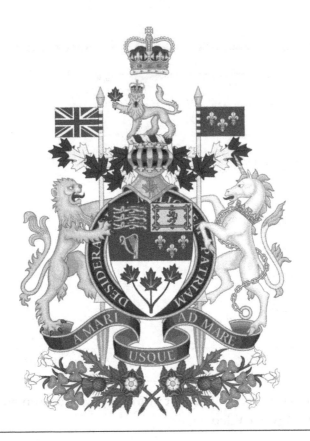

Figure 2.4: Rendition of the Royal Coat of Arms of Canada

Source: Jorge Compassio, Wikimedia Commons

Terminology

Canada is a liberal democracy structured as a federation of 10 semi-independent provinces and 3 territories, and governed collectively as a representative, parliamentary democracy under a constitutional monarchy, as described below. A key symbol of the nation, the Royal Coat of Arms, is shown in Figure 2.4.

Liberal Democracy

Along with other wealthy Western nations, Canada is often described as a liberal democracy. Collins Dictionary defines the term as "a democracy based on the recognition of individual rights and freedoms, in which decisions from direct or representative processes prevail in many policy areas."[28] In his essay on the topic, Plattner described the two words separately, pointing to the origins of democracy as "the rule of the people" and saying, "As the rule of the many, it is distinguished from monarchy (the rule of one person), aristocracy (the rule of the best), and oligarchy (the rule of the few)."[29] He argues that the term *liberal*, above all, implies "that government is limited in its powers and its modes of acting. It is limited first by the rule of law, and especially by a fundamental law or constitution, but ultimately it is limited by the rights of the individual."[30]

These principles are all reflected in Canada's constitution. As others have done, Plattner argued that as authoritarian regimes have fallen over the past 25 years, many have been replaced by some version of a democracy, but certainly they cannot all be called liberal democracies.[31] Canada, the United States, the Commonwealth of Australia, New Zealand, the United Kingdom, and many western European nations would fall under the *liberal democracy* moniker.

The Federation

The Oxford Dictionary defines *federation* as "a group of states with a central government but independence in internal affairs."[32] In this structure, both the central (or federal or national) and individual state governments have defined authority, rights, and responsibilities, and in general, none of them is subordinate to another.[33] A unitary state, on the other hand, primarily has one centralized level of government; examples include the United Kingdom, New Zealand, Japan, the French Republic, the People's Republic of China, and the Republics of Chile, Turkey, and South Africa.

Canada is a federal state. Note the difference between the use of *confederation* to describe the process of creating the Canadian federation during the 1860s, and *confederation* as an actual governance structure, such as the collective of the 28 nations of the European Union. The European Union is not officially identified as such, but behaves as a confederation in its governance—in its own words, "pooling sovereignty" and sitting "between the fully federal system found in the United States and the loose, intergovernmental cooperation system seen in the United Nations."[34]

It is important for nurses and other students of public policy to understand from the outset that Canada's provinces do not report in some hierarchical way to the federal government. That misperception reveals itself in letters to federal officials, for example, from citizens—and sometimes from health care providers, including nurses—imploring them to intervene in an unresolved provincial, regional, or even employer issue. Even planned lobbying efforts seem sometimes to be misdirected to the wrong level of government. As shown in Figure 2.5, the common unifying structure in the Canadian federation, in a hierarchal sense, is not the federal government or the prime minister, but the sovereign—the head of state—and the Constitution. As it is worded in the founding agreement establishing the Council of the Federation, "Under the Constitution, Canada's two orders of government are

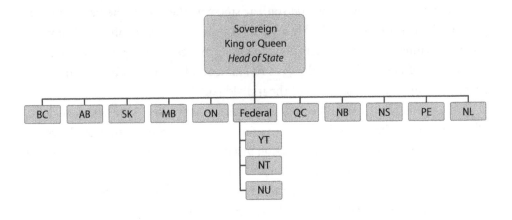

Figure 2.5: A High-Level Representation of the Canadian Federation

of equal status, neither subordinate to the other, sovereign within their own areas of jurisdiction."[35] That concept is explored further in this chapter.

Canada shares the North American continent with two other large nations—Mexico and the United States—each of which is a federal presidential constitutional republic with an elected president who serves as head of state and head of government. In his extensive examination of Canadian federalism, Smith argued that modern federalism—"associated with a geographical division of power"[36]—in fact began with the Constitution of the United States, written in 1787.[37] Canada and Australia are federations with some traits in common with the United States; however, their governance structures are more similar to each other than to that of the United States, with both being federal parliamentary constitutional monarchies, and, of course, sharing the same head of state.

Canada, Mexico, and the United States[38] have constitutions that spell out structures, rights, and responsibilities around a division of powers between federal and state levels—and in the case of Mexico the municipal level as well. Each of these nations also has a federal governance structure that includes executive, legislative, and judicial branches. Examples of other large federated nations include the Federative Republic of Brazil, the Federal Republic of Germany, the Republic of India, and the Russian Federation.

Parliamentary Democracy

A parliamentary democracy is a system of government wherein "the law is the supreme authority."[39] In this model, governance is grounded in bodies elected freely by the people to represent them (hence the term *representative democracy*), and the executive structures derive their authority from the elected legislatures and the Constitution. Canada's federal Parliament includes the Crown (i.e., the sovereign head of state) and a bicameral—two chambers—legislative structure made up of the appointed Senate (or Upper House), and the elected House of Commons (or Lower House).

In a parliamentary democracy, the executive and legislative branches of government are therefore deeply interrelated and interdependent, and one may not act unilaterally without authority of the other. This structure means that the head of government (i.e., prime minister of the country or premier of a province or territory) and the cabinet ministers are all accountable to the elected parliament or legislature (representing the people), and vice versa. With many checks and balances built into the system, in theory no one person or group in a parliamentary democracy has a right to take over or make unilateral policy decisions.

Constitutional Monarchy

In a constitutional monarchy, the head of state is separate from the head of government, and both take their authority from the constitution. This structure differs from an absolute monarchy, where the head of state is also head of government and has unrestricted authority over the people and even above courts—the Nation of Brunei, the United Arab Emirates, the State of Qatar, and the Kingdom of Saudi Arabia, for example. In a constitutional monarchy the head of state may not exert any power or action beyond what is provided in the constitution, typically assumes an apolitical stance on affairs of the nation and does not appoint politicians. However, she or he may exercise a number of functions, including giving royal assent to federal policy and legislation and dissolving and opening parliaments. In some nations, the constitutional monarch is more directly involved in governing: the Hashemite Kingdom of Jordan and State of Kuwait are two examples of constitutional monarchies where the monarch (the king and the emir, respectively) wields significantly more legislative and executive power compared to the heads of state in Canada or Denmark.

Canada's monarch (or sovereign), Her Majesty Queen Elizabeth II, has been head of state and head of Canada's executive, legislative, and judicial branches since 1952. The Royal Style and Titles Act formally conferred upon her the title Queen of Canada in 1953.[40] She "personifies the state and is the personal symbol of allegiance, unity and authority for all Canadians. Legislators, ministers, public services and members of the military and police all swear allegiance to the Queen."[41] Queen Elizabeth II also serves as queen and head of state of the United Kingdom, Australia, New Zealand, and 12 other nations.[42]

The queen's role as head of state is sometimes misunderstood to mean that

Canada remains under the legislative or judicial control of the United Kingdom. The Constitution Act (1982) severed all remnants of this relationship and, in truth, Britain had been advocating for such a separation for more than 50 years. Other than the fact that the queen we share predominately resides in London, there is no other legislative relationship with the United Kingdom.

The queen also is head of the Commonwealth of Nations, made up of 53 countries around the globe banded together to promote "democracy, rule of law, human rights, good governance and social and economic development."[43] Most Commonwealth member nations were once part of the British Empire, which at one time covered nearly a quarter of the globe. Canadian nurses were represented in the Commonwealth Nurses and Midwives Federation from its founding in 1973 until the middle of the past decade, when membership was discontinued by the CNA. In 1980, a past CNA president, Helen Taylor, was elected to lead the federation. Membership in the federation is one structure that allows member associations to be included in ministerial and other meetings in which policy is debated and developed across the Commonwealth.

The Governor General of Canada

The queen is represented in Canada by an 11-member vice-regal team that includes the governor general at the national level, and lieutenant governors in each of the 10 provinces. The governor general is appointed by the queen on the advice of the prime minister, who is head of Her Majesty's Government. Since the powers of the office were redefined during the reign of King George VI in 1947, the governor general has "daily and fully exercised the duties of the Head of State, not only in Canada, but also abroad."[44] This governance model is similar in the other major Commonwealth federation, Australia, where the queen is head of state and is represented by a federal governor general, governors in each of the six states, and administrators in certain territories.

Canada's governor general has responsibilities in several areas. For example:

- Constitutional duties, which include the responsibility to ensure that a prime minister and government are in place and the right to "advise, caution or warn" that prime minister.[45]
- Appoints the provincial lieutenant governors on the advice of the prime minister.
- Presides over swearing-in ceremonies for prime ministers and their cabinets.
- Delivers the speech from the throne.

- Confers royal assent to parliamentary acts—the final step in the legislative process.
- Serves as commander-in-chief of Canada's military.
- Represents Canada in visits abroad, hosts visiting heads of state, and promotes Canadian sovereignty.
- Leads a broad program of awards of excellence to honour Canadians and hosts a variety of events intended to bring Canadians together.
- Leads the Canadian Heraldic Authority.

The two official residences of the governor general—and the queen when she is in Canada—are Rideau Hall, located at 1 Sussex Drive in Ottawa, adjacent to the homes of the prime minister and leader of the opposition, and at the Citadelle de Québec, at Cape Diamond in Quebec City. The governor general generally serves for a term of five years, but that may be extended. The incumbent holds the title of His or Her Excellency while in office and, after leaving office, is called "the Right Honourable" for life.

The Constitution and the Charter of Rights and Freedoms

Malcolmson and Myers defined *constitution* as "a set of rules that authoritatively establishes both the structure and the fundamental principles of the political regime."[46] Put more simply, the constitution is the rule book by which the structure of the country is laid out alongside a description of the powers that govern it. It is the supreme law of Canada and stands above all others. Originally titled the British North America Act, the renamed Constitution Act (1867) established the Dominion of Canada on July 1, 1867, as the confederation of the founding provinces of Ontario, Quebec, New Brunswick, and Nova Scotia (see Figure 2.6). It laid out legislative, executive, and judicial structures and authority, and described the division of powers among the federal government and the provinces.

While much of the act reflected Canada's British parliamentary roots, other elements, including the relationships among federal and provincial governments, were more strongly shaped by the American constitution. The United States had been a functioning democratic federation since 1776, but that was a model with which the United Kingdom had no real experience. The confederation of Australia would not follow until 1901, and indeed experience with the Canadian governance model was "in the psyche of [Australia's] founding fathers" during the negotiation of that country's formation.[47]

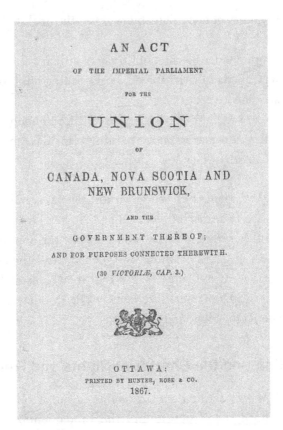

Figure 2.6: Front Page, British North America Act, 1867

Source: Library and Archives Canada

The act describes the distribution of legislative powers of federal and provincial governments as shown in the examples cited in Table 2.1. These divisions are important because they define the areas in which federal and provincial governments have authority to create laws—and where they do not. And here, with the "establishment, maintenance, and management of hospitals"[48] and other health-care structures delegated exclusively to the provinces, lies the source of what would become the seemingly relentless tussle between the federal and provincial governments around health care and its funding and delivery for 150 years.

Under the Constitution Act (1867) the United Kingdom retained ultimate authority over Canada and its foreign policy, with the Judicial Committee of the British Privy Council being the final court of appeal in Canadian legal matters.[49] The British government had begun to urge patriation of the Canadian constitution at least as early as 1927[50]—that is to say, that Canada should be a

Table 2.1: Distribution of Legislative Powers, Constitution Act, 1867

EXAMPLES OF EXCLUSIVE POWERS OF THE FEDERAL PARLIAMENT	EXAMPLES OF EXCLUSIVE POWERS OF PROVINCIAL LEGISLATURES
Public debt and property	Management and sale of public lands
Regulation of trade and commerce	Direct taxation
Taxation	Education
Postal service	Establishment, maintenance, and management of prisons
Census and statistics	
Militia, military, naval service, defence	Establishment, maintenance, and management of hospitals and other health-care structures
Quarantine and the establishment and maintenance of marine hospitals	
Beacons, buoys, and lighthouses	Shop, saloon, tavern, and other licenses
Navigation and shipping	Municipal institutions
Seacoast and inland fisheries	Incorporation of companies
Currency and coinage	Property and civil rights within the province
Banks	Administration of justice within the province
Indians and land reserved for the Indians	
Marriage and divorce	
Criminal law	
Old age pension and benefits	

fully independent nation with its own constitution. The Statute of Westminster (1931) had effectively granted independence to the various realms and nations of the British Empire, but politicians across Canada remained deadlocked on amendment processes for 50 years.

Things came to a head during the late 1970s and early 1980s when the prime minister, the Right Honourable Pierre Trudeau, threatened to proceed with unilateral federal action to repatriate the constitution, to some degree buoyed by a complicated (and split) Supreme Court decision on the issue. After rancorous debate, in the end all provinces except Quebec signed on and the Constitution Act (1982) finally established Canada as a nation fully independent from the United Kingdom. In London, the Canada Act (1982) received Royal Assent on March 29, 1982, ending the United Kingdom's role in amending Canada's constitution. The queen proclaimed the Constitution Act (1982) in force on April 17, 1982, at which time the original British North America Act became known as the Constitution Act (1867).

The Constitution Act (1982) includes the Canadian Charter of Rights and Freedoms and addresses fundamental legislative issues including the Rights of the

Aboriginal Peoples of Canada, Equalization, and Regional Disparities, as well as procedures to amend the constitution. Quebec has its own Charter of Human Rights and Freedoms that has a quasi-constitutional status in the province. However, the Canadian charter still stands above the Quebec Charter because, although Quebec did not sign the Constitution Act, the laws of Canada still apply in the province.

As in many areas of life for Aboriginal Peoples, legal rights are a mix of imposed and negotiated concepts and structures. In law, Aboriginal rights "refer to Aboriginal peoples' historical occupancy and use of the land. Treaty rights are rights set out in treaties entered into by the Crown and a particular group of Aboriginal people. The Constitution recognizes and protects Aboriginal rights and treaty rights."[51]

Some protections of rights apply to all people inside Canada—for example, freedom of conscience and religion; freedom of thought, belief, opinion, and expression; freedom of the press; freedom of peaceful assembly; freedom of association; the right to life, liberty, and security; and the right to equality without discrimination based on race, national or ethnic origin, colour, religion, sex, age, or mental or physical disability. Other rights are reserved solely for Canadian citizens and/or permanent residents—for example, the right to vote, the right to leave and re-enter Canada, and the right to live and work in any province or territory.

It is important to note that the provinces and territories also have rights legislation. The Canadian charter speaks only to the behaviours of governments, "meaning to the provincial legislatures and Parliament, and to everything done under their authority"[52] and "not to private individuals, businesses or other organizations."[53] These rights fall under provincial and territorial human rights legislation, which in general "prohibits discrimination in employment, housing and in providing goods, services, and facilities to the public."[54]

Governance of the Nation

Expanding on the high-level representation of the Canadian federation shown earlier in Figure 2.5, Canada's main governing structures are depicted in greater detail in Figure 2.7 and discussed in the following section.

How Well Do You Know Your Rights?

Read the Charter of Rights and Freedoms here: http://laws-lois.justice.gc.ca/eng/const/page-15.html.

Look up the bill or charter of rights for your own province or territory. What are your rights in your home jurisdiction?

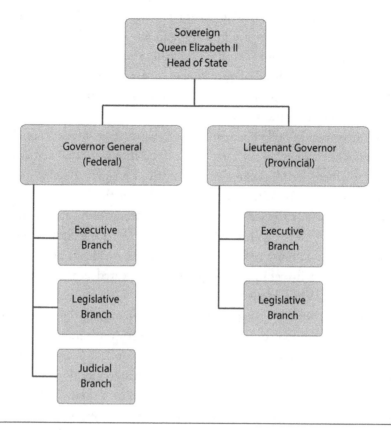

Figure 2.7: Summary of Governing Structures, Canada

Federal

Canada's governance at the federal level rests in three bodies—the executive, legislative, and judicial branches. The queen, represented by the governor general, is the head of all three branches, but the head of state has a role only in the executive branch. The legislative branch makes or changes laws, the executive branch administers and enforces laws, and the judicial branch "resolves disputes according to law—including disputes about how legislative and executive powers are exercised."[55]

The Executive Branch

"While there are obviously profound differences between the management of a government and the running of a business, the prime minister is still the chief executive officer of the largest and most complex corporation in the country."

—*Eddie Goldenberg, CM, former senior political advisor to Canadian Prime Minister Jean Chrétien*[56]

The executive branch of the federal government, depicted in Figure 2.8, is made up of the governor general, the prime minister and his or her office, the cabinet, and the Queen's Privy Council for Canada—typically shortened to the Privy Council. The prime minister is the head of government, chair of the cabinet, and a member of the Privy Council. The prime minister is addressed as "the Right Honourable" while in office and thereafter for life.

The prime minister's office is made up of the team of advisors, analysts, and administrators he or she chooses to appoint. The office is located across the street from the Parliament buildings in Ottawa, in the Langevin Block. This physical arrangement of power is quite different from that of the United States and the United Kingdom, where the seat of government power is associated with the home of the elected leader—the White House and 10 Downing Street, respectively. While some state functions are held there, the official residence of Canada's prime minister at 24 Sussex Street in Ottawa generally is treated as a much more private residence than the White House, for example.

The cabinet is chosen by the prime minister from among the elected members of the House of Commons to help him or her govern the country; occasionally a cabinet minister is chosen from among the members of the Senate. The members are called ministers, and collectively the prime minister and his or her cabinet are responsible for a) the departments of the government, usually called ministries; b) First Nations; and c) the three territories. Each minister usually is responsible for one department, although sometimes for more than one. Together the ministers are accountable to Parliament for their actions as a government.[57] Cabinet ministers are appointed by the governor general as advised by the prime minister. Cabinet ministers, who all belong to the Privy Council, hold the title of "the Honourable" while in office and thereafter for life.

How Canadians Govern Themselves

The Parliament of Canada provides an excellent summative timeline of the country's governance; go to Time Travel—Discover How Canadians Govern Themselves at http://www.parl.gc.ca/About/Parliament/SenatorEugeneForsey/time_travel/index-e.html.

To read the Honourable Eugene Forsey's comprehensive original document, visit http://www.parl.gc.ca/About/Parliament/SenatorEugeneForsey/book/preface-e.html.

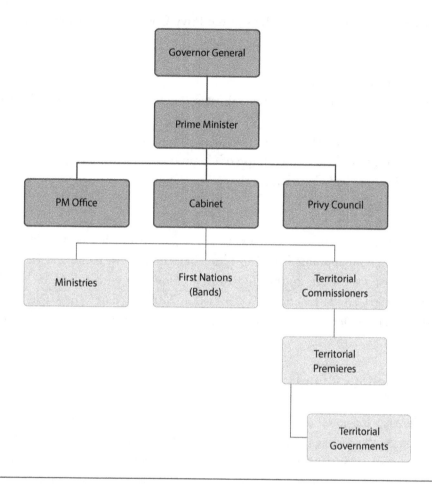

Figure 2.8: Executive Branch of Federal Government, Canada, and Related Governance and Support Structures

Junior ministers, variously titled over the years as a minister or secretary of state, or a minister without portfolio, have less authority than full ministers; for example, generally they do not lead government departments (ministries) and do not have authority to sign legislation. A minister of state may be assigned specific duties and/or areas of responsibility that may include assisting a more senior minister. Since this category was created by the government of Pierre Trudeau in 1971, prime ministers have used the different titles and assigned responsibilities in many different ways—including abolishing them altogether at some times.

The Privy Council Office is intended to be "the hub of non-partisan, public service support to the Prime Minister and Cabinet and its decision-making structures."[58] The Privy Council is led by a clerk—the most senior bureaucrat in the government —who serves as deputy minister to the prime minister, secretary to the cabinet, and head of the federal public service.[59] Members of the Privy Council are appointed for life to advise the Crown on state and constitutional issues, and include:

- former governors general,
- current and former cabinet ministers, including the current and former prime ministers,
- the current chief justice of Canada and former chief justices,
- former speakers of the House of Commons and the Senate, and
- distinguished Canadians.

The Legislative Branch

The legislative branch, the Parliament, is made up of the elected House of Commons and an appointed Senate. Federal elections must be held at least once every five years according to the Constitution. However, with Bill C-16, An Act to Amend the Canada Elections Act, passed in 2007, the date is now fixed as the third Monday in October every four years. The prime minister may call an election

The Senate Scandal

Interest in the power of the team in the Prime Minister's Office likely has never been greater among the general public than it was during the public squabbling over a $90,000 payment made by the former prime minister's then chief of staff, Nigel Wright, to cover expenses of the Honourable Senator Mike Duffy (Conservative, representing Prince Edward Island). In the court case that unfolded beginning in August 2015, Duffy faced 31 criminal charges largely related to expense claims, including claims related to his province of residence. Three other senators also faced questions about expenses around their primary residences—former Liberal Senator the Honourable Mac Harb, and two Conservative senators, the Honourable Pamela Wallin and the Honourable Patrick Brazeau, who were suspended without pay. Questions about who works in the office, who holds power, and who knew what drew significant ongoing media and public attention during Duffy's trial. He was acquitted of all charges in April 2016 and charges against Wallin and Brazeau were dropped. But the process had done significant damage to all of their reputations, to the Senate itself, and of course to the people who worked in the Prime Minister's Office. The entire process, which dragged out over four years, fuelled long-standing calls for Senate reform or outright abolition.

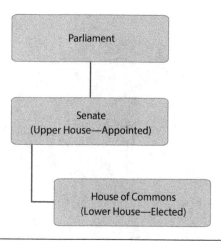

Figure 2.9: Legislative Branch of Federal Government, Canada

earlier than the four-year limit, and the governor general can do the same. The first fixed-date federal election was held in October 2015.

As of the October 2015 federal election there were 338 electoral districts (or ridings) across Canada. Redistribution of ridings usually follows a review of population numbers and patterns, based on the national census.[60] Canadians must be age 18 or older to vote in federal elections. Results of the 2015 federal election are shown in Figure 2.10.

Canadians do not vote directly for the prime minister the way Americans, for example, vote separately for their local representatives and for the president. In Canada, only the registered members of political parties vote for their party leader, typically during conventions held well ahead of an impending election. In the federal election, Canadians vote only for a local representative of a party (or an independent candidate) in that riding. In Canada's first-past-the-post system, the candidate who receives the most votes is elected as the Member of Parliament (MP) for that constituency (electoral district); there is no need for the winning candidate to secure a majority of votes—just the most votes from among all the candidates. This system is also called single-choice voting or a simple plurality. The party winning the most seats across the country forms Her Majesty's Government, and that party's leader normally becomes prime minister. Similar to the riding level, the winning party does not require a majority of the seats, but simply the most seats. If the leading party wins more than half of the seats, then it forms a majority government; with less than half—a simple plurality of seats—it forms a minority government.

Responding to pressure from Canadians and the Law Reform Commission, Justin Trudeau made a commitment that if he was elected he would lead electoral

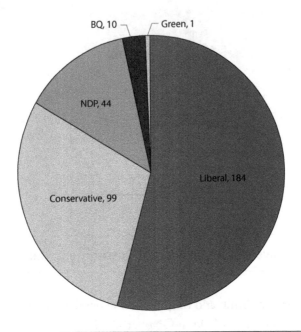

BQ, 10 ⌐   ⌐ Green, 1

NDP, 44

Liberal, 184

Conservative, 99

Figure 2.10: Federal Party Standings Following the October 2015 Election, Canada

---

reform before the next federal election. Commenting that Canada is "one of the few remaining countries that has not undertaken the needed reforms," Broadbent, Himelfarb, and Segal explained that a "central problem with our winner-take-all system is that the composition of our elected parliament does not reflect how we actually voted. A candidate who receives a plurality of the votes wins, even if a majority of the voters chose others."[61] But of course, in our system all those other votes have no impact, as Broadbent and colleagues noted, and they concluded that the system has "fed a democratic malaise." They call for a proportionality model as the needed fix for Canada. The Fraser Institute (a politically conservative public policy think tank), on the other hand, has presented evidence to argue that "proportional electoral rules are linked with higher public spending than plurality/majoritarian systems" and they note a connection "between proportional representation and deficits."[62] Finally, the Fraser Institute argued that the more fractured a government (e.g., as a result of large, unstable coalitions), "the more difficult a time it will have responding to fiscal crises."[63]

The party with the next-greatest number of seats forms Her Majesty's Loyal Opposition. More commonly known simply as the Official Opposition, the leader normally is allowed the first opportunity to speak after the Government during

Question Period and is expected, in essence, to oppose the Government in its daily work by asking questions, pushing for details, and recommending improvements. Usually the Opposition appoints critics from among its members for the various Government ministers' files and portfolios, in a sort of shadow cabinet that allows the Opposition to develop expertise in its role—but also to be prepared in the event that it might for some reason become the Government on short notice.

A minority government is a more precarious position for a leader and government than a majority government. In the case of a minority parliament, the governing party is obliged to negotiate with other parties and/or independent sitting members of the House of Commons in order to pass legislation. Despite the rancour witnessed in some minority parliaments, they may be very effective in passing transformative legislation. The two consecutive Liberal minority governments led by the Right Honourable Lester Pearson, 1963–1968, serve as famous examples. Among a long roster of landmark pieces of legislation during those years, Canada established two of its flagship safety net programs—medicare (universal health care) and the Canada Pension Plan—as well as abolished capital punishment and raised a new national flag. Those achievements and many more were possible only

What Is a Political Party?

Canada's electoral system has a long tradition of being structured around political parties at the federal and provincial levels. Collins Dictionary defines a political party as "an organization of people who share the same views about the way power should be used in a country or society (through government, policy-making, etc.)."[64] At the federal level, Canadians typically hear about the five major political parties: the Bloc Québécois, the Conservative Party of Canada, the Green Party of Canada, the Liberal Party of Canada, and the New Democratic Party. Differing from some other nations, Canada's federal political parties may or may not have formal links with their provincial counterparts. For example, there are no formal links between the Conservative Party of Canada and the provincial conservative parties, but there are links between the Liberal Party of Canada and some of its provincial cousins. The New Democrat Party is fully integrated at the federal and provincial levels.

As of the 2015 election, there were 18 political parties registered with Elections Canada and vying for seats in the Parliament of Canada. To learn more about Canada's federal political parties, visit http://www.elections.ca/content.aspx?dir=par&document=index&lang=e&section=pol.

through constant negotiation by Mr. Pearson and his team with the other party members sitting in the House—Progressive Conservatives under the leadership of the former prime minister, the Right Honourable John Diefenbaker, and the fledgling New Democratic Party and its leader, Tommy Douglas.

A minority parliament introduces the possibility of a motion of no confidence, wherein the other parties vote down a piece of the Government's proposed legislation and bring down the Government, forcing another election. This strategy does not apply to all bills before a parliament, but it always applies to the federal budget. Therefore, in the case of a minority parliament, if the other parties align to vote down the proposed budget, and their collective votes are greater than the number of votes from the sitting minority government, then that government has lost the confidence of the House.

To oversee the business of the House and its rules and decorum, a Speaker of the House is elected by secret ballot from among all the elected members other than the party leaders, the prime minister, and cabinet ministers. He or she is expected to "interpret these rules impartially, to maintain order, and to defend the rights and privileges of Members, including the right to freedom of speech."[65] The Speaker retains a seat in Parliament but votes only in the event of a tie; otherwise the Speaker is expected to maintain a neutral stance.

Differing from the elected House of Commons, the Senate (Canada's Upper House) is an appointed body. Members of the Senate review legislation from the House of Commons and may suggest amendments, or vote to either pass or defeat any bill. The Senate also takes on a number of its own activities, including providing valuable perspectives on a number of population health and health care issues important to nurses, such as mental health,[66] palliative care,[67] and the landmark review of the 2004 to 2014 Health Accord.[68]

The Constitution provides for 105 senators, representing the four major regions of the country: the western provinces, Ontario, Quebec, and the Atlantic provinces. Each of the four regions has 24 Senate seats, and in addition there are seats for Newfoundland and Labrador and the three territories. A senator may serve to the age of 75. A sitting senator is addressed as "Senator, the Honourable" and thereafter for life as "the Honourable."

There has been long-standing debate about reforming or even abolishing the Senate. Why does Canada need the Upper House? Its intention was, in part, to respond to Canada's unique geographical challenges discussed earlier in this chapter. Imagine that Party X is elected to lead a majority government. Party X wins most of the seats in vote-rich Ontario and Quebec, a few seats in the Maritimes, and only a handful of seats in the west and the territories. In this situation, there is a risk that legislation could be shaped to favour the centre of the country, its needs and its ideologies, while ignoring the needs of the rest of the country. To add context, Ontario has more than a third of all the House of Commons seats in the country; Prince Edward Island has four and New Brunswick just ten. With the existence of the Upper House, there are senators representing every region of Canada. It is their duty to examine all proposed legislation with an eye to its impact on the provinces or regions that may not be well represented in the House. This important check—sometimes known as "the sober second thought"—is designed to be a counterbalance to representation by population in the House of Commons.[69] The Parliament of Canada also notes that, in the way it is able to respond to Canada's geographic challenges, the Senate also can be used to increase under-represented groups, such as visible minorities and Aboriginal Peoples.

The idea of sober second thought has a downside, however, and to some its very existence seems anti-democratic. If the duly elected members of Parliament create and pass a piece of legislation, one may well ask why a sometimes-partisan, non-elected body should have an opportunity to render any opinion on the legislation. On the other hand, the Senate may more closely represent and advocate for the public. For example, during the legislative process around Bill C-14, the Government's proposed legislation on medical assistance in dying, the House of Commons did accept "most of the Senate's seven amendments" to its bill and agreed to study several issues—but they but stood firm in rejecting the Senate's proposal to remove the need for a person requesting assisted death to be facing death imminently.[70] In this situation, the Senate was indeed representing public opinion more closely than the House of Commons was, (i.e., the belief that people who are suffering but are not considered immediately terminally ill should be able to request assisted death in advance). Ultimately in this case, senators backed down, and deferred to the House of Commons, with some saying they hoped unresolved issues would make their way to the Supreme Court. The law was passed, and indeed, a constitutional challenge based on that very issue was launched in British Columbia almost immediately following its Royal Assent.

The Judicial Branch

The judicial branch includes the court system, which interprets and applies the laws of Canada.[73] At the head of the branch is the Supreme Court of Canada, established in 1875. The Supreme Court is in every sense the court of last resort in Canada. It "adjudicates on all areas of the law and on all cases from both the provincial/territorial courts and from the federal court system" with its decisions being "binding on all other courts in Canada."[74]

Canada has two law systems, common law and civil law, and is therefore known as having a bijural system. Originating in England, the common law (or case law) system applies across Canada, with the exception of Quebec. *The Economist* called common law "a peculiarly English development" going back a thousand years, when laws were first drawn from customs around the country and were not written down.[75] Common law is based in precedent rather than in codes or legislation; it relies on understanding past decisions.[76] The European, and particularly French, tradition of civil law applies to private legal matters in Quebec. This tradition is based in civil codes—specifically the Napoleonic Code—made up of comprehensive rules and broad general principles.[77] At the federal level, "bills and regulations must respect both types of systems, and the legal concepts within these laws must be expressed in both English and French."[78]

The Supreme Court is led by a chief justice and eight associate judges. The present chief justice, the Right Honourable Beverley McLachlin, was appointed in 2000, and is the first woman to have held the role. The chief justice also serves as

A Few Words on Senate Reform

Former Prime Minister Harper was a long-standing advocate for what is called a Triple E Senate—equal, elected, and effective. Such a model would maintain the notion of counterbalancing the House of Commons by having senators representing all regions of the country, but they would be elected rather than appointed. In July 2015 he announced his decision to refuse to appoint further senators until the Senate is reformed. The Supreme Court has ruled that Senate reform is not possible without the consent of seven provinces and at least half the nation's population—a tough target to achieve. The Official Opposition leader at the time, the Honourable Thomas Mulcair, promised to abolish the Senate if his party was elected, a change that the Supreme Court ruled requires unanimous consent of the provinces.[71] The new prime minister, Justin Trudeau, said he would appoint a panel of experts to recommend senators in an attempt to avoid the partisanship of what is in theory meant to be a more neutral body. Within the first six months of his mandate the new Independent Advisory Board was formed and in March 2016 the first seven senators were appointed under the new process. As Thomas Axworthy—policy chair at the University of Toronto's Massey College—noted in a March 2016 commentary, Trudeau's appointment model for senators comes with some challenges, but marks a major advance in "fundamentally changing the institution."[72] The chair of the Independent Advisory Board on Senate Appointments is Huguette Labelle—a former Principal Nursing Officer for Canada and former CNA president.

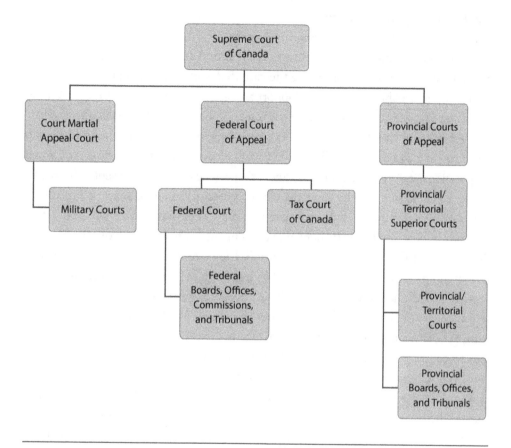

Figure 2.11: Judicial Branch of Federal Government, Canada, and Related Structures

deputy of the governor general and administrator of Canada in the absence of the governor general for a prolonged period of time. The appointment of federal judges is addressed in the Constitution, with provincial laws applying to provincial judicial appointments. Judges typically are chosen to represent the different regions of the country, and the court always includes at least three from Quebec, who are familiar with the province's civil law tradition.[79] Supreme Court justices are appointed by the governor general on the advice of the prime minister. They hold the title "the Honourable" while in office, with the exception of the chief justice, who is addressed as "the Right Honourable." In July 2016, the prime minister announced his decision to establish an independent advisory panel to receive applications from individuals interested in being appointed to the Supreme Court of Canada. The intention was to create more transparent and less partisan processes. A former prime minister, the Right Honourable Kim Campbell, was selected to lead the panel.

The Public Service of Canada

Discussing his new book[80] during an August 31, 2015, interview on CBC's *The Current*, Donald Savoie, Canada Research Chair in Administration and Governance at the University of Moncton, made the case that a vibrant democracy is dependent on a "top flight public service." To support and act on the decisions of the governing branches, Statistics Canada reported the total number of people working for the federal government in 2011 to be 427,000, including all members of the military and reservists, at a cost of $31.1 billion.[81] They work across some 200 departments, Crown corporations, commissions, boards, and other agencies of government. The public service exists to support and serve the elected government and is supposed to adhere to a code of ethics that includes non-partisan support of that government's policies.

Savoie described government departments as monopolies or quasi-monopolies, insulated from competitive pressure.[82] They may grow out of control in size, and with no competition this can lead to inertia, just as in any other industry. He argued that Canada's renowned public service, along with cabinet-driven government, began to be whittled away during the Pierre Trudeau era when the prime minister came up against barriers across some areas of the public service and began to centralize control by strengthening his own offices and instruments (i.e., the Privy Council and Prime Minister's Office). The wrenching away of control from ministries and public servants in favour of more centralized decision-making reached perhaps unprecedented levels during the Harper administration. In a commentary for the Caledon Institute of Social Policy, Torjman likened the Harper government to "the Wizard of Oz—the all-powerful, but rarely seen, player behind the scenes."[83] It was during this era that the power and activities—perhaps even the existence—of the Prime Minister's Office were exposed in ways most of the public would not previously have seen.

There may be many layers of hierarchy in a federal government department, depending on the scope and complexity of the ministry. The most senior civil servant is the clerk of the Privy Council, who is the head of the public service. As shown in Figure 2.12, the most senior member of a government department (e.g., Health Canada) holds the title of deputy minister (or equivalent). The deputy is responsible for daily operations of the department, while the minister is accountable to Parliament for his or her portfolio. The deputy does not report to the minister per se, but in practice holds a dual accountability to the head of the public service (the clerk of the Privy Council) and to the minister. Depending on the size of the department, the deputy may be supported by an associate deputy minister, who may hold a portfolio of special projects or lead one or more assistant deputy ministers. An assistant deputy minister typically leads a branch of the department. From that level, the hierarchy may include an associate assistant deputy minister,

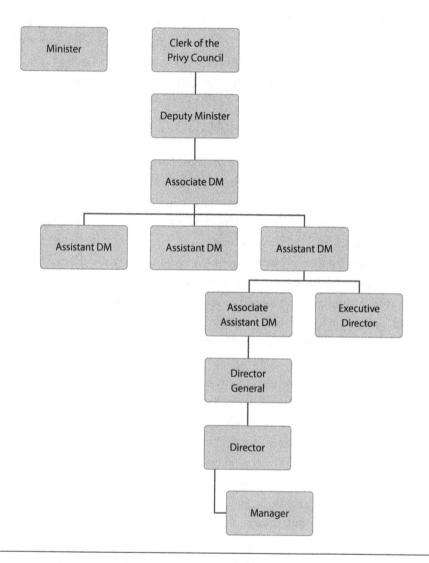

Figure 2.12: Example of Hierarchy of the Public Service within a Federal Government Department, Canada

who may lead teams or special projects, and the assistant deputy often would have one or more directors generally leading directorates within a branch, each in turn led by a director and then a manager. This federal hierarchy is fairly similar in the bureaucracies of the provinces and territories.

The Canadian Government Abroad

While it is not part of the nation's governance, students of policy should be reminded that the Government of Canada is represented through a network of some 260 offices in roughly 150 countries.[84] These include full-service embassies located in national capitals (called High Commissions in Commonwealth capitals) and a roster of permanent missions, consulates general, consulates, consular agencies, and offices that may offer a more limited range of consular and other services than an embassy.

PROVINCIAL AND TERRITORIAL GOVERNANCE

While it was not a new idea, the notion of a federated Canada emerged more seriously during the 1840s, when the United Kingdom then oversaw three provinces in North America, mirroring its Westminster model: the Province of Canada (consisting then of Canada West, or Upper Canada, and Canada East, or Lower Canada), New Brunswick, and Nova Scotia. Once provincial legislatures were established, political leaders on both sides of the Atlantic began to discuss the notion and logistics of establishing Canada as a new and separate country.

Talks were formalized and moved to action at the Charlottetown Conference in September 1864, which originally was intended to include the four Maritime provinces (New Brunswick, Nova Scotia, Prince Edward Island, and Newfoundland). Representatives of the Province of Canada asked to be included and were invited to join the meeting. However, while Newfoundland was described as "heartily" supporting the movement, in his notes about the 1864 meeting, Upper Canada's George Brown recorded that the province's leaders were "not notified in time to take part in the proceedings."[85] While Prince Edward Island was strongly resistant to confederation, generally it was thought by the others that uniting would be beneficial.

A second major conference on confederation, the Quebec Conference, would follow just a month later, resulting in 72 resolutions that would become the backbone of the Canadian Constitution. Significant debate during the meetings focused on the governance model, divided largely between those in favour of a federation like the United States that would maintain strong provincial powers, and those who favoured the unitary model of the United Kingdom that was familiar to them. Perhaps foreshadowing a Canadian trait, compromise won out: Canada would be a federated state, with a division of powers between central and provincial governments. And in addition to an elected legislative body (the House of Commons), to protect regional and cultural rights and interests there would be an appointed Senate with representation from each region of Canada.

With most of the resolutions accepted by the provinces over the following two years, the British North America Act was drafted at the London Conference of 1866, and the new nation of Canada began to take shape. Many names for the nation were proposed, with the Kingdom of Canada favoured by some. Concerns in London and in Canada about agitating the bordering United States with the *kingdom* moniker, where many still felt bruised by the events of the War of 1812, contributed to the decision to abandon that title.

The legislation to establish the new nation was ratified by the British Parliament on March 29, 1867.[86] At confederation on July 1, 1867, the former Province of Canada became the two new provinces of Ontario and Quebec, united in the federation with New Brunswick and Nova Scotia as the Dominion of Canada (see Figure 2.13).

Canada's internal borders changed significantly over the subsequent years as provinces and territories joined the federation as follows:

1870	Manitoba and the Northwest Territories (created from the unification of Rupert's Land and the North-Western Territory)
1871	British Columbia
1873	Prince Edward Island
1898	Yukon Territory (split from the Northwest Territories)
1905	Alberta and Saskatchewan
1949	Newfoundland (renamed Newfoundland and Labrador in 2001)
1999	Nunavut (split from the Northwest Territories)

Whose Land Is It?

The entire process of Canada's early formation and colonization was contingent upon a belief that the lands were in fact the United Kingdom's to claim—or at least to settle, use, occupy, and/or sell. Differing from some other countries, where one nation invaded and simply took over another, early settlers in what became the Dominion of Canada negotiated a series of treaties with Aboriginal Peoples in the name of the Crown, then Queen Victoria. In his discussion of Aboriginal rights and the Crown, Slattery cited the Supreme Court of Canada ruling that such treaties served to "reconcile pre-existing Aboriginal sovereignty with assumed Crown sovereignty, and to define Aboriginal rights."[87] Furthermore, the court stated that it "is always assumed that the Crown intends to fulfil its promises" and that promises would be delivered "through the process of honourable negotiation."[88] While treaties, on paper, seem to be two-way agreements, many Aboriginal Peoples in Canada argue that they have not been negotiated or operationalized as honourably as intended, including negotiations around the key issue of sovereignty over land. That sovereignty, of course, relates directly to the long and troubling issue of Aboriginal governance, including imposed and highly controversial colonial structures such as the Indian Act (1876).

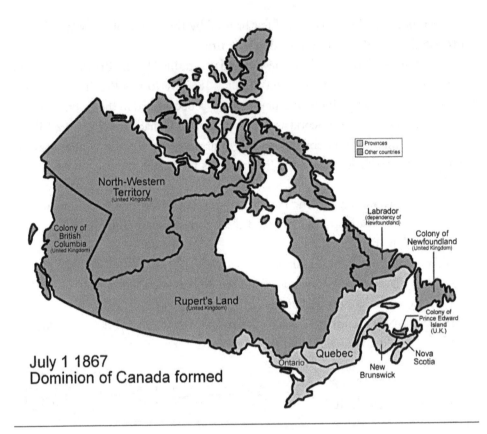

Figure 2.13: Map of Canada at Confederation, July 1, 1867

Source: Wikimedia Commons

The area known as Rupert's Land, shown in Figure 2.13, encompassed much of the land west of Hudson Bay, between the Arctic Circle in the north to the 49th parallel in the south, as well as much of what is now northern Ontario and Quebec—essentially all the lands that drain toward Hudson Bay and James Bay. The Hudson's Bay Company had been granted a monopoly on trade throughout that region by an agreement with the Crown since 1670. That charter was based, of course, on the disputable assumption that the land was the Crown's to take over or give away in the first place. With no consultation with the First Nations, Métis, or Inuit already living on the lands, the territory was transferred to the Dominion of Canada in 1870. Rupert's Land was later divided to enlarge Ontario and Quebec and, along with part of the North-Western Territory, to create Manitoba, Saskatchewan, and Alberta. In 2017 the Canadian federation consists of 10 provinces that derive their authority, rights, and responsibilities from the Constitution Act (1867), three territories whose legislative power falls under the authority of the federal government, and more than 700 First Nations, Métis settlements, Inuit communities, and the Inuit Nunangat lands.

The Provinces

Mirroring the federal model, Canadian provinces each have executive and legislative branches (see Figure 2.14). However, while most provinces originally had bicameral structures like the federal government, the provincial parliaments now are all unicameral, meaning they have only one (elected) legislative chamber. The line of accountability for the judiciary in the provinces is to the Supreme Court of Canada, described earlier; hence there is no judicial branch in the provincial governments.

The executive branch of each provincial government includes a lieutenant governor, representing the sovereign; the elected premier (or in the case of Quebec, prime minister); and the cabinet. The structure is similar to the federal parliament, with the premier selecting cabinet members from among the elected members of the legislature; they hold the title of minister and lead the various government departments or ministries. Lieutenant governors are addressed as "the Honourable" while in office and thereafter for life; the premier and cabinet ministers are addressed as "the Honourable" while in office only. The legislative branch includes the elected members, who are called members of the Legislative Assembly, with the exceptions of Ontario (members of Provincial Parliament), Quebec (members of the National Assembly), and Newfoundland and Labrador (members of the House of Assembly). Legislatures have a maximum term length fixed in the Constitution, and in many cases provinces themselves have laws requiring elections every four years. Like in federal governance, the provinces have electoral districts (ridings) that change over time as populations shift and move. In a political party system similar to the federal parties noted earlier, elections are held using a first-past-the-post system, and so there can be majority or minority governments in the provinces too. Each provincial parliament appoints a Speaker to oversee the business, traditions, and rules of the legislature.

The provincial bureaucracy supporting the governing branches is organized in hierarchies very similar to the federal civil service. According to Statistics Canada, there were 348,084 people working for Canada's provincial governments in 2011.[89]

The Territories

The massive lands that occupied all of Canada outside the three founding provinces and Newfoundland were originally called Rupert's Land and the North-Western Territory by settlers. Originally claimed by the Hudson's Bay Company, the lands

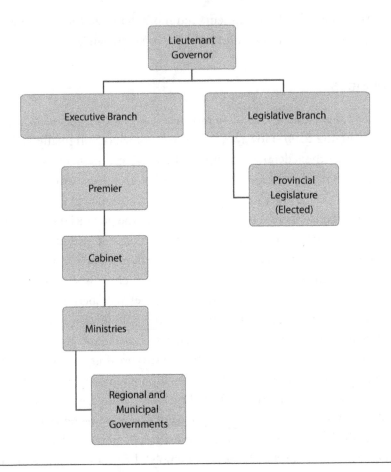

Figure 2.14: Executive and Legislative Branches of Provincial Governments, Canada, and Related Structures

were sold to Canada in 1870. The size of Canada was increased even further when Britain turned over more than 36,000 Arctic islands to Canada in 1880.[90] Once merged, these lands were at first all called the Northwest Territories by British and French settlers. Their borders changed considerably as they became parts of provinces over the decades. The Yukon Territory split from the Northwest Territories in 1898, and Nunavut did so a hundred years later in 1999, resulting in the three northern territories we know today.

Differing constitutionally from the provinces, the territories originally were each governed by a commissioner—not unlike a provincial lieutenant governor—who represented the federal government (not the queen) and administered the territory. As a result, "While provinces exercise constitutional powers in their own right, the territories exercise delegated powers under the authority of the

Parliament of Canada."[91] Those delegated powers now include an elected legislature and an Executive Council, as "province-like powers are increasingly being transferred" to the territories in the interest of local accountability and control.[92] Territorial commissioners, premiers, and cabinet ministers all are addressed as "the Honourable" while in office.

Powers were devolved to the Yukon beginning in the late 1970s when the territory adopted a governance model very similar to the provinces (i.e., a responsible government model that included political parties). Since the Yukon Act was passed in 2003, the territory has held much of the same power and accountability as a province.

Under self-government since the 1980s, the Northwest Territories and Nunavut, and more recently the government of Nunatsiavut, choose a leader in a consensus government model. In this system there are no parties; all elected members of the Legislative Assembly in the two territories are independent.[93] Through discussion, formal presentations, question-and-answer sessions, and finally secret votes, those elected members choose a Speaker, a premier, and 6 ministers, leaving the remaining 11 regular members holding the balance of power. All legislation proposed by the Executive Council passes through the regular members as part of the consensus government model. Supporting the legislative decisions of these governing bodies, there were 8,265 people employed in territorial governments in 2011.[94]

The Council of the Federation

The council of the Federation is a policy table that brings together the premiers. Formed in 2003, its goals are:

- promotion of interprovincial-territorial cooperation and closer ties between premiers, to ultimately strengthen Canada;
- fostering meaningful relations between governments based on respect for the Constitution and recognition of the diversity within the federation; and
- showing leadership on issues important to all Canadians.[95]

The council takes on a range of policy issues in areas including health care, fiscal arrangements, energy, internal trade (i.e., trade within Canada and across provincial/territorial borders), water, and economic productivity. The prime minister is sometimes invited to attend what then becomes a first ministers' meeting.

Municipal and Regional Governments

Municipal governments may be based in districts, counties, large cities, or tiny towns. Municipalities are given authority from provinces and territories for a range of services including public transit, local water systems, public parks, libraries, and local emergency services, including police.[96] Of importance to nurses, public health services normally are based in municipalities. In larger urban areas, such as Montreal, Toronto, Hamilton-Wentworth, and Vancouver, provinces may establish metropolitan governments, a complex unifying regional structure wherein the metropolitan and municipal governments coexist.

Members of municipal governments are elected just like in the federal, provincial, and territorial governments, with many having fixed terms. In some cases, school trustees and other officials may also be elected at the same time as members of the municipal government. Most municipal elections within a province are held on the same day, and most of these elections involve independent candidates, although there are political parties in some municipalities.

At the municipal level, a group of elected members typically joins a council, with the head or chief executive usually titled as mayor or reeve. Mayors in Canada are elected at large (i.e., to represent an entire city or district and not just one area within it) and have limited power independent of the council.[97] The mayor is addressed as His or Her Worship while in office.

Council decision-making is supported by public servants who are divided into departments; their work is often informed by decisions emerging from a number of council committees. Local governments (not including local school boards) employed roughly 608,000 Canadians in 2012, with salaries and wages costing some $21.2 billion.[98] Apart from provincial or territorial funding, municipalities have some powers of taxation to raise funds, including through

A Working Day in the Senate and House of Commons

Check out this link for an animation of a typical day in the House and the Senate, including seating arrangements, roles, protocols, a typical order of business, and links to live streaming of the House and Senate:

http://www.parl.gc.ca/About/Parliament/SenatorEugeneForsey/inside_view/parliament_in_action-e.html.

property taxes and revenue from issuing permits, such as building permits. Occasionally the federal government also may provide direct funding to a municipality for a special project or program development.

ABORIGINAL GOVERNANCE: FIRST NATIONS, INUIT, AND MÉTIS PEOPLES

The governance of First Nations, Inuit, and Métis peoples includes a complex mix of treaties, agreements, and structures where members may have rights and responsibilities within an Aboriginal governance arrangement while also retaining all the privileges and duties of citizens of the country and a province or territory. The notion of a nation-to-nation relationship between Canada and First Nations is complicated by the Indian Act, which tethers them to (and beneath) the Government of Canada. The department of Indigenous and Northern Affairs Canada (formerly Aboriginal Affairs and Northern Development Canada) remains deeply involved in the governance and lives of Aboriginal Peoples. Its role is to negotiate and implement acts, agreements, treaties, and land claims for the federal government, and to support Aboriginal Peoples working toward self-government.

The smallest group of Aboriginal Peoples are the Inuit—59,445 in number in 2011.[99] There are another 100,000 Inuit living in Greenland, northern Alaska, and Russia. Within Canada, Inuit participate in the governance of their provinces and territories like other Canadians. Consensus is the primary tool of governance, which relies heavily on consultation with community elders within individual Inuit communities. The consensus model of territorial governance in Nunavut and the Northwest Territories was described earlier.

Inuit belong to many national and international (especially circumpolar) associations, and are represented by Inuit Tapiriit Kanatami, which identifies itself as an advocacy organization and "the national voice of 55,000 Inuit living in 53 communities" across Inuit Nunangat.[100] As the national leader of Inuit, each president of Inuit Tapiriit Kanatami is elected to a three-year term and governs with an elected board of directors representing the four regions of the Inuit Nunangat, as well as representatives of the Inuit Circumpolar Council (Canada), National Inuit Youth Council, and the Pauktuutit Inuit Women of Canada.

Under four land claims agreements, Inuit were granted title to regions covering some 40 per cent of the landmass of Canada.[101] Nunavut Tunngavik Incorporated is an example of a separate organization involved in the governance of Nunavut. Its mandate is to coordinate and manage "Inuit responsibilities set out in the Nunavut Land Claims Agreement" and to ensure that "federal and territorial governments fulfill their obligations."[102]

The next largest group, the Métis Nation, includes 452,000 members. Like Inuit, Métis share privileges identical to other Canadians in their participation in federal and provincial or territorial elections. They also have rights within the Métis Nation, which describes its central goal as securing "a healthy space for the Métis Nation's on-going existence within the Canadian federation."[103] A landmark and unanimous Supreme Court decision in April 2016 ruled that the federal government has constitutional responsibility for Métis and non-status Indians, opening the door to future negotiation of rights and benefits by the two groups.

The governing body, the Métis National Council, includes a democratically elected president as well as the presidents of its member nations: the Métis Nation of Ontario, the Manitoba Métis Federation, the Métis Nation—Saskatchewan, the Métis Nation of Alberta, and the Métis Nation British Columbia. The individual Métis nations also hold democratic elections for their local or community councils and provincial bodies. At the time of this writing, a key objective of the current leadership is the development of a Métis constitution. The Métis Nation Protocol, an agreement between the Métis Nation and the Government of Canada renewed in 2013, identifies certain priorities, including "more flexible funding agreements and reduced administrative burden" and ongoing efforts to "strengthen national policy support for Métis economic development and participation in major development projects."[104]

At 851,560 in number, First Nations make up the largest proportion of Aboriginal Peoples in Canada.[105] Although some identify explicitly as being sovereign nations, like Inuit and Métis they also share the same voting and citizenship privileges as all other people within Canada. As some First Nations assert themselves as sovereign, there has been reluctance among some leaders to participate in Canadian governance structures. Others—including the Assembly of First Nations—advise that First Nations peoples should assume a stance similar to dual citizenship, urging citizens to participate (and vote) in both structures.

As the Canadian government has said, these complicated governance structures "are at different stages of maturity and development," from minimal governance to self-governance.[106] The recent First Nations Elections Act (2015) is intended to support "the political stability necessary for First Nations governments to make solid business investments, carry out long term planning and build relationships, all of which will lead to increased economic development and job creation for First Nations communities."[107] Opting into the new legislation is optional for First Nations.

At the national level, the Assembly of First Nations is an advocacy body representing all the chiefs of First Nations across Canada, each being elected by the members of their respective communities. The executive body includes a national chief (who is elected every three years by all the other chiefs), 10 regional chiefs, and chairs of the elders, women's and youth councils.[108] As directed by all the chiefs, the national Assembly takes on work that includes advocacy efforts and campaigns, legal and policy analysis, and communication, relationship building, and negotiation with governments.

Within individual First Nations—also called reserves or bands—the members of each community elect chiefs and their band councils. Through a wide range of

The Indian Act

To gain an appreciation for the perspective from which some First Nations view Canadian governments, in any discussion of governance it is important to acknowledge the contentious Indian Act (1985). First passed in 1876, this far-reaching legislation affects Indian status, bands, and reserve lands—and, some would say, nearly every aspect of the lives of First Nations peoples. There is no shortage of acrimony among many First Nations regarding the act, which has been described as "highly invasive and paternalistic" throughout its history of "oppression and resistance."[109] The opening words of the final report of the Truth and Reconciliation Commission are less ambiguous:

> For over a century, the central goals of Canada's Aboriginal policy were to eliminate Aboriginal governments; ignore Aboriginal rights; terminate the Treaties; and, through a process of assimilation, cause Aboriginal peoples to cease to exist as distinct legal, social, cultural, religious, and racial entities in Canada. The establishment and operation of residential schools were a central element of this policy, which can best be described as cultural genocide.[110]

Canada has been accused of doing a poor job "educating its young people about federal policies that forced Indigenous tribes onto reserves [and] the pass system that imprisoned them there"—and that these policies are in part responsible for the "enormous gulf of distrust between communities."[111]

To read the *Summary of the Final Report of the Truth and Reconciliation Commission of Canada,* go to http://www.trc.ca/websites/trcinstitution/File/2015/Honouring_the_Truth_Reconciling_for_the_Future_July_23_2015.pdf.

To read the Indian Act (1985), go to http://laws-lois.justice.gc.ca/eng/acts/i-5/.

governance agreements with the federal government, they may administer services and programs much like many municipalities do, from basics including water, sewage, and garbage collection to a full range of health care services in the case of some bands operating under a self-government model. The chief and council are the final authority within First Nations, although they may come together with other bands in tribal councils—a regional structure, to which they may delegate some measure of governance authority. Chiefs in First Nations and Métis nations are always addressed as "Chief," while band councillors have no formal title.

The three national First Nations associations just described are joined by two other important national Aboriginal associations, whose governance and policy work bring them into regular contact with Canadian governments—and can impact health care and the nurses delivering it. The Congress of Aboriginal Peoples represents the interests of Métis and non-status Indians as well as "all off-reserve status and non-status Indians, Métis and Southern Inuit Aboriginal Peoples."[112] The organization has affiliates across the provinces and territories. Finally, the mandate of the Native Women's Association of Canada is to "advance the well-being of Aboriginal women and girls, as well as their families and communities through activism, policy analysis and advocacy."[113]

SUMMARY AND IMPLICATIONS

The country's governance may feel remote to the daily practice of nurses, who are busy delivering care and other services, but it is critical to be aware of the country's structures and players—and to know something of their spheres of control and levels of influence. Simply knowing the levels of governance of the nation, provinces, and territories can help nurses to appropriately target policy efforts.

In all this work, gender frequently arises as a factor influencing power and decision-making among nurses. In a now famous TED Talk, Sheryl Sandberg argued

Test Yourself

Test your learning about the governance hierarchy of Canada with this quick online puzzle: http://www.parl.gc.ca/About/Parliament/SenatorEugeneForsey/inside_view/puzzle-e.html.

Challenge yourself with this simple animation: http://www.parl.gc.ca/About/Parliament/SenatorEugeneForsey/touchpoints/index-e.html. Can you identify the services provided by each level of government?

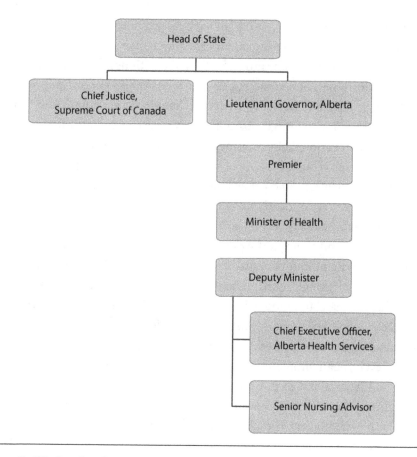

Figure 2.15: Senior Governance Structure of Alberta and Its Health Care System, 2015

that "women are not making it to the top. A hundred and ninety heads of state; nine are women. Of all the people in parliament in the world, 13 per cent are women. In the corporate sector, women at the top—C-level jobs, board seats—tops out at 15, 16 per cent."[114] Nursing is something of an occupational oddity in that there are more women in senior roles, so the gender situation is complicated. Consider the example shown in Figure 2.15—the senior governance structure of the province of Alberta and its health care system in 2015. What these roles have in common is that, in 2015, all of them were occupied by women. Moreover, the most senior, operational decision-making roles in the health system—the deputy minister and chief executive officer of Alberta Health Services—were filled by registered nurses. Figure 2.15 should provoke thought around the concerns of some nurses that they do not personally have power, or that nurses at large do not have power. On paper, the example of the Alberta governance structure might challenge that notion, and in fact there are a lot of nurses, nearly all women, positioned in similar senior deci-sion-making roles across most Canadian health systems.

Appointing women and/or nurses to formal positions of power in governance is an important signal, of course, but anyone who studies gender and power will know that it is only one of many structures required to create equity and em-powerment; indeed, the formal position on its own may be nothing but a set-up for failure. Organizational charts aside, the sharp divide between the ways some nurses see themselves at the point of service and how they view governments, administrators, scientists, and other formal nurse leaders is an ongoing problem. Despite a half century of social change, many nurses, most of whom are women, retain traditional, primary responsibilities for providing family care and man-aging a home beyond their paid work. Many nurses encounter a lack of reliable, full-time employment and benefits, forcing them to cobble together a full-time equivalent salary through multiple part-time jobs. Nurse leaders may face some or all of the same social realities, but they have higher salaries (with which they can purchase help outside work), more predictable schedules, and typically have at least some supports (e.g., clerks or assistants) to manage their paid work. Their roles may even mean simple comforts such as being able to afford a vehicle to travel to and from work, and, once there, having a place to park it. These gen-dered realities of nurses' lives—and women's lives in general—are an important variable in understanding the challenge inherent in adding yet more work to their lives in order to involve more nurses in influencing policy.

Keeping gender, role, and power issues in mind, those involved in policy work will return again and again to governance structures during the planning, devel-opment, and implementation of policy. Nurses must become familiar with the structures and the human beings leading them—hence the positioning of this topic near the beginning of this book.

DISCUSSION QUESTIONS

1. How effective is Canada's governance structure? What enablers and bar-riers does it put up in the development of public policy?
2. Describe potential health care delivery challenges associated with the distribution of the population across Canada. How are these challenges additionally affected by population demographics such as ethnic diversi-ty, average age, and Indigenous status?
3. How do the Canadian Constitution and Charter of Rights and Free-doms potentially affect the health of Canadians?
4. What are the potential implications of the intersection of the governance

structures of Canada's federal, provincial, territorial, and Aboriginal governments? How do these create and/or resolve conflicts?

5. How does gender in nursing affect politics, policy influence, and public life?

ADDITIONAL POLICY RESOURCES

FEDERAL/NATIONAL GOVERNANCE AND POLITICAL STRUCTURES

Government of Canada

The Queen, Head of State	http://www.royal.gov.uk/monarchandcommonwealth/canada/canada.aspx
Governor General	http://gg.ca
Office of the Prime Minister	http://pm.gc.ca
Privy Council Office	http://www.pco-bcp.gc.ca
Parliament of Canada	http://www.parl.gc.ca
Departments and Ministers	http://www.parl.gc.ca/Parlinfo/Compilations/FederalGovernment/TheMinistry.aspx
Supreme Court of Canada	http://www.scc-csc.gc.ca

Leading Federal Political Parties

Bloc Québécois	http://www.blocquebecois.org
Conservative Party of Canada	http://www.conservative.ca
Green Party of Canada	http://www.greenparty.ca
Liberal Party of Canada	https://www.liberal.ca
New Democratic Party	http://www.ndp.ca
Canada's registered and eligible federal political parties	http://www.elections.ca/content.aspx?dir=par&document=index&lang=e&section=pol

Provincial and Territorial Governance and Political Structures

Canada's provincial lieutenant governors and territorial commissioners	http://www.parl.gc.ca/Parlinfo/compilations/ProvinceTerritory/LieutenantGovernors.aspx
Canada's provincial and territorial premiers	http://www.parl.gc.ca/Parlinfo/compilations/ProvinceTerritory/PremiersTerritorialLeaders.aspx
Canada's provincial and territorial governments	http://www.cic.gc.ca/english/newcomers/before-provincial-gov.asp
Council of the Federation	http://www.canadaspremiers.ca

National Indigenous Governance, Policy, and Advocacy Organizations	
Assembly of First Nations	http://www.afn.ca
Congress of Aboriginal Peoples	http://abo-peoples.org
Inuit Tapiriit Kanatami	https://www.itk.ca
Métis National Council	http://www.metisnation.ca
Native Women's Association of Canada	http://www.nwac.ca

CHAPTER 3

Canadian Health Systems Today: Governance and Organization

CHAPTER HIGHLIGHTS

- How Are Health Care Systems in Canada Organized?
- Beyond Health Ministries: Other Legislation Influencing Health Care
- What Services Are Covered by Public and Private Payers?
- The Federal Role in Health Care
- Provincial and Territorial Roles in Health Care
- Aboriginal Health Care
- Summary and Implications
- Discussion Questions
- Additional Policy Resources

LEARNING OUTCOMES

1. State examples of key initiatives and pieces of legislation leading to the establishment of universal health care (medicare) and the Canada Health Act (1984).
2. State the purpose and key conditions of the Canada Health Act (1984).
3. Describe the governance, major institutions, and structures of Canada's health systems today.
4. Differentiate among federal, provincial, territorial, and Aboriginal division of roles and responsibilities for health care delivery.
5. State five examples from each of the categories of services delivered in Canada's public and private health care systems.

Policy Influencer: Kamal Khera

One of the youngest members of Canada's House of Commons (and the youngest Liberal), Kamal Khera, RN, BSc, BScN, was elected to Parliament in October 2015 representing Brampton West. Born in Delhi, India, Khera immigrated to Canada as a child and went on to become a registered nurse, where she quickly expanded her interests in political activism. Before running for Parliament she gained professional experience in the Greater Toronto Area with the Centre for Addiction and Mental Health, Peel Family Shelter, William Osler Health System, and St. Joseph's Health Centre, in addition to her numerous volunteer positions.[1] She was appointed in 2015 as the parliamentary secretary to the minister of health, the Honourable Dr. Jane Philpott. While she is new to Parliament, Khera's social media shows her being a very active member of Parliament, taking on activities related to immigration settlement, mental health services, and broader issues around trade and innovation, the tax system, and gaps in skills and training.

"Canadians view medicare as a moral enterprise, not a business venture.... Canadians want their health care system renovated; they do not want it demolished."

—Commission on the Future of Health Care in Canada

HOW ARE HEALTH CARE SYSTEMS IN CANADA ORGANIZED?

As noted in Chapter 1, records of organized health care in Canada date to the 1600s, with the arrival of Jeanne Mance and the construction of the first small hospital in Montreal. Whether there were any formal structures among First Nations at the time of contact is uncertain. It is understood through oral history that spiritual healers, also known as shamans, were common and that care, comfort, and support for illnesses or injuries would have been provided by family and community members in home settings.[2]

It goes without saying that health care in Canada today has evolved into a much more comprehensive and complicated affair. It encompasses a broad range of services across a continuum of every possible age, culture, gender, and care need— "from sperm to worm" as Vicki Kaminski, one of the members of the National

Expert Commission, famously said during one of the commission meetings in 2012. Canadian provinces and territories offer a rich mix of health promotion and illness prevention services, the full range of primary, secondary, tertiary, and quaternary treatment services, rehabilitation, long-term care, and palliative and hospice care—each of which may treat persons suffering from the broadest possible range of physical and emotional illnesses and injuries. And while nurses are highly concentrated in institutional settings, they are positioned at nearly every point in that continuum and in every corner of the country, from isolated Inuit and First Nations nursing stations to the largest urban teaching hospitals.

It is challenging to separate the ways health care is organized from the issue of cost. But this chapter endeavours to focus on the governance and structure of health care to enable a better understanding of who does what and who pays for what, leaving the exploration of the actual costs and allocation decisions for later chapters.

The Development of Medicare

The universal health care system in which the majority of nurses work in Canada—medicare—evolved from a basic belief that health care should be available to Canadians based on need and not on their ability to pay. It took decades to be fully implemented in Canada, despite the landmark policy precedent that had been set in the United Kingdom with the National Insurance Act (1911). That law provided most working people with their first measure of health and unemployment insurance, with workers, employers, and the government of the United Kingdom each contributing portions to the fund. Although the coverage was fairly limited, Heller describes the legislation as causing a seismic shift "in the relationship between state and individual which laid the basis for future reform." He argues that the scope of the legislation was not as important as "the principle it enshrined," describing it as "one of the most important pieces of legislation of the 20th century."[3]

Of course, with news of the act in Great Britain, discussion of the need for a similar program spread across Canada during World War I—fuelled by welfare issues such as poverty and poor housing, health issues including "high maternal and infant mortality rates[,] ... and high rates of industrial accidents and trauma in addition to war casualties."[4] But the talk did not prompt much action in response; then, as now, there was tremendous resistance in some quarters to governments being involved in funding or providing health care in any sort of universal and/or not-for-profit model. These debates reveal evidence of a fundamental difference in the founding values, purpose, and organization of health care systems; Decter, as noted earlier, described this difference as ability-to-pay versus ability-to-benefit, where necessary care is provided when it is needed without the potential barrier raised by individual, out-of-pocket payment.[5] These concepts are discussed further in Chapter 11.

In the lead-up to the creation of the first federal health department in 1919, Hansard (the record of Parliament) recorded that Peter McGibbon, Liberal member of Parliament for Argenteuil, Quebec (1917–1921), was landing on the ability-to-benefit side, advocating strongly in the House of Commons in favour of "giving every poor man, woman and child in this country free medical service from the cradle to the grave."[6] Awareness of public health issues was growing among Canadians and was described by some as "sweeping" across the continent[7]—and the need to tackle and pay for care to respond to them began to move more forcefully onto formal government policy tables.

Cost pressures on individual Canadians mounted steadily over the first half of the 20th century in lockstep with the evolving range, complexity, and promise of new health care services. Nurses at the time, still largely providing private home and community care, were paid directly by those using their services. The basic cost just to be treated by a general practitioner had always been a barrier for some, but by setting medical fees on something of a sliding scale, wealthier patients had been subsidizing some of the costs for access to physicians for the less wealthy. Of course, churches and charities had always contributed in some measure to help pay for the care of the poor—and still do. But paying out of pocket for care in the rapidly growing urban and rural hospital sector introduced a whole new level of costs that could be catastrophic for all but the wealthiest Canadians. Nursing costs were included in hospital bills, but physician costs were not.

By hosting a number of prominent national conferences on the topic after the war years, the Canadian Medical Association asserted its position as a leader in early discussions about public access to care and payment for it. From those early days, many physicians were opposed to what they perceived as government oversight of their relationships with patients.[8] That resistance would continue throughout the life of the medicare debate, and still does in some cases. That is not to say there were not many physicians in support of medicare from the beginning, and the official stance

The History of Medicare in Canada

The Canadian Museum of History provides an extensive online history of the development of health care and medicare in Canada. To explore the topic, see http://www.historymuseum.ca/cmc/exhibitions/hist/medicare/medic-1h01e.shtml.

of the association today is one of strong support; in fact, the Canadian Medical Association joined with the CNA in 2011 to urge an expansion of medicare to make the program more comprehensive.[9]

The debate evolved very differently in nursing, where from "the earliest discussions on universal health insurance … to the passage of the Canada Health Act in 1984, and at countless commissions and conferences in between and since then, CNA has demonstrated consistent political support for the philosophical underpinnings of socialized medicine."[10] The opposing value sets that sometimes drive the policy positions of nursing and medicine—socialism versus capitalism, respectively—have been a long-simmering philosophical flashpoint that periodically rears its head between the two professions.

The consequences of a global war, followed in a decade by an unprecedented economic depression and then another global war, all contributed to growing public health needs, and the possibilities introduced by advancing diagnostics and hospital care. Together these dynamics drove a growing roster of health care cost issues that required a more sustainable solution for most Canadians.

After World War I ended in 1918, several provinces began exploring and testing various models and programs to manage payment for physician and other health care services. The province of British Columbia, for example, launched its own Royal Commission in 1919 around health care insurance, but uptake of its 10 recommendations—including establishment of mandatory health insurance for all wage earners below a certain salary, and voluntary insurance for everyone else[11]—was limited and the payment debate raged on. There were also experiments with municipal-level hospital insurance plans in the western provinces during the 1920s.

The federal government was watching as the provincial debates unfolded over the years—and nurses were watching too. During a meeting of federal, provincial, and territorial ministers of health in April 1935, CNA leaders presented their *Outline on Health Insurance and Nursing Services* to the acting prime minister, the Right Honourable Sir George Perley, and health minister, the Honourable Donald Sutherland.[12] The nursing intervention was so effective that the association was later included in the planning of a Royal Commission that would be struck to investigate health care in Canada for the purpose of gathering evidence on state medicine and health insurance.[13] In 1938, CNA briefed the Royal Commission on Dominion-Provincial Relations, advocating for a study of the state of health services nationally and calling for nursing to be included in the "development, administration and regulation of any new health insurance plan."[14] From the outset, it was the position of CNA that insured services should not just be for physician and hospital costs, but should apply to other providers and settings; that battle, too, continues today.

While that Royal Commission was underway, Saskatchewan was positioning itself ahead of the curve, pushing the idea of universal coverage for all citizens and not just the poor. The Municipal and Medical Hospital Services Act (1939) allowed Saskatchewan municipalities "to levy either a land tax or a personal tax to finance hospital and medical services."[15] Led by the Honourable Reverend Thomas Clement "Tommy" Douglas, a Baptist minister, the Saskatchewan Co-operative Commonwealth Federation—later the New Democratic Party—was elected to power in a landslide in 1944, partly on a platform calling for comprehensive health insurance. It was to be the first democratically elected socialist (or, as some at the time said, communist) government in North America.

Douglas made good on his campaign promise with another new precedent: despite considerable political opposition, in what has been described as the most sweeping reform on the continent to that date, the Hospital Insurance Act (1947) was passed, guaranteeing "every citizen of the province hospital care without a fee."[16] Alberta would follow with similar legislation in 1950. And so the scene was set for a broader introduction of public insurance and universal health care; debate about public health insurance and the roles of governments and the private sector in health care intensified in every province and at the federal level over the ensuing decade. The National Health Grants Program (1948), put in place under Health Minister, the Honourable Paul Martin, Sr., exerted the spending power of the federal government, providing conditional grants to the provinces for a range of health initiatives largely aimed at building physical and human resources capacity across health systems (e.g., building hospitals, education, and research). This spending power allows the federal government to make payments in areas where it otherwise "has little or no regulatory authority." [17] Some observers consider the 1948 legislation as the first stage in establishing public health care in Canada.[18]

The Hospital Insurance and Diagnostic Services Act (1957) was passed into legislation under the Liberal government of the Right Honourable Louis St. Laurent. Herein can be found the origins of some of the language of the Canada Health Act (1984), and as well the roots of the ongoing debate about federal funding of health care. Under this legislation the federal government agreed to "reimburse, or cost share, one-half of provincial and territorial costs for specified hospital and diagnostic services." The program could effectively provide universal coverage under public (government) administration for a defined roster of health care services given that certain conditions were met.[19] All provinces signed on by 1961—and like the ongoing battle to expand medicare beyond doctors and hospitals, the debate around what the financing commitment of the federal government should be rages on nearly 60 years after the legislation passed.

In 1960, Progressive Conservative Prime Minister John Diefenbaker announced that the Honourable Justice Emmett Hall would lead a Royal Commission on Health Services. Established in 1961, the Hall Commission, as it came to be known, was struck to "inquire into and report upon the existing facilities and the future need for health services for the people of Canada and the resources to provide such services, and to recommend such measures, consistent with the constitutional division of legislative powers in Canada, as the commissioners believe will ensure that the best possible health care is available to all Canadians."[20] Nurses were active throughout the lead-up to and execution of the Commission, with Alice Girard, dean of the nursing school at Université de Montréal, sitting as a member. The brief by CNA on behalf of Canada's nurses made 25 recommendations to improve nursing services in order to strengthen the nation's health care systems, and was well received. A discussion of nursing reform efforts is included in Chapter 6.

Back in Saskatchewan, although Douglas had left his role as premier to help establish the New Democratic Party of Canada, his reputation as one of the fathers of Canadian medicare was sealed with passage of the Saskatchewan Medical Care Insurance Act (1962), which laid out a program of universal medical insurance. Physicians had been strongly opposed to any compulsory plan and, on Canada Day that year, some 90 per cent of the province's doctors walked off the job in response to the legislation. It was a notoriously acrimonious strike, with physicians bolstered by the backing of the American Medical Association and its rabid fear of the spread of socialized medicine. In a 2007 interview, Shirley Douglas described the situation as the "propaganda department from Washington" swarming Saskatchewan in tandem with insurance companies and medical associations from both countries—all united in opposition to universal medicare.[21]

Over the next three weeks, physicians threatened the public that socialized health care—precisely what nurses had long been advocating for—would cause most physicians to leave Saskatchewan. There was mixed support for this position, but the public certainly was attentive and understandably worried. In the end the government capitulated on a critical issue that still shapes Canadian health care today: physicians could opt out of medicare. That model continues across the country today, with most providers in the public health care system working as salaried employees, while most physicians operate as private entrepreneurs who work around the system and bill it in a fee-for-service (or fee-for-visit) model.

Setting aside the contentious physician payment issue, medicare was established in Saskatchewan, and although many politicians across the country were vehemently opposed, it was only a matter of time before all Canadians would want the same. In its final report in 1964, the Hall Commission identified the need to resolve a range of issues, including costs, financing, quality of care, and the human resources required to support the system. But most importantly, it recommended that the nation should adopt the Saskatchewan model of universal health care.

With the Diefenbaker government defeated in April 1964, it fell to his successor, Lester B. Pearson, and his Liberal minority government to complete the work of establishing universal medicare. The Canada Pension Plan (1965) and Canada Assistance Plan (1966) were passed into legislation under Mr. Pearson, providing a social safety net through a cost-sharing arrangement with the provinces and territories. After bitter debate and a number of delays, the Medical Care Act (1966) came into force on Canada Day, 1968, providing a 50/50 cost-sharing agreement for provincial and territorial medical insurance plans. Universal health care in Canada was finally a reality. Saskatchewan and British Columbia joined the program immediately and all other provinces and territories joined the program over the following four years, the last being the Yukon in April 1972. The federal acts of 1957 and 1966 are considered by some to be "the second stage of a national health insurance system for Canada." [22]

The Canada Health Act (1984)

A decade after the Medical Care Act came into force, concerns were being expressed about whether medicare was effectively fulfilling its intended objectives. In her discourse on the topic, Chenier argued that by 1979 the federal government was concerned "that federal funds allocated for health were being diverted by the provinces into non-health activities such as road building." [23] Justice Emmett Hall was summoned back into action by the federal government in 1979 when he was asked to act as a special commissioner and to lead a time-limited Health Services Review. By August 1980 Justice Hall tabled his report, *Canada's National-Provincial Health Program for the 1980s*. [24]

The submission to the Health Services Review by CNA—*Putting Health Back Into Health Care*—reintroduced a long-standing organizational theme by including policy proposals "for the introduction of new entry points into the health-care system through which the public could access qualified personnel who were not necessarily physicians." [25] The brief attracted particular attention from Justice Hall: a chapter of his report was devoted just to the CNA recommendations, with which Hall said he generally agreed, and he recommended that the association's work be given "the most serious consideration" by governments. Hall recommended the abolition of hospital user fees and extra billing by doctors because they were barriers to universal access; a House of Commons Task Force on Federal-Provincial Fiscal Arrangements concurred in 1981 "that extra-billing and user fees were detrimental." [26]

Fuelled in part by Hall's 1980 report, a bill for a new health act was tabled in 1983. Ginette Lemire Rodger and Helen Preston Glass—then the executive director and president of CNA, respectively—and their teams intervened forcefully and strategically with the health minister, Monique Bégin, and with parliamentarians and legislators across the country to amend the bill. Among their 11 suggested amendments was a shift away from the singular focus of medicare on acute care to include coverage for insured services outside hospitals and institutions. In addition, they recommended that nursing and other providers beyond physicians should be included as insured points of access to the health care system, and that all extra billing and extra fees should be abolished. In the end they were not successful in the battle on extending services beyond hospitals, but "they did manage to have the description of potential providers of insured services broadened to include health-care practitioners and not just physicians."[27] An example of a pluralist theory of public policy in action, nurses were the only group successful in forcing an amendment of the Canada Health Act, and their success is still seen as another turning point in the policy influence of strategic, well-organized nurses.

The Canada Health Act (1984) was passed by the federal government and given Royal Assent on April 1, 1984, replacing the previous federal hospital and medical insurance acts, prohibiting extra billing and user fees, extending coverage to nurses as entry points to health care, and consolidating long-standing principles in a set of funding criteria.[28] Passage of the Canada Health Act may be seen as the final major piece of legislation during the first wave of health reform in Canada in the hospital era—the era of establishing universal health care coverage across the country.

Contrary to the perceptions of some, the Canada Health Act does not direct provinces and territories regarding the operation or specific services of their health care systems. Rather it is a fiscal transfer agreement setting out the conditions under which each jurisdiction is eligible to receive the full federal financial contribution. There are a number of other conditions in the act, but the five principles of the Canada Health Act most often discussed—and with which provinces and

The Canada Health Act

To learn more about the policy work of CNA leading up to Royal Assent of the Canada Health Act, explore the Canada Health Act in Chapter 6 of the history of CNA, pages 105–106. Go to http://www.cna-aiic.ca/html/en/CNA-ONE-HUNDRED-YEARS-OF-SERVICE-e/index.html.

principles

territories must comply—are public administration, comprehensiveness, universality, portability, and accessibility (see Figure 3.1), explained by the Parliament of Canada as follows:[29]

- *Public administration* (section 8 of the act) requires that each provincial and territorial insurance plan be administered on a not-for-profit basis by a public authority—a single payer model, as it is commonly known. Public administration should not be confused with public delivery. Other than those who are working in organizations where they are paid a salary, physicians bill the publicly administered insurance plan but are private providers, which is private delivery. Many laboratories and medical imaging clinics provide insured services to patients who pay nothing out of pocket—again, public insurance and private delivery. In fact, the hospitals in which most nurses work are only quasi-public institutions, managed by regions or boards, and not unlike physicians, nurses are reimbursed under a variety of formulae by governments for the services they deliver. But for the purposes of this discussion, public general hospitals are considered to be public institutions.
- *Comprehensiveness* (section 9 of the act) means that each insurance plan must provide insurance for all medically necessary services. The Canada Health Act does not define what medically necessary services are, hence the unevenness of some services across Canada.
- The *universality* condition (section 10 of the act) requires that there be access to public health insurance, based on uniform terms, for every resident of a province or territory.
- The *portability* clause (section 11 of the act) requires that each province and territory provide insured services for its citizens when they access care in another province or territory, or outside the country. For care received in another jurisdiction within Canada, the provincial and/or territorial governments involved negotiate payment. For care outside the country, the amount insured must be at least equivalent to what the province would cover for services inside its borders.
- *Accessibility* (section 12 of the act) means that residents "must have reasonable and uniform access to insured health services, free of financial or other barriers" and that "no one may be discriminated against on the basis of such factors as income, age, and health status."

In addition to these five principles, the federal Parliament noted that "free access to insured health services is the key factor of the *Canada Health Act*. The two

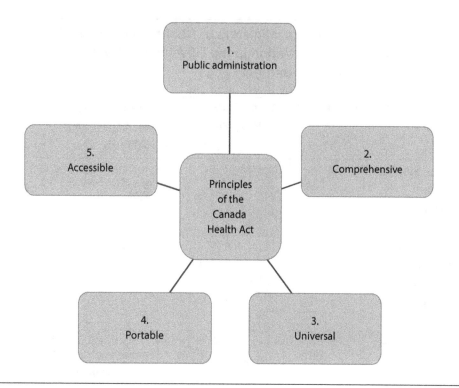

Figure 3.1: Principles of the Canada Health Act (1984)

provisions of the Act specifically discourage financial contributions by patients, either through user charges or extra-billing, for services covered under provincial health care insurance plans."[30] Despite heated and significant debate among the federal, provincial, and territorial governments about these conditions, all jurisdictions ending extra billing and user fees by April 1, 1987, as set down in the law. The main pieces of legislation and related federal/pan-Canadian initiatives leading to the Canada Health Act are summarized in Table 3.1.

BEYOND HEALTH MINISTRIES: OTHER LEGISLATION INFLUENCING HEALTH CARE

Beyond health ministries, a number of acts and agreements at the national level between and among the federal, provincial, and territorial governments may directly or indirectly influence health care in Canada. Some of these are part of ongoing attempts to acknowledge and respond to Canada's geographic challenges, as introduced earlier. The various health accords and other reform initiatives are introduced in the discussion of system reform in the next chapter and so will not

Table 3.1: Prime Ministers, Ministers of Health, and Federal/Pan-Canadian Legislation in the Development of Medicare and the Canada Health Act

PRIME MINISTER	YEARS	MINISTER(S) OF HEALTH	MAJOR HEALTH LEGISLATION AND INITIATIVES
Louis Stephen St. Laurent (Liberal)	1948–1957	Paul Martin, Sr.	Hospital Insurance and Diagnostic Services Act (1957)
John George Diefenbaker (Progressive Conservative)	1957–1963	Alfred John Brooks (acting) Jay Waldo Monteith	Royal Commission on Health Services established, 1961
Lester Bowles Pearson (Liberal)	1963–1968	Judy Lamarsh Allan MacEachen	Royal Commission on Health Services reports, 1964 Canada Pension Plan (1965) Canada Assistance Plan (1966) Medical Care Act (1966, in effect 1968)
Pierre Elliott Trudeau (Liberal)	1968–1979	Allan MacEachen John Munro Marc Lalonde Monique Bégin	(National) Committee on Costs of Health Services, 1970 *A New Perspective on the Health of Canadians* (Lalonde), 1974 Established Programs Financing Act (1977)
Charles Joseph Clark (Progressive Conservative)	1979	David Crombie	
Pierre Elliott Trudeau (Liberal)	1979–1984	Monique Bégin	*Canada's National-Provincial Health Program for the 1980s* (Hall), 1980 Task Force on Federal-Provincial Fiscal Arrangements, 1981 Canada Health Act (1984) Federal Task Force on the Allocation of Health Care Resources reports, 1984

be covered here. But there also exists a broad slate of legislation within each province and territory that may affect health care within each jurisdiction.

Important in the discussion of legislation impacting health and social funding is A Framework to Improve the Social Union for Canadians—typically shortened to the Social Union Framework Agreement or SUFA. This agreement among the federal, provincial, and territorial governments was signed in 1999 on the federal side by the Right Honourable Jean Chrétien, prime minister at the time.[31] The principles of the agreement were intended to promote a more communal approach to a number of social and health policy and program areas, including:

a.   equality, equity, and fairness across the country;
b.   access to essential programs of reasonably comparable quality across the country, respect for the principles of medicare, and provision of appropriate supports for people in need;
c.   adequate, affordable, stable, and sustainable social program funding; and
d.   the treaty and other rights of Aboriginal Peoples.

The agreement also was intended to support the mobility of Canadians by removing barriers, and spoke to joint planning and collaboration. It raised the often-prickly issue of federal spending power, whether through conditional transfers—medicare, for example—or direct transfers to organizations or individuals in pursuit of the goals and principles of the agreement. In the words of the agreement: "The use of the federal spending power under the Constitution has been essential to the development of Canada's social union. An important use of the spending power by the Government of Canada has been to transfer money to the provincial and territorial governments. These transfers support the delivery of social programs and services by provinces and territories in order to promote equality of opportunity and mobility for all Canadians and to pursue Canada-wide objectives."[32] With a federal commitment to limit spending power, it increased its cash contribution by more than $11 billion through the Canada Health and Social Transfer and provinces agreed to use the funds for health care reform activities.

Such direct and conditional transfers can be a very thorny issue for governments. For example, imagine that the federal government decides it would like to create a new $20 million fund to provide scholarships for students entering nursing schools over the next three years. Those schools, of course, are all in provinces or territories and overseen by their respective governments. Those governments are just as apt to balk at that sort of program as praise it, the reasoning being that if the federal government has funds to turn over, then it should turn those funds over with no conditions for the province (or territory) to use as it sees fit for the needs it has identified in its area of jurisdiction. If Province A has an urgent need for road repairs, and Province B needs help building more public schools, they may not see the nursing scholarship as a priority. This is a very simple example, but points to the kind of challenge the federal government may face any time it chooses to exert its conditional spending power.

WHAT SERVICES ARE COVERED BY PUBLIC AND PRIVATE PAYERS?

Common in the language around health care is the notion that health care is free in Canada. Of course, it is not free; Canadians pay mightily for health care through their personal income taxes and other taxes and charges. What is inferred by *free* is that necessary care is accessible without an out-of-pocket payment—also known as first-dollar coverage.

There is no national health care insurance scheme in Canada. Rather, there is a national plan with principles entrenched in the Canada Health Act (1984), discussed above. According to that plan, Canadians may access a range of

A Charter Challenge

Brian Day, a physician who owns two private, for-profit health care facilities in British Columbia, has challenged the legislation stopping physicians from billing both the public and private systems and from extra billing. He has argued that "because the publicly-funded system compels some patients to wait for the delivery of some medically necessary services (in particular, elective surgery), patients should have the right to obtain such services more quickly by paying privately, either out-of-pocket or through private insurance."[33] Because they do not have that right, Day has alleged that the Canada Health Act and its companion framework in British Columbia "infringe patients' rights to life, liberty and security of the person under Section 7 of the Canadian Charter of Rights and Freedoms."[34] After numerous delays, at the time of writing the case has yet appear before the British Columbia Supreme Court. Whatever the decision in British Columbia, the case is expected to come before the Supreme Court of Canada. Depending on the final decision, this case could change the face of health care in Canada and bears close attention by nurses and their political allies.

medically necessary services with first-dollar payment covered under one of the 13 publicly funded provincial and territorial insurance schemes. Generally, there are no additional fees.

Canadians also may choose to access services that are compensated fully or partially by private insurers or through direct payment by the patient. Some of the same services may appear in both the public and private payment and delivery realms, and/or may be partially compensated by both payment systems at the same time. To cite a simple example, a resident may be eligible to receive post-surgical home care from licensed practical nurses covered under the provincial health insurance plan, while at the same time paying the same agency privately to provide nursing care to a frail parent in the same home. While they may not bill aspects of the same specific service to both systems, nurses (in all the regulated categories), physicians, and other providers may work within either or both payment systems. Nothing stops a registered psychiatric nurse, for example, from working in a public hospital during the week and also providing private, for-profit care while employed in another agency. A home care nurse may deliver publicly funded care to one client and privately funded care to the next one, all while she or he is employed and paid by the same private agency.

Medicare: What Is Covered Under Public Insurance Schemes?

It is important to differentiate what services are provided under public and private payment systems. For any resident of Canada covered under a provincial or territorial health insurance plan, insured coverage minimally must be provided to cover:

1. All medically required physician services that are delivered by medical practitioners and, for the most part, wherever they are provided; this clause includes family physicians, surgeons, and the full range of medical specialists, whether seen in a hospital, emergency room, clinic, or private office.
2. All in- or out-patient hospital services that are "medically necessary for the purpose of maintaining health, preventing disease or diagnosing or treating an injury, illness, or disability"[35] and including "accommodation and meals, physician and nursing services, drugs and all medical and surgical equipment and supplies."[36]
3. All necessary dental surgery procedures that must be provided in a hospital (typically services requiring general anesthesia and/or some level of nursing care).

Similarly insured services are also provided to Canadians who access emergency care while travelling in another country, reimbursed at the same rate as the home province or territory's insurance plan. Elective procedures taking place in another country, including surgery, may be covered by a provincial or territorial plan, but only on the condition of prior approval.

Beyond these minimally required services, optional additional benefits provided by provinces and territories may include partial or full coverage for:

- prescription drugs
- services provided by dental surgeons, optometrists, and chiropractors
- ground and/or air ambulance services
- assistive devices
- various medical and surgical procedures, including routine circumcision of newborns, breast reduction or augmentation, tattoo removal, reversal of sterilization, and many more.[37]

Any of these additional services provided by a province or territory are negotiated, delivered, and funded in each individual jurisdiction; such services may be targeted to vulnerable groups, and are not subject to the terms of the Canada Health Act. As expressed by the Canadian Foundation for Healthcare Improvement, it is important to be cautioned that "a service that is publicly insured in one province may not be in another. Likewise, care provided in a hospital may not be covered if provided in the community or the home, and physician services billable to the province may not be covered if provided by other health professionals, such as psychologists."[38]

Although the places care happens have changed—as have the providers who deliver it—the focus of the services provided on the public side of the system in Canada remains strongly centred on physicians, hospitals, and treatment. These evolutions in care have given rise to long-simmering concerns. When the Standing Senate Committee on Social Affairs, Science and Technology reported in 2002 on a comprehensive review of health care in Canada, its authors noted that "many more health services can be provided safely and effectively on an ambulatory basis or at home. Hospital stays are shorter; drug therapy often enables people to avoid hospital-based care altogether."[39] Similarly, a report by Parliament warned about the creep of passive privatization, finding that "many services that are deemed medically necessary today are not publicly insured because they are not provided in hospitals or by physicians," suggesting that the definition of *medically necessary* is out of date.[40] It was to address these exact concerns that CNA had lobbied so stridently in 1983 and 1984 to have care beyond hospitals included in the Canada Health Act.

What is more, the Senate Standing Committee was critical of the "sharp contrast between Canada and other OECD countries in terms of the scope of its public health care coverage"[41] and cited numerous examples of fellow OECD member nations that have much broader coverage than Canada. In the end, the Senate review recommended expanding medicare and the Canada Health Act to cover catastrophic prescription drug costs, post-hospital home care costs, and palliative home care costs. These system reviews are discussed further in Chapter 5.

Private Payment

Private insurance, direct (out-of-pocket) pay by individuals, or some combination of the two normally provides payment for services not included under provincial or territorial public insurance schemes; some services may also be covered by charities or municipal governments in facilities such as homeless shelters. There is a range of extended care services that are not subject to the Canada Health Act, and they may include:

- prescription and non-prescription pharmaceuticals
- medical supplies
- equipment outside hospitals
- dentistry outside hospitals
- ambulatory care
- home care
- adult residential care
- long-term care, nursing homes, and retirement homes
- child care
- rehabilitation care outside a hospital
- non-urgent (i.e., non-ambulance) patient transfers
- diagnostic and treatment services provided privately by any regulated or unregulated provider, including nurse practitioners and physicians who choose to work in private clinics and other care settings.

In addition, hospital and physician services not covered by public insurance include:

- preferred accommodation in a hospital (unless ordered by a physician, such as when a patient with a communicable infection requires a private room)
- private duty nurses or attendants
- charges for personal items such as televisions and telephones in a hospital

- physician services, including the provision of letters for employers, schools, insurance companies, or fitness clubs; court testimony; cosmetic procedures; and the renewal of prescriptions by telephone.[42]

THE FEDERAL ROLE IN HEALTH CARE

There is a fairly clear federal and provincial/territorial division of responsibilities for population health and the delivery of health care services. Much more contentious is the perpetual debate about how much federal, provincial/territorial, and even municipal governments should contribute to funding health care services. Remembering that the fiscal issues are tackled in more detail in Chapter 7, this chapter focuses more directly on the governance story.

After significant lobbying by the Canadian Public Health Association (CPHA) and other health associations, Canada's first federal health department was established in July 1919, just before the end of World War I. Prior to 1919, federal health duties fell under the Agriculture Department. The first policy imperative of the new department was the development and implementation of "federal shared-cost funding programs to deal with tuberculosis and venereal disease, scourges that were feared among returning troops."[43] This was also the year that the Spanish flu was raging throughout the world; some 50,000 Canadians were among the 40 to 50 million people believed to have died around the world, and unusually, many of them were young people in the prime of their lives. Child welfare had also emerged over the preceding years as a national issue to which the department was tasked to respond. So the new department started with a pressing and full slate of policy and program needs.

While there has been some back and forth around the division of authority between the federal government and the provinces and territories since 1919, from the outset the health care powers and responsibilities of the federal government have been limited to areas and people over which it has had jurisdiction—for example, quarantine and food and drug standards have always been under the federal umbrella. But the role has grown over the years to include a broader range of services, including pensions, general welfare, and public and population health more broadly.

The federal government has used its spending powers to invest in health systems through conditional funding arrangements—that is to say, to transfer funds to offset the costs of health care based on the provinces and territories achieving an agreed-upon set of conditions; the Canada Health Act is a good example. As Dunsmuir noted in her discussion of the topic for Parliament, federal spending is a fairly new development, and is "the main lever of federal influence in fields that are legislatively within provincial jurisdiction, such as health care, education, welfare, manpower training and regional development."[44] It has, at times, proven to be a contentious policy instrument, and of course governments generally prefer fiscal transfers with no conditions. The steady chipping away of the original 50 per cent federal contribution to offset medicare costs has been an ongoing flashpoint in all conversations about our universal, public health care system.

As the federal role has evolved, the name of the department responsible has changed accordingly. When the federal government took on health and other services for war veterans in 1928, for example, the name was changed to the Department of Pensions and National Health.[45] As World War II was ending in 1944, the federal government turned its focus to standards of living as much as health. The new Department of National Health and Welfare was established under the leadership of the Honourable Brooke Claxton, its first minister. Revealing very different priorities than the first federal health department at the end of the previous world war, one of Claxton's priorities was to establish and roll out the universal Family Allowance program.

The department maintained its dual health and welfare function until 1993 when, during the brief tenure of the Right Honourable Kim Campbell's (Progressive Conservative) government, health functions were allocated to Health Canada and social welfare functions to a new department called Human Resources and Labour Canada—now titled Human Resources and Skills Development Canada.

Today, most of the health focus of the federal government continues to be vested in Health Canada; however, there are health services delivered in several other departments. In addition to Health Canada, as of 2010 the federal government employed some 3,500 health care providers across Citizenship and Immigration Canada, Correctional Service Canada, the Department of National Defence, the Public Health Agency of Canada, the Royal Canadian Mounted Police, and Veterans Affairs Canada. Together they deliver health care services to First Nations and Inuit, eligible veterans, refugee protection claimants, inmates of federal penitentiaries, and serving members of the Canadian Forces and the Royal Canadian Mounted Police.[46]

Health Canada now plays the roles of a leader, partner, funder, guardian, regulator, service provider, and information provider as depicted in Figure 3.2. Its powers and responsibilities are described as:

- helping Canadians to maintain and improve their health;
- preserving Canada's health care system by "looking for ways to improve the system and ensure its sustainability";

- enhancing the health of Canadians, including disease surveillance, prevention, and control, as well as monitoring safety and risks related to food, drugs, chemicals, pesticides, and medical devices;
- partnering with federal and provincial/territorial government departments and health organizations to meet the needs of all Canadians, "including specific at-risk groups"; and
- communicating with Canadians about health promotion, disease prevention, and safety.[47]

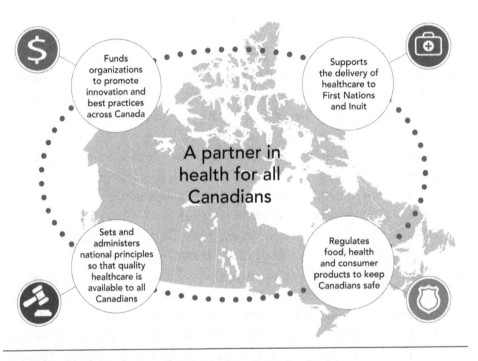

Figure 3.2: Key Roles Played by Health Canada, 2014

Source: Health Canada. (2014). *Health Canada: A partner in health for all Canadians.* Ottawa: Health Canada, p. 2. Retrieved from http://www.hc-sc.gc.ca/ahc-asc/activit/partner-partenaire-eng.php

In Figure 2.12, a typical generic hierarchy for a federal ministry was introduced. Figure 3.3 outlines the complexity of the hierarchy for Health Canada. There are 12 branches and bureaus reporting up to the associate deputy minister and deputy minister—and in addition to the deputy's areas, the minister is accountable for activities in three other large departments: the Public Health Agency of Canada, the Canadian Institutes of Health Research, and the Patented Medicines Prices Review Board. Arm's-length agencies of Health Canada include:

- Canada Health Infoway
- Canadian Agency for Drugs and Technologies in Health
- Canadian Blood Services
- Canadian Centre for Substance Abuse
- Canadian Foundation for Healthcare Improvement
- Canadian Institute for Health Information
- Canadian Partnership Against Cancer
- Canadian Patient Safety Institute
- Mental Health Commission of Canada

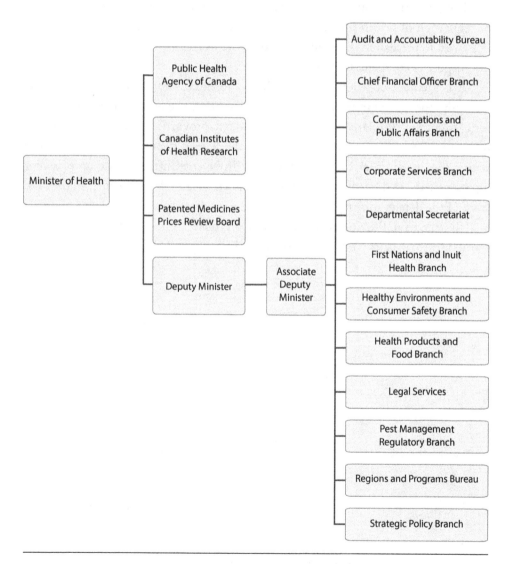

Figure 3.3: Organization Chart, Health Canada, 2015

PROVINCIAL AND TERRITORIAL ROLES IN HEALTH CARE

All 13 provinces and territories participate in the national health care plan, delivering public health services in each of their jurisdictions consistent with the principles of the Canada Health Act. Together they oversee, administer, and ensure delivery of the vast majority of health care services across the country. They administer their respective insurance plans and put in place mechanisms to plan, fund, implement, and evaluate health promotion, public health, and care in hospitals—including some 73,000 hospital beds across the country[48]—and other related organizations. Significantly, the provinces and territories also are the seat of regulation of health professionals, with the privilege of self-regulation largely delegated to professions like nursing and medicine, with which governments must also negotiate compensation and fees.

A conference of federal, provincial, and territorial ministers of health meets annually. The federal minister serves as co-chair with one of the provincial or territorial ministers. Similarly, a conference of federal, provincial, and territorial deputy ministers of health meets biannually, with the federal deputy serving as co-chair with a provincial or territorial counterpart. Three committees, made up of senior representatives of the federal/provincial/territorial health departments, support the work of the deputy ministers and, in turn, the ministers; see Figure 3.4.

The Federal/Provincial/Territorial Committee on Health Workforce—formerly the Advisory Committee on Health Delivery and Human Resources—was

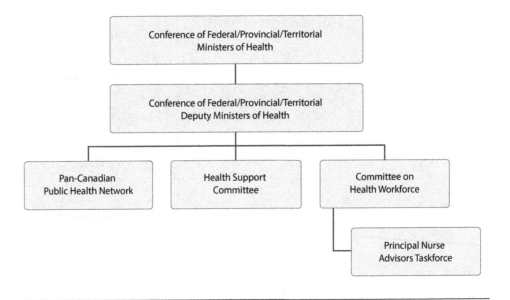

Figure 3.4: Federal/Provincial/Territorial Health Committees

established in 2002 to be a standing committee reporting to the conference of deputy ministers of health. The committee is made up of senior representatives of each jurisdiction, which over the years have included leaders such as assistant deputy ministers and provincial principal nursing advisors (see also Chapter 11).

Regional Health Authorities and Boards

Most provinces administer health services through a variety of arm's-length structures that are usually based closer to the recipients of care than the ministries of health would be—in most jurisdictions, a nod again to the geography issue. A model of regional health authorities has replaced hospital and other organizational boards in most jurisdictions. In theory these structures mean that with funding brought closer to points of care, the services delivered in Prince George, British Columbia, for example, may be slightly differently planned and organized than they would be in Surrey. When governments conducted all planning and funding themselves, there was often criticism that they failed to understand and were unable to meet the unique needs of populations outside the capital city.

The type and number of these structures continues to change. For example, Alberta has just one agency that oversees the entire province, employing more than 100,000 staff working in six zones. Similarly, Nova Scotia also now has one authority for the province plus a special governance structure for the IWK Health Centre in Halifax, which serves as a regional specialty centre for children's health in the Atlantic provinces. Manitoba has five regions and British Columbia has six. Ontario's complex mix includes 14 Local Health Integration Networks and maintains many of its hospital boards. The Local Health Integration Networks "plan, fund and integrate hospital, home and community services" but like other health regions in Canada "they lack responsibility for primary care services, pharmaceuticals and other complex provincial programs like cancer and transplantation."[50]

Boards of directors in health care organizations typically provide an oversight role with fiduciary responsibilities around key areas including balanced budgets, safety, and quality of care. The chief executive officer is normally recruited and

Provincial and Territorial Health Care Governance

Visit the following website to view a summary of health care governance in your province or territory:

http://www.ipac.ca/documents/ALL-COMBINED.pdf[49]

hired by the board, and is its only employee. Made up of community members with a variety of skills, board members provide links to communities and can help to engage them to support the organization, including providing fiscal support.

The staggering number of hospital and other boards has been drastically reduced across Canada—at one time Saskatchewan had 400. Although the structures continue to evolve, Ontario now has the most health care organization boards in the country, including some 150 hospitals, 14 regional Community Care Access Centres, and myriad other care delivery organizations.[51]

Public Health

At the federal level, the Public Health Agency of Canada was established at Health Canada in the wake of the severe acute respiratory syndrome (SARS) outbreak in 2003–2004. With a mandate to help protect public health and safety, its activities "focus on preventing chronic diseases, preventing injuries and responding to public health emergencies and infectious disease outbreaks.[52] A Pan-Canadian Public Health Network, which includes federal, provincial, and territorial public health officials and partners such as the Canadian Public Health Association, brings the parties together to collaborate and share information on a range of public health issues of common interest. The Public Agency of Canada becomes directly involved in public health activities if a health emergency grows to the point of crossing provincial and territorial borders. The agency may contribute supplies and/or human resources, and make connections as necessary with the WHO.

Each province and territory has the primary responsibility to ensure that a variety of public health services are delivered in its jurisdiction. These services may be administered and funded solely by the province/territory at the ministry level (in some cases including more than one ministry), but in some jurisdictions public health may be delivered and partly funded by municipalities. In Ontario, boards of health made up of elected municipal officials oversee public health in 36 units, which may include a region with a number of towns or smaller cities. Boards are considered autonomous corporations;[53] each unit is led by a chief medical officer. In British Columbia, public health is administered within each of the province's six health regions and services are delivered through a network of public health units and health centres.

A typical hierarchy would include a provincial or territorial chief medical officer linked to local chief public health officers or chief medical officers of health situated in regions, units, or municipal departments with public health nurses and others. As noted by the Public Health Agency of Canada, public health activities may be delivered by a broad range of providers including nurses, physicians, and other health professionals who may work in partnership with school teachers, community leaders, sports associations, families, and a variety of health and social organizations.[54]

Municipal Roles in Health Care

Municipal governments typically are delegated authority over policy and program issues related most immediately to the local community or a merged group of small towns or counties. Depending on the model in the province, they may or may not have authority over actual health services. Municipalities may have health and social issues that typically require public health and other local health services, social assistance services, and services related to health including water security, water treatment, and other sanitation measures. Most importantly, municipalities are the first line of defence in response to public health emergencies; depending on the nature and scope of the emergency, a municipality may seek assistance from one or more health units, a regional authority, and/or the province or territory. Newfoundland and Labrador's Department of Health and Community Services, for example, lists the following publicly funded services at the community level:

- health promotion
- community correction
- health protection
- child care services
- mental health and addictions services
- intervention services
- community support program
- residential services
- community health nursing services
- satellite renal dialysis services
- medical clinics
- community clinics.[55]

Deber and her colleagues were critical of decisions to base public health "locally without adequate provisions for higher level oversight and coordination."[56] Citing the 2003 SARS outbreak, they called into question the earlier Ontario decision to hand over funding responsibility for public health to municipal governments, arguing that doing so forced "such services into budgetary competition with the 'hard' services traditionally provided by local government." They concluded by calling for national, provincial, and territorial public health standards.

ABORIGINAL HEALTH CARE

Care in Aboriginal communities is delivered by a mix of Aboriginal and non-Aboriginal providers who may be based in the community, as well as health professionals—nurses, oral health providers, physicians, and others—who move into communities and provide care in a range of facilities. In terms of direct delivery of care to Aboriginal Peoples by the federal government, Health Canada's largest responsibility lies in the health of First Nations and Inuit. The health of First Nations and Inuit originally fell under the Department of Indian Affairs when it began to develop programs in 1904. Much later, in 1962, various medical services under the Indian Affairs and Health and Welfare ministries were consolidated under the new Medical Services Branch.[57]

Renamed as the First Nations and Inuit Health Branch in 2000, the department now employs nurses and other providers in 76 nursing stations and nearly 200 health centres across the country.[58] Roughly half of the health facilities are managed by Health Canada and the nurses working there are employed or deployed by the federal government; the rest are managed by Bands and communities who employ nurses and other health care providers directly.

Usually situated in isolated communities that may be accessible only by air (or by an ice road in the winter), nursing stations normally include a mix of staff including Aboriginal Community Health Representatives who have health training and professionals who live on site (or very nearby) such as registered nurses and dental hygienists. Nursing stations are able to provide 24-hour care in the event of emergencies and also provide health promotion, primary care, and a variety of specialty clinics. Physicians, oral health providers (e.g., dentists, dental therapists, and dental hygienists), and other providers may hold special clinics several times a year; family physician care may be available as often as one or more weeks per month. Occasionally, patients may be admitted for short stays if observation and nursing care are required.

An example of a particularly sophisticated level of remote health care can be found in Forth Smith, Northwest Territories, where the Fort Smith Health and Social Services Centre offers primary, emergency, and acute care; birthing rooms; a number of clinics; diagnostic services; and social services. In addition, there is a midwifery program, a multi-level care home that provides long-term, respite, and day care, as well as meals for disabled persons, two child welfare facilities, a safe facility for women and children seeking protection from violence, a program for healthy babies and families, and a wellness centre, home to addiction and mental health services.[59] Instrumental in the planning, delivery, and evaluation of all these services are nurses, nurse practitioners, and midwives. Among them is Julie Lys, a policy-savvy nurse practitioner who was a member of the National Expert Commission and who brought the great breadth of her community care knowledge to bear on the policy recommendations of the commission. The commissioners could all see the value of a strong community-based, nurse-led model where the people delivering services know the community, its people, and their health and social needs. They could also see the value of a model where the providers were not entirely confined to buildings and existing programs, but moved out into the community and were creative in developing programs and bringing them to the people. ← outreach

Less-isolated communities are more likely to have a health centre that provides some of the same services as a nursing station but does not provide 24-hour care or admit patients; it is assumed that residents of these communities can travel a reasonable distance by ground or air to a hospital for emergency treatment.

SUMMARY AND IMPLICATIONS

Canada's health care system has evolved over the past century to include a rich tapestry of services responsive to all major health concerns, and it provides universal access to medically essential services based on need and not the ability to pay. Public, not-for-profit services are provided by all three levels of government as well as Aboriginal governments, but the bulk of formal health care falls under the jurisdiction of provinces and territories. A significant amount of care also is provided through private, for-profit payment, including dentistry and a number of elements of home care and long-term care. Having an understanding of system governance, we next turn to Chapter 4, which identifies major governance structures in nursing, while the financing and performance of Canadian health care are explored in Module II.

DISCUSSION QUESTIONS

1. What is the role of the state in shaping population health in Canada? What should be the role?
2. What are the expectations of Canadians regarding their governments' roles in health care?
3. Should the federal government have a stronger role in health care, or should its role be further distanced from that of the provinces? Discuss what the respective division of responsibilities should be.
4. What is universal health care as defined in Canada? What is our collective obligation to provide health care as needed versus the ability to pay?

5. The Canada Health Act is an effective instrument to drive improved population health in the 21st century: defend your position for or against this proposition.
6. What is the *right* model of health system governance? How do we determine that and how can we know?
7. What services now covered in the public system could be provided safely on the private side? And in reverse, what current private services should be publicly funded and delivered? What would be the benefits and risks of implementing those changes?
8. Why not treat health care as a commodity and leave the rest to market influences? What are the risks and benefits? What does the evidence tell us, as opposed to the ideology?

ADDITIONAL POLICY RESOURCES

FEDERAL, NATIONAL, PROVINCIAL, AND TERRITORIAL HEALTH SYSTEM STRUCTURES	
Health Canada	http://www.hc-sc.gc.ca
Provincial and Territorial Health Systems	
Links to provincial and territorial ministries of health	http://healthycanadians.gc.ca/health-system-systeme-sante/cards-cartes/health-role-sante-eng.php
Links to provincial and territorial health care resources online	http://www.hc-sc.gc.ca/hcs-sss/medi-assur/links-liens-eng.php
Health Systems Organizations	
Canadian Alliance for Long Term Care	http://www.caltc.ca
Canadian Association for Health Services and Policy Research	http://cahspr.ca
Canadian Health Information Management Association	https://www.echima.ca
Canadian Home Care Association	http://www.cdnhomecare.ca
HealthCareCAN (a merger of the Association of Canadian Academic Healthcare Organizations and the Canadian Healthcare Association)	http://www.healthcarecan.ca
Canadian College of Health Leaders	http://www.cchl-ccls.ca
Canadian Public Health Association	http://www.cpha.ca
World Health Organization	http://www.who.int

CHAPTER 4

Health Human Resources and Nursing: Structures, Regulation, and Professional Organizations

CHAPTER HIGHLIGHTS

- Health Human Resources
- Nursing Structures, Organizations, and Networks: From Local to Global
- Summary and Implications
- Discussion Questions
- Additional Policy Resources

LEARNING OUTCOMES

1. State the purpose and goals of the Pan-Canadian Health Human Resources Planning Framework.
2. Describe the basic tenets of competency-based health human resources planning.
3. Describe the governance of regulated nurses in Canada, including the names and functions of the key regulatory, professional, union, and speciality structures at the national level and in your home province or territory.
4. Understand the purposes and roles of professional nursing associations and nurses' unions.
5. Describe the purpose and key pillars of policy and program activity of the International Council of Nurses.

Policy Influencers: Gail Tomblin Murphy and Walter Sermeus

Dr. Tomblin Murphy, RN, PhD, is a professor in the School of Nursing, Faculty of Health Professions, and Department of Community Health and Epidemiology in the Faculty of Medicine at Dalhousie University in Halifax. She is director of Dalhousie's World Health Organization/Pan-American Health Organization Collaborating Centre on Health Workforce Planning and Research and the inaugural director of the School of Nursing's Centre for Transformative Nursing and Health Research. She is also a co-investigator at the Faculty of Nursing, University of Toronto, and is the co-principal investigator and eastern hub lead for the Pan-Canadian Health Human Resources Network. For over a decade, Tomblin Murphy's leadership and extensive program of work has informed health human resources policy development across the country and beyond. Her contribution to developing the concept of competency-based health human resources planning is a transformative policy innovation that has helped make the idea of *the right care by the right provider at the right place and time* a reality.

On the other side of the Atlantic, Dr. Walter Sermeus, RN, BA, MSc (biostatistics), MSc, PhD, FEANS, is a full professor in the School of Public Health, Faculty of Medicine at the Leuven Institute for Healthcare Policy, University of Leuven, Belgium. He also serves as program director of the Master in Health Care Policy and Management. From 2015 to 2016, Sermeus was the Frances Bloomberg International Distinguished Visiting Professor at the Lawrence S. Bloomberg Faculty of Nursing, University of Toronto. From 2009 to 2011, he was coordinator of the RN4CAST project, "one of the largest nurse workforce studies ever conducted in Europe," conducted to "add to accuracy of forecasting models and generate new approaches to more effective management of nursing resources in Europe."[1] Sermeus publishes and presents widely around the world and serves as a member of Strategic Advisory Committee of the European Health Management Association.

"Nursing creates the culture of the healthcare organization; if nurses don't drive change, it won't happen, and if nurses don't change, it doesn't matter who else does."

—*Timothy Porter–O'Grady, APRN, FAAN, Professor of Practice and Leadership Scholar, College of Nursing and Health Innovation, Arizona State University*

HEALTH HUMAN RESOURCES

From among the more than 3.6 million Canadians working in the public sector in 2012, nearly 860,000 (23.7 per cent) were employed in health and social services institutions across the provinces and territories at a cost of nearly $45.2 billion.[2] This figure does not include providers, such as nurses, employed in federal government health services. When those providers and people working for private health organizations and across the social sector are included, Statistics Canada pins the total number in the range of 2.2 million in 2014.[3]

The Canadian Institute for Health Information collects data on the 32 health professions shown in Table 4.1. Professional health care is dominated in numbers by nursing and medicine, which together represent about 57 per cent of the 26 professions shown in Table 4.2. The next largest professions in order of numbers are social workers, paramedics, and pharmacists.

Despite years of research and experimentation, landing on the right number and mix of health human resources has remained elusive for Canadian health care planners and employers. Nurses interested in this area of policy should be aware of structures that have been put in place to help governments and providers resolve this dilemma. The CNA and the Canadian Medical Association released a green paper in 2005, *Toward a Pan-Canadian Planning Framework for Health Human Resources*, to describe core principles and strategic directions for a pan-Canadian health human resources plan.[4] Some of CNA's positions

---

Table 4.1: Health Care Providers Tracked by the Canadian Institute for Health Information

Audiologists	Licensed practical nurses	Opticians
Cardiology technologists	Nurse practitioners	Optometrists
Chiropractors	Registered psychiatric nurses	Paramedics
Dental assistants		Pharmacists
Dental hygienists	Registered nurses	Pharmacy technicians
Dentists	Medical laboratory technologists	Physicians
Dietitians		Physician assistants
	Medical physicists	
Environmental public health professionals	Medical radiation technologists	Physiotherapists
Genetic counsellors		Psychologists
	Midwives	Respiratory therapists
Health information management professionals	Naturopaths	Social workers
	Occupational therapists	Speech-language pathologists

Table 4.2: Number of Providers in 26 Health Professions, 2012

CATEGORY	NUMBER
Audiologists	1,701
Chiropractors	8,493
Dental assistants	26,256
Dental hygienists	27,653
Dentists	21,292
Dietitians	10,478
Environmental public health professionals	1,603
Health information management professionals	4,763
Medical laboratory technologists	19,664 (2011 data)
Medical physicists	435
Medical radiation technologists	18,295
Midwives	1,080
Occupational therapists	13,830
Opticians	7,444
Optometrists	5,356
Paramedics	38,248
Pharmacists	33,458
Physicians (excluding residents)	75,142
Family medicine	38,156
Specialists	36,986
Physiotherapists	18,469
Psychologists	16,853
Regulated nurses	365,494
Licensed practical nurses	88,280
Nurse practitioners	3,286
Registered nurses	268,521
Registered psychiatric nurses	5,407
Respiratory therapists	10,775
Social workers	41,845
Speech-language pathologists	8,624
TOTAL	**777,251**

Source: Canadian Institute for Health Information. (2012). *Canada's health care providers: Provincial profiles—2012.* Ottawa: CIHI.

were informed by the technical reports prepared for the nursing sector study discussed in Chapter 6.

The framework was endorsed in 2006 by the Health Action Lobby—a coalition of 41 national health organizations[5]—and was used in the development of the *Framework for Collaborative Pan-Canadian Health Human Resources Planning* released by the federal, provincial, and territorial Advisory Committee on Health Delivery and Human Resources, now the Committee on Health Workforce, in 2007.[6] Greater self-sufficiency, identified as one of the principles of effective health human resource planning—and traditionally defined almost exclusively in terms of numbers—was important to developing the framework.[7] The committee recognized that there were a number of weaknesses in traditional health human resources planning, which "relied primarily on a supply-side analysis of past utilization trends to respond to short-term concerns."[8] Goals of the plan were to:

- Improve all jurisdictions' capacities to plan for the optimal number, mix, and distribution of health care providers based on system design, service delivery models, and population health needs.
- Enhance all jurisdictions' capacity to work closely with employers and the education system to develop a health workforce that has the skills and competencies to provide safe high-quality care, work in innovative environments, and respond to changing health care system and population health needs.
- Enhance all jurisdictions' capacity to achieve the appropriate mix of health providers and deploy them in service delivery models that make full use of their skills.
- Enhance all jurisdictions' capacity to build and maintain a sustainable workforce in healthy safe work environments.[9]

More recently, the Pan-Canadian Health Human Resources Network, funded by Health Canada and the Canadian Institutes for Health Research, was established to support health human resources planning, management, and evaluation across the country by:

- Providing access to the latest information and evidence on innovative approaches to health human resources development, training, financing, regulation, recruitment, and retention.

- Gathering, sharing, exchanging, and building capacity in high-quality health human resource research and provide access to ongoing research and model development at pan-Canadian, provincial/territorial, and local/regional service delivery levels.
- Connecting experts, researchers, and policy/decision makers to better coordinate research and support the development and implementation of high-quality, evidence-based policies and best practices.[10]

The network's lead is Ivy Bourgeault, who is the Canadian Institutes of Health Research Chair in Gender, Work and Health Human Resources at the University of Ottawa. She is supported by co-leads from the western region (Morris Barer, professor of Health Services and Policy Research at the University of British Columbia) and eastern region (Gail Tomblin Murphy, a nurse scientist and director of the World Health Organization Collaborating Centre on Health Workforce Planning at Dalhousie University).

Nurse scientists have been at the forefront of health human resources research and have informed policy development in Canada for the past quarter century. Tomblin Murphy has been a leader in the development of the Service Based Planning Framework, which has emerged as a dominant model in Canadian health human resources planning, and is used in Canada's Health Human Resources Strategy.[11] This competency-based approach to human resources planning in some ways flips traditional planning on its head—it is driven not by existing providers and what range of services they can deliver, but rather by identifying population service needs, what competencies are required to meet them, and which provider(s) could deliver services. As Tomblin Murphy and her colleagues described the approach, "Within the broad category of needs-based planning methods, competency-based approaches are designed to allow policy makers to move beyond profession-centred plans and consider the specific combinations of knowledge, skills and judgment (competencies) required to meet healthcare needs."[12] They go on to say that it offers "increased flexibility to planners compared with typical profession-specific models and [is] of particular value in cases where healthcare resources (human or non-human) are especially scarce, where the health needs of the population to be served are not well understood, or where the respective roles of the provider groups involved in service delivery are not well-defined."[13] This approach to planning asks, Who here is competent to deliver this service? It is a useful model to inform staff decisions within the nursing family, from unregulated support workers to advanced practice nurses.

NURSING STRUCTURES, ORGANIZATIONS, AND NETWORKS: FROM LOCAL TO GLOBAL

The four separately regulated categories of nurses in Canada (see Preface) collectively represent nearly half of all the regulated health care providers in Canada.[14] With the exception of registered psychiatric nurses—who are regulated only in the four western provinces and the Yukon—all categories of nurses are regulated and work in all 13 Canadian jurisdictions. The practice of nursing is broad and may include health care planning, delivery, management, evaluation, and/or education. In many settings, nurses are responsible for more than one of these overlapping areas of practice.

Depicted in Figure 4.1 is the complex matrix of regulatory, professional, specialty practice, and union structures supporting nursing; nurses have many masters and divided loyalties. Each of these arms of nursing may be fully or partly replicated for each of the four regulated categories and may exist in some or all of the provinces and territories. With the broadest scope and range of

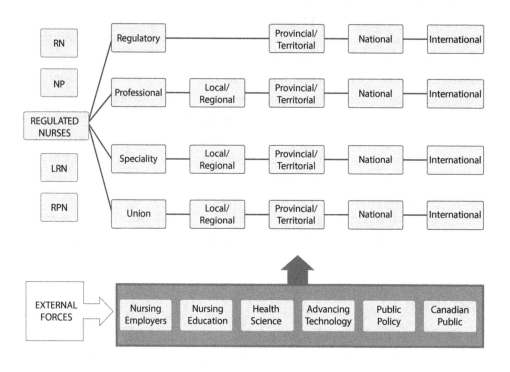

Figure 4.1: Overview of Regulated Nursing Governance and Practice Structures, and Examples of External Forces

practice settings, more of the pillars and levels apply to registered nurses and nurse practitioners than to registered psychiatric nurses and licensed practical nurses. Adding to the complexity is that within each category, an individual nurse may have affiliation or formal membership at local/regional, provincial/territorial, national, and international levels. Any individual nurse may belong to a number of nursing associations—the web of nursing associations and organizations across Canada numbers well over 100.

In the organization of professional nursing, the challenges of geography and governance again come into play. The Constitution delegated health care to the provinces, almost by default setting up a piecemeal system within and across professions, and within and across health care. Yukon, with its 400 registered nurses, and Prince Edward Island, with about 1,750, have many of the same needs and obligations—and hence, corresponding organizations—as Manitoba and Ontario, which have more than 12,000 and 97,000 registered nurses, respectively. The large number of small nursing organizations, often poorly resourced, means that many of them are not nearly as effective as they could be if their efforts and funds were consolidated. This pattern has plagued nursing and many other health professions, jeopardizing their access to policy decision-making power structures and their effectiveness when they are included. Certainly leaders of registered psychiatric nursing have struggled tremendously with this long-standing challenge, especially given what can seem like the disproportionate power of registered nursing.

Beyond the regulations, policies, rules, and conditions by which the practice of nursing is shaped, there are of course many external forces that constantly affect the practice of nurses and all other health providers—including, but hardly limited to, employers and their management structures, the education sector, advances in health science and technology, changing public policy, and most urgently, the needs and expectations of Canadians. The following section provides a brief exploration of these structures; examples of forces influencing nursing structures are discussed throughout the text.

Regulation

The early fight for the regulation of nurses was a long and bitter one. Despite her push to raise other aspects of nursing professionalism, safety, and quality, Florence Nightingale dug in doggedly against registration. In what has been described as a "thirty year war,"[15] her opposition was so absolute that she "contributed to delaying the enactment of legislation for nursing registration."[16]

The most transformative force in nursing regulation in Canada came in the form of Mary Agnes Snively (1847–1933). Snively had trained at Bellevue in New

York City—the first school of nursing in North America built on the Nightingale model.[17] She brought that experience to her role as superintendent of nurses at Toronto General Hospital, where for 25 years she shaped and led what would become one of the most renowned nursing departments in the world. Despite her reverence for Nightingale, they disagreed on the issue of registration. Regulation to protect the public (and frankly, employers) was a high priority for Snively. She served as the founding president of the Canadian Society of Superintendents of Training Schools for Nurses (later the Canadian Association of Nursing Education and eventually CASN) and then as founding president of the Canadian National Association of Trained Nurses—renamed the Canadian Nurses Association (CNA) in 1924. Much of her work outside Toronto General during the first two decades of the last century was directed at developing standards of nursing education and standards of practice, and the creation of regulatory structures. For her far-reaching policy influence in organizing Canadian nursing education, standards of practice, regulation, professional behaviour, and the link to international nurses and health, Snively is sometimes called the "Mother of Canadian Nursing."

The first nursing legislation in Canada was passed in Nova Scotia in 1910 and allowed for voluntary registration by nurses. The first registration act was passed in Manitoba in 1913, and by 1922 all nine existing provinces had some form of nursing legislation. In order to practice today, all regulated nurses must be licensed or registered by a provincial or territorial regulator annually. Self-regulation is a privilege granted by provinces to established and credible professions like nursing and medicine. Nursing regulatory bodies establish the requirements for entry to practice (including the review of education programs in the various categories of nursing), set and enforce standards and scope of practice and codes of ethical professional conduct, and provide quality assurance programs. With their focus on protecting the public, regulatory associations do not take part in advocacy activities around health systems or nursing.

Other than in Ontario, where the College of Nurses of Ontario and Registered Nurses' Association of Ontario have been separate organizations since the early 1960s, registered nurse associations in the provinces and territories have historically housed both regulatory and professional divisions. British Columbia (2010) and Manitoba (2015) have recently moved to a model like Ontario, with both now having separate regulatory and professional organizations, and some other provinces are considering the same change. British Columbia is moving even further toward the model seen in Ontario, announcing in June 2016 that its three nursing regulators (College of Licensed Practical Nurses of British Columbia, College of Registered Nurses of British Columbia, and College of Registered Psychiatric Nurses of BC) were "working to co-create a new nursing body that will replace our existing colleges" to regulate their three categories of regulated nurses, including nurse practitioners.[18]

A national regulatory group, the Canadian Council of Registered Nurse Regulators (CCRNR), was formed in 2011, made up of representatives of the regulatory and/ or professional associations from each province and territory. With the exceptions of Ontario and Quebec, the presidents of the provincial/territorial mixed regulatory and professional associations sit as jurisdictional representatives at the CNA board of directors table, and their executive directors make up the members of the CCRNR.

The Registered Psychiatric Nurse Regulators of Canada represents the four western provincial jurisdictions and the Yukon, and oversees the Registered Psychiatric Nurses of Canada Examination. The four provincial jurisdictions each have a regulatory mandate; only the Registered Psychiatric Nurses Association of Saskatchewan maintains a dual regulatory and professional function. There is no association in the Yukon Territory.

Similarly, the Canadian Council of Practical Nurse Regulators is the national regulatory body for licensed practical nurses in the provinces, and it oversees the Canadian Practical Nurse Registration Examination. All 10 provinces are members; the territories are not part of the council. All members have solely regulatory mandates, with the exceptions of the Ordre des infirmières et infirmiers auxiliaires du Québec (the practical nurses association in Quebec) and the Association of New Brunswick Licensed Practical Nurses, which both maintain dual regulatory and professional functions.

Adult and pediatric nurse practitioners write the American Academy of Nurse Practitioners Certification Program's Adult-Gerontology Primary Care Nurse Practitioner Exam and the Pediatric Nursing Certification Board's Pediatric Primary Care Nurse Practitioner Exam, respectively.[19] The primary health care group of nurse practitioners (family/all ages) still write a Canadian examination offered through Assessment Strategies, Inc.

Entry-to-Practice Testing for Registered Nurses: Unrest in the 21st Century

For registered nurses, the national licensing examination—the Canadian Registered Nurse Examination (CRNE)—was developed, owned, and overseen by CNA starting in 1970. It was used by all jurisdictions outside Quebec. In addition, CNA was a facilitator in the development of the pan-Canadian approach to nurse practitioner exams through the CNA Nurse Practitioner Exam Program for the family/all ages category.

After issuing a call for proposals to select a new entry-to-practice examination that would incorporate "state-of-the-art best practices,"[20] the Canadian Council of Registered Nurse Regulators announced in December 2011 that it would terminate its relationship with CNA's testing company and the Canadian Registered Nurse Examination. The contract for the new examination was awarded to the National Council of State Boards of Nursing in the United States, which develops and administers the National Council Licensure Examination for Registered Nurses (NCLEX-RN) using computer-adaptive testing. The examination is now used by all Canadian jurisdictions other than Quebec and the Yukon.

The Canadian Council stated that, although based in the United States, the NCLEX-RN examination would not be an *American* examination but rather would test Canadian nursing and health system content. Still, the move provoked considerable upset and debate across Canadian nursing at large, and certainly within nursing education circles. Concerns were voiced about whether Canadian nursing curricula, designed to meet CRNE standards, would enable writers to pass the NCLEX-RN examinations. After a mapping exercise conducted by the CASN, Kirsten Woodend, president of the association, concluded in October 2015 that the fit between the NCLEX-RN and the Canadian context was poor.[21] The executive director of the CASN further stated that "one third of the competencies expected of a Canadian nurse are not addressed at all by the NCLEX-RN and over a quarter are only partially tested. This represents more than half of the competencies." She cited national guidelines related to patient safety, interprofessional collaboration, client-centred care, and cultural safety as examples of missing competencies.[22]

Administration of the new examination was effective January 2015. Early outcomes did nothing to dampen the anxiety: in a blunt commentary published in the *National Post* in December 2015, Woodend and Jennifer Medves—both leaders of Ontario university nursing schools—stated that, despite positive intentions, "the bodies that regulate nursing in Canada have made a big mistake." They went on to cite examples such as the case of the Université de Moncton, where the pass rate dropped from 93 per cent for the CRNE to 39 per cent for the NCLEX-RN. As they pointed out, since the education of those writers didn't change in that time, one assumes that most would have passed the original Canadian examination.[23]

Speaking to the *Globe and Mail* in May 2016, the CASN charged that "Canadian regulators adopted the U.S. licensing test without consulting non-regulatory nursing organizations in Canada," and said that "Canadian members of the harmonization team were drawn solely from provincial regulatory bodies, who are working with American partners without the knowledge of Canadian nursing educators or other professional nursing groups in Canada."[24] In the same piece, Linda Johnston, dean of the Lawrence S. Bloomberg Faculty of Nursing at the University of Toronto, added that "an American-style system that licenses nurses to practice without requiring a university degree may not foster the academic career pathways that have made Canada a world leader in nursing education."

In a letter to the *Globe and Mail*, Anne Coghlan, then president of the Canadian Council of Registered Nurse Regulators, denied that there were efforts to harmonize testing. She countered that she was "mystified by CASN executives' ongoing and aggressive campaign to misinform the public and discredit the public safety efforts of Canada's nurse regulators," calling the comments "alarmist" and saying they wrongly portray the position of the regulators.[25] But despite assurances from the Canadian Council of Registered Nurses Regulators that there was no concern about process or outcomes of the examination, students, new graduates, and educators who spoke out at length at the CNA annual meeting in June 2016 remained on edge. Students especially expressed significant distress about the examination issue, citing their fear of personal failure based on the first year of Canadian NCLEX-RN results, including:

- From among all graduates of Canadian baccalaureate programs in 2015, 9,048 wrote the NCLEX-RN English examination; 69.7 per cent of those passed the test on the first writing, ranging from 50.3 per cent in New Brunswick to 94.2 per cent in the Northwest Territories. First-time pass rates for the CRNE, on the other hand, were 87 per cent for Canadian-educated graduates, according to the Canadian Council of Registered Nurse Regulators.[26]
- The number ultimately passing in 2015 was 84.1 per cent (ranging from 71.4 per cent in New Brunswick to 94.7 per cent in the Northwest Territories).[27]
- For those writing in French, the first-time pass rate was 27.1 per cent and ultimate pass rate was 50 per cent.

These outcomes prompted significant concerns among some health human resources planners, including those based in governments, who depend on a fairly reliable supply of new graduates licensed to practice each year. The results were challenged right across the country; the French language issue sparked particular uproar. The perception that there was a lack of transparency in the process fuelled some of the backlash. It also was not lost on observers that if there was not a conflict of interest, it was at least strange that the decision to change the exam was made by executive directors of the very organizations that make up the CNA jurisdictional members. And the change to the NCLEX examination may have hit a nerve not just because it moved Canadian testing to another country, but particularly because it was to the United States, around which there are well-known cultural sensitivities underlying the long-standing cross-border friendship (see Chapter 1). The results sparked letters to the Canadian Council of Registered Nurse Regulators, as well as governments, asking for the process to be reviewed or even reversed. In letters to provincial ministers, CFNU was harsh in demanding a systemic review of the situation, citing "high NCLEX failure rates, the inequities created by the lack of nation-wide harmonized regulatory standards (re: number of writes, working when failed, length of temporary licenses, etc.), the lack of student supports (to help with prep costs, stress, etc.), particularly for francophone students, and perhaps most regrettably, the lack of acknowledgement from provincial/territorial nursing regulatory bodies that the transition to the NCX has been a failure."[28]

As a result of the fallout, some regulators decided to allow graduate nurses to write the examination as often as needed until they pass (where initially only three attempts were allowed). At the CNA annual meeting in June 2016 there was lengthy discussion and debate on a motion tabled by the Canadian Nursing Students' Association asking that the CNA "support urgent constructive dialogue and resolution of the issues and concerns associated with the current licensing exam, specifically to advocate and call for action to the current entry-to-practice exam by collaboration with provincial associations, regulatory bodies and Canadian nursing students, until issues are fully resolved."[29] The motion was carried. Resolutions are for the consideration of the board and are not binding on the organization. At the time of writing the response of CNA is not known, but at its national conference in January 2017, the Canadian Nursing Students' Association ramped up its political action with a three-pronged social media and letter-writing campaign targeting Canada's nursing regulators as well as the National Council of State Boards of Nursing in the United States.

Professional Representation

Professional associations exist to represent the professional voices of their members. For nurses, that mandate means they are the focal point for advocacy and policy in nursing—and in some cases are the only players actively involved in this work. With their relative size and funding, they often are also the only groups in nursing other than unions equipped to mount effective political responses to nursing, health system, and broader societal issues, and to develop platforms and tools to involve nurses meaningfully in policy and political activities such as election campaigns. As Peter noted, compared to individual efforts, "Organized professional groups stand to have the most success in sustained collective action at the level of policy, given the opportunities they have to pool resources of all kinds, including talent and will."[30] In addition, of course, they provide valuable guidance and expertise to nurses around practice and policy issues, and to non-nurse organizations taking on work that requires a nursing perspective or contribution.

The largest and oldest national professional nursing association in Canada is CNA—which is the voice of registered nurses, including nurse practitioners. The organization was founded in October 1908, initially as a strategy to link Canadian nurses to the newly forming International Council of Nurses, which it joined in 1909. All nine existing provinces were members of CNA by 1922 and the Newfoundland association would join later when the province joined Canada. From then, until the 1980s when Quebec withdrew,[31] all ten provincial professional nursing associations sat as CNA's jurisdictional members. The Northwest Territories joined in 1975 and Yukon in 1982, so there were three years when all Canadian jurisdictions had member organizations at the CNA table.

There is no comparative national professional association for registered psychiatric nurses. For licensed practical nurses, the Canadian Practical Nurses Association, established in 1974, became Practical Nurses Canada in 2006; at the time of writing, the latter is undergoing restructuring. When the national (or cross-provincial) organizations for the two categories both evolved to a regulatory mandate, professional issues were left unmet, or not fully met, at a pan-Canadian level.

Having moved around the country, CNA settled its headquarters in Ottawa in 1954, where it remains today. The organization has been intensely active in a wide range of health, social, and economic policy activities over its history; examples are explored throughout this book. With members in all 13 provinces and territories, CNA remains the only nursing association with a truly pan-Canadian reach. As of 2017, CNA had five different membership categories/groups, including provincial/territorial jurisdictions, independent members in Ontario and Quebec, retired nurses, students, and specialty associations.[32]

Historically, CNA held mandates related to regulatory policy, the socio-economic welfare of nurses, and professional issues and advocacy. The association was originally the single national body representing all domains of nursing, except for the group of superintendents of nursing schools, which had a separate national organization, the Canadian Society of Superintendents of Training Schools for Nurses. That group eventually folded into CNA. Throughout the years, the education group came and went as structures changed, sometimes positioned within CNA as an arm of its work, finally settling as what is now the CASN. Unions broke away in 1981, and eventually most specialty groups also formed their own separate associations. However, CNA maintains the specialty certification program that first began in 1984, and 20 specialty certification examinations now are offered through the program.

At the provincial/territorial level, registered nursing regulatory and professional bodies have been arms of the same organizations since most were established. The exception is Ontario, where the College of Nurses of Ontario—the regulatory body for registered nurses and registered practical nurses (originally registered nursing assistants)—was established as a stand-alone organization, separate from RNAO, in 1963. More recently, British Columbia and Manitoba have moved to a similar model, as discussed later in this section.

For registered psychiatric nurses, the Association of Registered Psychiatric Nurses of British Columbia is a stand-alone professional association, and the Registered Psychiatric Nurses Association of Saskatchewan maintains a professional advocacy role along with its regulatory function. Alberta and Manitoba now have solely regulatory colleges for registered psychiatric nurses.

Four provinces maintain professional associations for licensed practical nurses; two of these, British Columbia (Licensed Practical Nurses Association of British Columbia) and Ontario (Registered Practical Nurses Association of Ontario), have stand-alone organizations. As noted in the discussion of regulation, Quebec (Ordre des infirmières et infirmiers auxiliaires du Québec) and New Brunswick (Association of New Brunswick Licensed Practical Nurses) both have dual regulatory/professional associations. There is no professional representation for licensed practical nurses in the other jurisdictions. *LPNs don't have prof repr. outside ON, BC, Qb, NB.*

Professional Associations and Membership: Turmoil and Change

Membership in registered nursing professional associations has become a somewhat prickly political issue in nursing over the past few years and is one that has far-reaching implications. Because provincial and territorial regulatory and professional bodies have been arms of the same organizations for much of the past century, nurses who register to practice have also enjoyed automatic membership in their provincial or territorial professional associations. In turn, members of the provincial and territorial professional associations automatically have membership in CNA and the International Council of Nurses. This universal membership model was sustained over the decades, with two exceptions:

1. During the 63 years that the Ordre des infirmières et infirmiers du Québec was the CNA jurisdictional member from Quebec (1922–1985), all nurses who registered in Quebec automatically had professional representation by their association and, in turn, membership in CNA and the

International Council of Nurses. After Quebec disaffiliated from CNA in 1985, CNA membership was no longer included in provincial registration. Since 2014, with the implementation of new bylaws, nurses in Quebec have been able to join CNA as independent members and thereby also access membership in the International Council of Nurses.

2. Since RNAO became a stand-alone professional association in Ontario after the establishment of the College of Nurses of Ontario (1963), membership has been voluntary. However, nurses who did join RNAO then had automatic membership in CNA and, in turn, the International Council of Nurses, because that aspect of membership was part and parcel of membership in RNAO.

The state of professional nursing association representation across Canada is very fluid today. Change has been driven in part by associations formerly holding a mixed regulatory and professional function divesting themselves of their professional mandates to become stand-alone regulatory colleges—British Columbia and Manitoba, for example, as discussed in the following section. But first there is the case of Ontario, where there are different dynamics at play.

Ontario

There could hardly be a starker example of politics seemingly trumping smart policy than in the very public decay of the relationship between RNAO and CNA that began early in the new century. Tensions had been simmering for some time when the RNAO board of directors brought a resolution to its own annual meeting in 2006 requesting a consultation with members on its relationship with CNA. Some RNAO members were concerned that something was afoot that would lead to withdrawal of the association from CNA. Members were reassured that this was not so, and in the subsequent member-wide consultation, support for CNA was very strong. At a special members' meeting held in January 2007, then-president of RNAO Mary Ferguson-Paré said, "Members made it clear they want nursing policy and practice and healthy public policy discussed on a national scale, and that a national organization should lead social activism on nursing and health issues by mobilizing nurses from coast to coast, and by speaking out on social determinants of health and defending Medicare."[33] She went on to say, "They also called on RNAO's board to continue to work with CNA to create change nationally."

In some ways echoing the discord between the Ordre des infirmières et infirmiers du Québec and CNA in the years leading up Quebec's disaffiliation from CNA, in response to issues raised before and during the consultation, CNA increased its activity significantly in areas important to RNAO. But tensions between the two associations continued to smoulder. They may be partially explained by the challenges of federated models where the national or central body has to juggle a broad roster of competing demands that do not always fully meet the expectations or needs of any one jurisdiction. CNA not only had professional obligations to fulfill, but also had a regulatory policy role to fulfill for all its members outside Ontario: until 2014, CNA was the seat of the national entry-to-practice examination, and the specialty certification program cited earlier remains one of the organization's core programs. As a result, some of the tension was simply the result of disagreements about activities, priorities, and style. It is important to remember that CNA policy directions flow from its board, which historically has been made up of the jurisdictions across the country. So they debate those decisions together and vote on them. Operational choices of leaders in Ottawa are intended to respond to those directions from the board as a whole.

Things escalated in April 2013 when RNAO advised CNA's board of directors of its intent to move to voluntary, rather than universal, membership of its members in CNA, effective 2014. What this meant was that when Ontario nurses joined or renewed membership in RNAO, they would no longer automatically become members of CNA. Efforts were made over the following year by CNA and individual members of RNAO to have the RNAO board revisit its decision and/or take the question to its members. Those efforts were unsuccessful. Subsequently, in March 2014, efforts were undertaken through establishment of a memorandum of understanding to co-market the two associations to Ontario nurses. By the end of that membership year, roughly 30 per cent of nurses joining RNAO also had chosen CNA membership—a significant drop in membership numbers for CNA and an exclusion of more than two-thirds of RNAO members from national and global representation.

In March 2015, CNA invoked the one-year notice clause to discontinue the memorandum of understanding established around the co-marketing of CNA and RNAO, effective March 31, 2016. The CNA board also supported a bylaw change confirming the decades-long practice of providing universal membership in CNA as a requirement to be the CNA jurisdictional member (i.e., the provincial and territorial associations) and advised RNAO of the same. The bylaw was openly debated and ultimately passed by the required two-thirds majority of members at the June 2015 CNA annual meeting. During 2015 and 2016, CNA advised RNAO that it needed to be compliant with those bylaws by the time of CNA's June 2016 annual meeting.

In July 2015, RNAO notified CNA and RNAO members of its board's decision to withdraw from the national association in October 2018. The RNAO president had stated in 2006 that "RNAO has grown into an association that is owned by its members" and that "the board believes members should be in the driver's seat."[34] In this case, however, RNAO members were notified of their board's decision in the July 2015 email edition of its *In the Loop* communication tool.

Ongoing lobbying of the RNAO president and board by representatives of its current and former members during 2015 and 2016—including past RNAO presidents, life members, and its former executive director—had no effect, even in the face of public resignations from RNAO by long-standing members. In a further attempt to compel RNAO to consult with its members on CNA-related decisions, early in 2016 members of one RNAO region, five chapters, and two interest groups—representing more than 25 per cent of registered nurse and nurse practitioner membership[35]—submitted a resolution requesting reversal of the board's decision. They asked that the resolution be openly debated and voted upon by members at the May 2016 RNAO annual meeting. The resolution was denied and therefore was not put forward to the members for a vote. Shortly thereafter, CNA again advised RNAO that to remain the CNA jurisdictional member for Ontario, it would have to comply with CNA bylaws by the time of the June 2016 CNA annual meeting.

The RNAO did not change its position and was ultimately advised in May 2016 of its impending termination as the CNA jurisdictional member from Ontario, assuming that nothing changed during a final, 20-day, "sober second thought" period built into the notice. There was no material response, and, for the first time in its history, RNAO was not the CNA jurisdictional member for Ontario. Through another board decision, RNAO also severed its relationship with the Canadian Nurses Protective Society in late 2015, when professional liability protection for members was moved to another provider.

Members of RNAO who had chosen the CNA membership option were kept informed of unfolding events through the Canadian Nurse journal, as well as through the CNA website and other tools. With membership in the independent category exceeding 2,000 nurses by March 2017 and increasing, structures for representation and meaningful engagement of individual CNA members in Ontario and Quebec were being put in place throughout 2016. Effective June 2016 a small transitional executive team composed of CNA Ontario nurses was established to oversee the development of a new governance and membership structure to bring Ontario nurses into CNA and to ensure that the voices of Ontario nurses continue to inform and influence CNA's work. By early 2017, Dr. Mary McAllister had been appointed to lead the Ontario independent nurses, coming together under the title CNA*Ontario*, and two vice presidents were in place by March 2017.

Given the historically important position of RNAO as one of only two founding provincial members of CNA (the other being Manitoba), and its long-standing position as a leading Canadian nursing organization, the reasons behind choosing to increasingly isolate Ontario nurses through a public power struggle with the national association are perplexing. The RNAO took this action at a time when the new Association of Registered Nurses of British Columbia and Association of Registered Nurses of Manitoba were both being established (see following discussion), and both of those associations are compliant with the universal membership condition common across CNA jurisdictional members.

Despite public rhetoric about collaboration and cooperation, the relationship between RNAO and CNA played out in one tense episode after another for over a decade. How much is related to personalities versus strategic organizational policy is unclear. But in the end, both organizations were weakened, the profession left more fragmented, and nothing was improved for nurses as a result of the expenditure of years of time, money, and angst—and none of it improved care delivery or other outcomes for those served by the members of either association. Reflecting on her time as chief executive officer of CNA and her own role in the history of membership struggles, Lucille Auffrey expressed deep personal pain about that period. She lamented that "the problems that were germane to our patients are still present and nurses at the entry level are no better off" as a result of it (L. Auffrey, personal communication, July 13, 2016).

British Columbia

The Registered Nurses Association of British Columbia, established in 1935, had maintained dual regulatory and professional mandates until umbrella legislation in 2005 "created a stronger demarcation between the regulatory and professional functions across the health professions."[36] The board "put into motion a series of incremental policy and organizational changes that led to the gradual attrition of most of its prior professional association and functions over a period of several years" and eroded nursing professional development and advocacy.[37] Ultimately taking on a purely regulatory function—repurposing itself, as Duncan and colleagues put it in 2015—the original, dual-function association became the new College of Registered Nurses of British Columbia (CRNBC). When the new college announced its decision to pull out of CNA membership, British Columbia nurses were left without provincial or national professional representation.

A network of nurses in the province received one-time funding from the new college to help launch and build a new professional association. Since 2010 the Association of Registered Nurses of British Columbia has emerged as a growing professional force in British Columbia. Assuming a collaborative approach to relationship building, the association has attracted interest from British Columbia nurses, been a strong supporter of CNA, and helped build a coalition of nursing groups in the province. The first of its kind in Canada, the BC Coalition of Nursing Associations brings together four provincial nursing associations representing registered nurses, registered psychiatric nurses, nurse practitioners, and licensed practical nurses, as well as the province's Nursing Education Council. Bringing these key nursing groups under one tent, the purpose of the "collaborative forum" is "to engage elected nurse leaders from across the professional nursing groups in discussion around topics, policy and directions that impact the nursing profession as a whole."[38]

Although the professional association representing registered nurses and nurse practitioners has the most resources and has taken on some fiscal responsibility to help other associations to take part effectively, representation among members of the coalition is equally distributed so as not to be weighted in favour of the largest group. It is intended to achieve "fair, objective discussion that benefits all nurses."[39] The process of coming together was not easy and raised many old issues, but the associations found a way to build something new together. As Joy Peacock, then executive director of the Association of Registered Nurses of British Columbia, said about the new coalition, "Nursing has a limitless potential to break down the old hierarchy and barriers in our profession—if we work together collaboratively. We can do this, and we need to do this. We must do this" (J. Peacock, personal communication, July 7, 2016).

Despite the good will and these successes, the professional association journey has not been entirely smooth in British Columbia. The British Columbia Nurses' Union (BCNU), which had withdrawn from the CFNU in 2011 after contravening the rules of the Canadian Labour Congress,[40] has launched two legal actions against the ARNBC since 2013. The first of these, set in motion by the BCNU and its previous president in 2013, was brought against the CRNBC and its chief executive officer and registrar, as well as the ARNBC's previous president, after the CRNBC had freed up a one-time $1.5 million grant "to help with ARNBC's start-up costs and to allow ARNBC to begin offering services to nurses that fall outside CRNBC's mandate."[41] The CRNBC has stated, "BCNU claims in its lawsuit that CRNBC had no authority under the *Health Professions Act* to make this grant to ARNBC. It also claims that the funds used for the grant were originally collected for the sole purpose of providing professional liability insurance coverage to nurses, and could not be used for any other purpose." The CRNBC disputes the BCNU's claims, saying that its board has full authority to allocate spending "for purposes consistent with the College's duties and determined to be in the public interest."[42]

In 2015, two union members, supported by the British Columbia Nurses'

Union, launched a second legal action against the Association of Registered Nurses of British Columbia. The ARNBC's president at the time said the second legal action "threatens to undermine the work the Association has done over the past four years on behalf of the profession and patients."[43] After the ARBNC noticed inconsistencies in its bylaws and called a special members meeting to rectify the situation, two members of the BCNU council—both members of the ARNBC as well—launched legal action "to declare null and void all previous activities of ARNBC."[44] They sought what is called a *short stay* from the court, asking, for example, that the ARNBC not be allowed to hold its May 2015 annual meeting. The court did not agree and the meeting went forward shortly thereafter.

At the time of this writing, both of these legal actions linger. As of mid-2015, the collective legal costs faced by the CRNBC and the ARNBC related to the two legal actions were approaching $500,000—all paid by nurses' registration and membership fees. As in the Ontario situation, there is no evidence that any of the public upheaval has done anything to benefit the associations, nurses, or people who need nursing services.

Manitoba

Under new umbrella health regulatory legislation in Manitoba, the College of Registered Nurses of Manitoba (CRNM) is no longer permitted to collect fees on behalf of other organizations. To facilitate that change and maintain a connection to CNA for Manitoba registered nurses, the CRNM worked collaboratively with a group of members who came together as the Manitoba Registered Nurse Network to address this change. With funding from the CRNM and CNA, the Manitoba Registered Nurse Network explored the feasibility of a new professional association to fill the gap created by the changing legislation. Through consultations with nurses, the network found overwhelming support for the creation of an association and the desire to once again have a professional voice for registered nurses in Manitoba. The network received further funding from the CRNM to develop a strategic plan and a business plan, and incorporate the new entity. In 2015, the CRNM's board of directors provided a loan to support the establishment of the Association of Registered Nurses of Manitoba (ARNM).

The new ARNM began operating in January 2016. As part of the transition, the CRNM transferred its membership in CNA (effective March 2016) and the Canadian Nurses Protective Society (effective January 2017, thereby providing professional liability protection) to the new organization. Similar to the long-standing model in Ontario before the events described above, membership in the ARNM is voluntary. For each member joining the association, membership in CNA and the International Council of Nurses is automatically included.

Future Implications

If the pattern of provincial and territorial registered nursing associations evolving to have solely regulatory functions continues, then funding for professional representation will continue to be a challenge. Historically, a significant portion of funding for provincial and territorial dual-mandate associations has come from licensing examinations and annual registration fees. There is understandable concern about the viability of stand-alone professional associations in the provinces and territories, as well as at the national level, if membership becomes entirely voluntary across the country. New models, missions, and mandates will have to emerge.

Specialty Practice in Canada

There are 46 associations affiliated with CNA through the Canadian Network of Nursing Specialties, representing the full scope of professional, clinical, administrative, education, research, social, and cultural interests of nursing (see Table 4.3). These organizations vary considerably in size and scope, but their work tends to focus on development and dissemination of knowledge, and standards and policy related to specialty. Differing from the professional voice of nurses expressed by organizations such as the Association of Registered Nurses of Prince Edward Island and CNA, which are focused on nursing and health systems more broadly, the Canadian Network of Nursing Specialties tends to narrow its focus to professional nursing interests within the topic area and to position each specialty area in relevant policy conversations. Many of these nursing groups are affiliated with global associations in the same specialty area.

Nurses' Unions

Advocacy for the compensation, safety, and workplace satisfaction of nurses was a pillar of activity within CNA dating back to its early days. As early as 1924, CNA was generating reports for the federal government using statistics to describe current trends and issues, and expressing concerns about recruitment, attrition, and deployment of nurses. In 1938 CNA formed a committee to advocate for 8-hour tours for student and graduate nurses, saying they should not exceed 96 hours every two weeks—and by 1943, CNA had put in place its first formal Committee on Labour Relations.

Throughout much of the 20th century, CNA maintained a position that labour relations activities for professional nurses belonged within provincial professional associations. But its stance on the details did waiver over time, sometimes in support of collective bargaining and at other times distancing

Table 4.3: Canadian Network of Nursing Specialties

Academy of Canadian Executive Nurses	Canadian Federation of Mental Health Nurses
Canadian Association for Enterostomal Therapy	Canadian Forensic Nurses Association
Canadian Association for International Nursing	Canadian Gerontological Nursing Association
Canadian Association for Nursing Research	Canadian Holistic Nurses Association
Canadian Association for Parish Nursing Ministry	Canadian Hospice Palliative Care Nurses Group
Canadian Association for Rural and Remote Nursing	Canadian Indigenous Nurses Association
Canadian Association for the History of Nursing	Canadian Nurse Continence Advisors
Canadian Association of Advanced Practice Nurses	Canadian Nurses for Health and the Environment
Canadian Association of Burn Nurses	Canadian Nursing Informatics Association
Canadian Association of Critical Care Nurses	Canadian Nursing Students' Association
Canadian Association of Hepatology Nurses	Canadian Occupational Health Nurses Association
Canadian Association of Medical and Surgical Nursing	Canadian Orthopaedic Nurses Association
Canadian Association of Neonatal Nurses	Canadian Society for Transfusion Medicine
Canadian Association of Nephrology Nurses and Technologists	Canadian Society of Gastroenterology Nurses and Associates
Canadian Association of Neuroscience Nurses	Canadian Vascular Access Association
Canadian Association of Nurses in AIDS Care	Clinical Nurse Specialist Association of Canada
Canadian Association of Nurses in Hemophilia Care	Community Health Nurses of Canada
Canadian Association of Nurses in Oncology	Infection Prevention and Control Canada
Canadian Association of Perinatal and Women's Health Nurses	Legal Nurse Consultants Association of Canada
Canadian Association of Rehabilitation Nurses	National Association of PeriAnesthesia Nurses of Canada
Canadian Association Self Employed Registered Nurses	National Emergency Nurses Association
Canadian Council of Cardiovascular Nurses	Operating Room Nurses Association of Canada
Canadian Family Practice Nurses Association	Practical Nurses Canada

itself from professional nurses undertaking union activity. Its public statement in 1946 opposing striking nurses was a prickly point of contention that, for some, never really healed.

In a recurring theme in this book, activity in Saskatchewan catalyzed a change across the country. In 1973, the Saskatchewan Registered Nurses' Association had applied to the Labour Relations Board to be the bargaining unit for registered nurses, which was also the model CNA favoured at that time—maintaining labour relations within professional associations in the provinces. The Service Employees International Union "opposed the application on the ground that the association was not a trade union because it was a company dominated organization, organized, formed and influenced in its administration by the Saskatchewan Registered Nurses' Association."[45] The Board dismissed the application, based in part on a perceived conflict of interest given the membership of the association, which was inclusive of managers, directors, and so on. The Saskatchewan Registered Nurses' Association applied to the Saskatchewan Court of Appeal—remember the governance structure described in Chapter 2—which ruled in its favour. The Service Employees International Union appealed that decision with the Supreme Court of Canada, which ultimately ruled against the association.

Nurses joined new union organizations throughout the provinces through the 1970s, and the National Federation of Nurses Unions was formed in 1981 to represent unionized nurses at the national level. The name was changed to the Canadian Federation of Nurses Unions (CFNU) in 1999. Nurses in most hospital settings (as well as other practice settings, such as long-term care) now join a provincial union, which sits as the member of the national union. These nurses

The Supreme Court of Canada Ruling on *Service Employees' International Union, Local No. 333 v. Nipawin District Staff Nurses Association et al.*

The Supreme Court of Canada's 1973 ruling on the Saskatchewan Registered Nurses' Association case makes for informative reading. It may be useful for nurses who are interested in policy to read through the court's thinking in reaching its decision. The case serves as an excellent example of the way a decision from the judicial branch of the government exerted a game-changing impact on nursing policy. See https://scc-csc.lexum.com/scc-csc/scc-csc/en/item/5342/index.do

are affected by local and central collective agreements negotiated with employers and the provincial government, respectively, and also hold membership in the national federation. The national body is not involved directly in the business of the provincial associations—in this case, collective bargaining—but rather serves as a unifying focal point and force for advocacy and other action by the collective membership. These structures mimic the governance structure of the country whereby the national (federal) body does not usurp or control the jurisdictions, but rather, with a national view and reach, brings different skills and opportunities that can rally the separate bodies across the country and support and boost their collective effectiveness. The CFNU also is the connection for its jurisdictional members to the federal government.

Depending on their category, employer, and province/territory of employment, nurses and nursing support workers may belong to unions that represent other workers. For example, nurses working in formal policy settings in a federal, provincial, or territorial government may belong to the Professional Institute of the Public Service of Canada. Many licensed practical nurses and non-regulated members of the nursing family, such as personal support workers, belong to large, multi-occupational unions such as the Canadian Union of Public Employees and Service Employees Union International.

But CFNU is Canada's largest union that only has nurses as members; it represents some 161,000 nurses and student nurses. The CFNU describes its work as "protecting the health of patients and our public health system, promoting nurses and the nursing profession at the national level—and doing it effectively."[46] While its individual members include registered nurses in each jurisdiction, the organization also represents licensed practical nurses, registered psychiatric nurses, and nurse practitioners in various provinces. As such, it is the only national nursing organization having all four categories of nurses as members—and is Canada's largest nursing organization. The difference between the national organization's opening statement about its role (above) and that of its member associations is revealing of their different roles. Consider Ontario and Newfoundland and Labrador, for example:

- "The Ontario Nurses' Association provides skilled staff to assist members in matters of contract interpretations, contract enforcement and patient care concerns."[47]
- "The Registered Nurses' Union Newfoundland & Labrador (RNUNL) is the official trade union for registered nurses in Newfoundland and Labrador. We represent over 5,700 members in forming a strong, unified voice for nurses working in Newfoundland and Labrador."[48]

In its language and public posture, the national body has positioned itself as one of the most credible, forceful, and effective players in Canada's nursing family—quite a change from the days when unions were cast as marginalized, confrontational self-interest groups. Some of the effectiveness of the CFNU reflects the benefit of expertise and the payoff of persistence and longevity: its president, Linda Silas, is the longest-serving current national leader not just in Canadian nursing but in any national health care organization. First elected in 2003, she has been re-elected seven times by voting delegates from across Canada at the organization's biennial conventions.

Leaders of CFNU have positioned the organization skilfully as a policy influencer through strategic use of evidence, rapid action on political timing opportunities, strong relationships with key decision makers, and linking its members with patient safety, quality, and value for taxpayer dollars. The impacts of professional associations and unions on policy are introduced further in Modules II and III. The CRNU is affiliated nationally with the Canadian Labour Congress and, in turn, the International Trade Union Confederation.

The national body's most direct international nursing connection is with Global Nurses United, which brings together 23 unions in 18 countries, including CFNU and Fédération interprofessionnelle de la santé du Québec. Global Nurses United was formed in 2013 to "fight against the harmful effects of austerity measures, privatization, and cuts in health care services that … are putting people and communities at risk across the planet" by working to "guarantee the highest standards of universal healthcare as a human right for all, to secure safe patient care, especially with safe nurse-to-patient ratios, and safe health care workplaces."[49]

THE INTERNATIONAL COUNCIL OF NURSES

Founded in 1899, the International Council of Nurses was the first international organization for health professionals and still has the widest reach. Formalizing the start of what would be a long tradition of global health leadership by Canadian nurses, the first executive of the new organization included its British founder, Ethel Bedford Fenwick, as the inaugural president; Lavinia Dock from the United States as inaugural secretary; and Canada's Mary Agnes Snively as inaugural treasurer—a role she held from 1899 to 1904 before going on to serve as vice president (1904–1908). Since then, a long list of esteemed Canadian nurses have held leadership roles in the International Council of Nurses, including vice president and the leader of several committees. Only two Canadians have ever served as president of the International Council of Nurses: Alice Girard (1965–1969) and Judith Shamian (2013–2017).

Today, members of the International Council of Nurses come from national nursing organizations that include a complex mix of professional, regulatory, and union functions. It is the focal point for nursing policy on a global level, describing its work as ensuring "quality nursing care for all and sound health policies global- ly" with a focus on professional practice, regulation, and socio-economic welfare.[50]

SUMMARY AND IMPLICATIONS

Figure 4.2 builds on the relationships shown earlier in Figure 4.1 to show some of the actual organizations that govern and shape the practice of registered nurses. As noted previously in this section, nurses are impacted by many forces external to these regulatory, professional, union, and specialty pillars, and these are explored through the remainder of this text.

Nurses may feel torn between their professional accountabilities, as defined in a regulator's standards of practice, and the realities of tight budgets and the resulting allocation choices nurses have to make in real practice. Liaschenko and Peter speak about the need to tackle "the oppressive master narrative of corporat- ism often present in health care institutions whose multiple purposes can conflict

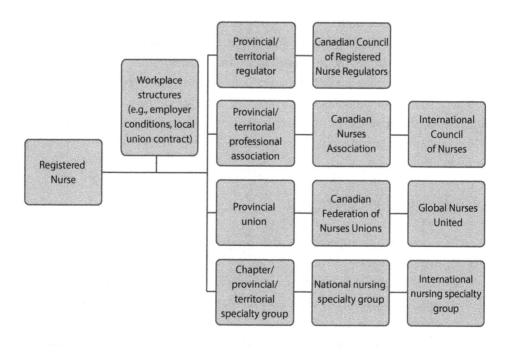

**Figure 4.2: Example of Registered Nurse Governance and Practice
Structures, Canada**

with patient care and damage nurses' identities and agency."[51] There are many other push-and-pull forces around nurses. For example, union rules may bump up against real-time employer needs, expectations, and pressures in a busy practice setting. Nursing education and the nursing and health science sectors generate an endless stream of new information with which nurses are expected to keep current; the same can be said of technological advances that require constant learning. And, of course, shifting public policy may impact fundamental issues, such as the amount of money available for any particular employer, or a new piece of legislation that may necessitate a change in who provides some aspect of care. In 2016, for example, nurses were faced with new practice challenges related to medical cannabinoids (or marijuana), assisted dying, and safe injection sites. (And to complicate the situation for health systems, the policy issue of medical use of cannabinoids was overtaken somewhat by the federal government's decision to legalize cannabis more broadly, or at least decriminalize its use.) Finally, nurses are constantly confronted with changing public needs and expectations, since in many places they are the first—and often most enduring—point of contact with patients, residents, clients, families, and communities; for example, think just of the influx of 25,000 Syrian refugees in 2015 and 2016.

Module I has focused on the basics—terminology, an introduction of theory, governance in the country, the history and current state of health systems governance and structures, and finally, in this chapter, the structures and regulation of the nursing profession. The book turns now, in Module II, to the reform, economics, and performance of Canada's health systems, all of which have direct and lasting impacts on the governance pillars that structure Canadian nursing—and all of which demand engagement in policy by nurses in order to shape those forces going forward.

DISCUSSION QUESTIONS

1. What are the impacts of Canadian governance structures on health human resources?
2. How might application of a competency-based human resources planning strategy impact the deployment, employment, and scope of nursing practice?
3. How do nursing governance structures in Canada facilitate or hinder effective nursing practice?
4. What are the strengths and weaknesses of Canadian nursing regulatory structures? What modifications should be implemented, and why?

5. What are the benefits and risks of the highly unionized nature of Canadian nursing?
6. Discuss possible implications of public disagreements (e.g., in popular media) among and across nursing organizations.
7. What are the risks and benefits to nursing organizations of merging memberships to include all regulated categories of nurses? What about including unregulated workers who provide aspects of nursing care?

ADDITIONAL POLICY RESOURCES

HEALTH PROFESSIONALS	
Medicine	
Canadian Federation of Medical Students	http://www.cfms.org
Canadian Medical Association	http://www.cma.ca
Royal College of Physicians and Surgeons of Canada	http://www.royalcollege.ca
Nursing	
Academy of Canadian Executive Nurses	http://acen.ca
Canadian Association for Nursing Research	http://canresearch.ca/contacts
Canadian Association of Advanced Practice Nurses	http://caapn-aciipa.org
Canadian Association of Schools of Nursing	http://www.casn.ca
Canadian Council for Practical Nurse Regulators	http://www.ccpnr.ca
Canadian Council of Registered Nurse Regulators	http://www.ccrnr.ca
Canadian Federation of Nurses Unions	https://nursesunions.ca
Canadian Nurses Association	http://cna-aiic.ca
Canadian Nurses Foundation	http://cnf-fiic.ca
Canadian Nurses Protective Society	http://www.cnps.ca
Canadian Nursing Students' Association	http://cnsa.ca
International Council of Nurses	http://www.icn.ch
Global Nurses United	http://www.nationalnursesunited.org/site/entry/global-nurses-united
Nursing specialty organizations affiliated with the Canadian Nurses Association	http://cna-aiic.ca/en/professional-development/canadian-network-of-nursing-specialties/whats-new-with-the-network/current-members

Registered Psychiatric Nurse Regulators of Canada	http://www.rpnc.ca
Other Leading Health Professions	
Canadian Association of Social Workers	http://casw-acts.ca
Canadian Dental Association	https://www.cda-adc.ca
Canadian Pharmacists Association	http://www.pharmacists.ca
Organisation for Economic Co-operation and Development: Health Human Resources	Organisation for Economic Co-Operation and Development. (2016). *Health workforce policies in OECD countries: Right jobs, right skills, right places.* Paris: OECD.

MODULE II

Population Health and Health Care in Canada

Module II moves the policy focus to population health and to the health care systems that have been built to respond to disease and injury. Canadians enjoy among the longest lives of any human beings in the 21st century. We have gained nearly a full decade of life just in the past half century, much of that thanks to improvements in sanitation and public health, which have reduced infant mortality and communicable disease. But the health and life quality of those longer lives is being called into question as the rates of chronic and non-communicable disease have risen dramatically across populations—not just in Canada but around the world.

The dynamic of rapidly growing numbers of older Canadians who are likely to move into older age with one or more chronic diseases has coincided with the worrying reality that Canada's health system spending was fully 50 per cent higher per capita in 2010 than in 1996.[1] Together, these forces—the aging curve, the rising prevalence of chronic disease, and soaring health care costs—have provoked two decades of unprecedented focus on the need for reform and transformation aimed at quality improvement and cost containment. Understanding Canada's shifting demographics and disease burden is vital to nurses, because so much of the care of aging, and the prevention and management of chronic disease, align perfectly with the practice of nursing; these areas of care will be the hallmarks of 21st-century nursing practice—should nurses choose to rise to the challenge.

Talking and learning about how health care is structured and how systems work may seem redundant for nurses. Once students and nurses start working in health care organizations, isn't it obvious how it all works? People get sick; go to a doctor, a nurse practitioner, a walk-in clinic, or the local hospital; care is provided; and physicians bill the government for their fees. Of course, the story is a lot more complicated than that. Most care providers typically quickly develop an understanding of how their immediate work settings function. But moving up to the larger organization, to the local community, the health authority, the provincial or territorial health ministry, the country, and society at large, the trail quickly becomes very murky. And how it all functions—how health care happens at a system level—is a puzzle to many experienced health professionals and to the public.

In an effort to demystify our health systems, Module II explores the evolution of health care in Canada, the values and political forces that drove development of health care policy, and our history of reform since the late 1990s. At the same time, it follows the parallel development and reform of nursing, changing scopes of practice, and the roles played by nurses and nursing organizations in Canadian health policy over the past 50 years.

If understanding the functioning of health systems is difficult, nurses and most Canadians certainly have heard the clear message that health care is very expensive. In fact, some think it is so expensive as to be unsustainable, and that survival of the public medicare system is threatened as a result. What are the facts behind the public messages we have all heard? The second part of this module explores the basics of health care funding so that nurses can be conversant in the general terms and concepts. It is clear that different actors spin statistics to suit their political interests and agendas. What does health care actually cost, and what are Canadians spending? It seems to depend on whom one asks. This section of the book explores how Canadians pay for health care, how much is spent, how health system funds are dispersed, and by whom.

Critical to any discussion of costs is their link to outcomes. There would be much less controversy about high health care costs if Canadians and their governments were happy with the results. There is a disconnect somewhere in the equation, and that gap merits investigation. In all these rising costs, what are Canadians investing in? What are the desired outcomes—and most importantly, what are citizens actually getting for those public and private investments? Module II wraps up by making links among investments of taxpayer and private dollars, the status of population health, and the performance of Canada's health systems. The views and expectations of governments who fund public health systems, the public who need health care, and professionals such as nurses who deliver the services are probed. And in all this, nursing must look inward to question the value nurses bring to population health and to health system performance: What is the return on public investments in nursing services?

CHAPTER 5

Health Systems in Canada: Development and Reform

CHAPTER HIGHLIGHTS

- Public Policy, Health Care, and Nurses in 20th Century Canada
- 21st Century Health Care in Canada: Reform and Transformation
- Life after Health Accords
- Summary and Implications
- Discussion Questions
- Additional Policy Resources

LEARNING OUTCOMES

1. Become conversant about milestones in Canada's health system evolution and reform initiatives over the past century.
2. Describe factors that led to health care reforms in the provinces and territories, including the various forms of regionalization of governance structures in each of the provinces, since the year 2000.
3. Describe the purposes and key outcomes of the health system reviews conducted by the Honourable Roy Romanow (2002) and the Honourable Michael Kirby (2002).
4. Discuss key actions funded in the federal/provincial/territorial health accords of 2000, 2003, and 2004.
5. Discuss the implications and effects of different waves of reform for nursing and health care recipients across Canada.

Policy Influencer: Marion Dewar (1928–2008)

Marion Dewar, CM, RN, BSc, graduated from the St. Joseph Hospital School of Nursing in Kingston, Ontario, in 1949 and practiced as a registered nurse with VON Canada and in Ottawa as a public health nurse starting in the late 1960s. She would go on to serve as an alderman in Ottawa and was then elected mayor, serving 1978–1985. After serving as national president of the New Democratic Party she was elected to the House of Commons in a by-election in 1987. Bringing her nursing and community background to her role as a federal member of Parliament, her policy work was focused on community economic development, employment, and the status of women.[1]

"If history were the past, history wouldn't matter. History is the present. You and me are history. We carry our history. We act in our history."
—*James Arthur Baldwin, American novelist, poet, playwright, and social critic*

FOLLOWING THE STORY OF HEALTH SYSTEMS REFORM IN CANADA

For the purposes of this book, the story of health systems reform is described as having evolved in three main waves:

1. The first major wave of health system reform in Canada is defined as the period from World War II through the period of major system growth from the 1950s through the 1970s. It includes all the efforts to create structures and legislation by which Canadians could afford to access all these new services, including the growth of a hospital system, medicare legislation and its implementation in the late 1960s, and culminating, finally, in the Canada Health Act (1984).
2. The second wave of health systems reform in Canada is described as the 30-year period following the Canada Health Act (1984), through the dramatic economic upheaval of the mid-1990s, and ending with the federal, provincial, and territorial system reviews and pan-Canadian health accords until 2014.
3. The third wave of health reform in Canada is cast in this book as the period starting in 2015 after the announcement of Justin Trudeau directing his health minister to begin negotiating a new pan-Canadian health accord and the initial funding commitment of $3 billion to strengthen home care over four years.

PUBLIC POLICY, HEALTH CARE, AND NURSES IN 20TH CENTURY CANADA

Mirroring the experiences of most wealthy nations, the development of formalized health care in Canada across the 20th century has been coloured sharply by two seminal discoveries: vaccines and antibiotics. While the history of health care in Canada is often framed around the implementation of medicare, in many ways the story is really one about the eras before and after these underlying scientific advances.

Canadians born today can expect to live an average of 82 years—80 for men and 84 for women. A century ago, the average life expectancies of Canadian males and females were 59 and 61 years, respectively.[2] But of course, most Canadians did not simply die around the age of 60. In the United States in 1900, for example, nearly a third of all deaths occurred before the age of five,[3] and the pattern was similar here. Apart from diseases like measles, pertussis (whooping cough), and tuberculosis, some 36,000 Ontario children died from

Public Health Achievements of the 20th Century

Strategically developed and implemented, public policy can exert massive impacts. The Centers for Disease Control and Prevention in the United States identified a list of the 10 greatest public health achievements of the 20th century[4]—each of them driven by policy changes:[5]

1. Immunizations
2. Motor vehicle safety
3. Workplace safety
4. Control of infectious diseases
5. Declines in deaths from heart disease and stroke
6. Safer and healthier foods
7. Healthier mothers and babies
8. Family planning
9. Fluoridation of drinking water
10. Tobacco as a health hazard

To learn more about each of these issues go to the Centers for Disease Control and Prevention website: http://www.cdc.gov/about/history/tengpha.htm.

diphtheria alone between 1800 and 1929.[6] But if children survived the rigours of childbirth, and later those of communicable diseases (including waves of typhus and cholera), then in the absence of traumatic injury or an incurable illness many lived into older age, much as Canadians do now. Public health and hygiene measures, including reliable access to clean water, improved food safety, and avoidance of causes of risk across the century—reduced smoking and the mandatory use of seat belts in cars, for example—have all added significantly to the longevity gains. The simple separation of drinking water from sewage, and later the pasteurization of milk, had dramatic effects on infectious disease and human health beginning in the late 19th century.

But few discoveries have had the disease-preventing impact of vaccines, which changed the course of history, dramatically reducing the rates of infant and child deaths and contributing significantly to a 20-year gain in life expectancy for men and 22-year gain for women from 1915 to 2015. While a number of vaccines have existed since the 19th century, their real impact on populations was felt in the wake of a key public policy decision: "the standard battery of childhood immunizations, including diphtheria, measles, mumps, and rubella" required for public school attendance starting in the mid-20th century.[7] Since its establishment in 1948, the WHO has featured vaccination programs as a prominent pillar of its public health efforts, and they have had a seismic impact on global health and longevity. The Centers for Disease Control and Prevention in the United States, for example, cite evidence that the current childhood immunization schedule in that country prevents 42,000 deaths and 20 million cases of disease in each US birth cohort—saving some "$14 billion in direct costs and $69 billion in total societal costs."[8] A great number of people who would have died in the past now need all the health and other services required during an average lifespan, increasing the population and the demand for the full range of public services.

Traumatic injury in Canada's early years brought different challenges. Being primarily a rural farming and natural resources economy in the pre- and early industrial era, injuries related to farming, logging, fishing, and mining were common. By the early 20th century, these were compounded by injuries arising in the unsafe work environments of the emerging industrial sector. Diagnostic and surgical techniques were crude by 21st century standards, but even in the hands of the finest surgeon, the effectiveness and safety of anaesthesia for patients was in its early days. These impediments meant that many patients did not survive injuries that are successfully treated routinely today.

But few of the technical challenges around trauma surgery were more damaging than post-injury and post-operative wound infection, which in the days before antibiotics could be a virtual death sentence. The same fate awaited many women following childbirth and patients needing elective surgeries, for example. Death was a potential outcome for anyone contracting pneumonia, tuberculosis, diarrhea, and enteritis, which together caused fully a third of all deaths in the United States in 1900.

Communicable diseases were especially devastating to Aboriginal Peoples when they encountered them, because they essentially had no immunity. As David Butler-Jones—then Canada's Chief Public Health Officer—put it in his 2008 report, "in some cases, whole communities all but disappeared" as Aboriginal people fell ill with smallpox, tuberculosis, and all the same diseases that were killing settlers.[9] Much more sinister than unintentional transmission is the evidence that some of the spread of disease among Aboriginal people—through contaminated blankets, for example—was initiated purposefully by settlers, even before germ theory was fully understood.

If vaccines were the most important advancement in the history of public health and disease prevention, then antibiotics surely are their equivalent in the history of health care. Fleming's discovery of penicillin in 1928, and the subsequent testing and rapid spread of the use of antibiotics during the World War II era, meant that hundreds of thousands of soldiers and civilians who previously would have died could now survive infections related to injuries or disease.

In the United States, the high death rate in 1900 among children under the age of five had dropped to 1.4 per cent by 1997, driven largely by the combined effects of sanitation, immunization, and treatment of infectious disease. Antibiotics, antivirals, and other antimicrobial drugs opened up new possibilities in medical and surgical care. Those discoveries triggered a sea change that, over the 20th century, shifted the focus of global health efforts away from communities, public health, and preventing injuries and disease to a mindset dominated by treatment, rescue, and cure—and by extension in Canada, to doctors, drugs, and hospitals. It is a pattern that has become very difficult to disrupt, despite a generation of conclusive evidence about the proven greater fiscal return on investments in health promotion, attention to broad determinants of health, and disease and injury prevention.

The Growth of Hospitals in Canada

"A hospital is a complicated institution, and a teaching hospital is the most complicated healthcare institution of all. It is the apex of Canadian healthcare."

—*Jeffrey Simpson, National Affairs Columnist, Globe and Mail*[10]

Early hospitals in Canada—as in many other nations—were dedicated largely to care of the poor, in part because that population was more susceptible to communicable diseases and lacked affordable, reliable access to nursing or medical care in their homes. A century ago, most care in Canada still was provided at home and most nurses were based in community and home care (sometimes called private duty) settings. Of course, a large part of the work of nurses in the early part of the 20th century was focused on public and community health measures, including teaching and monitoring basic hygiene.

But as hospital structures and sanitation improved and surgery and other treatments advanced, the popularity of hospital treatment began to flourish among more affluent Canadians. In addition to growing demand, the skewed distribution of Canada's population drove growth in the number of urban and rural hospitals after Confederation. Distance to hospitals and emergency care is still an issue in rural Canada, to say nothing of remote and northern settings. The pressure of access was of even greater concern in the era before rapid transit by a motorized ambulance, and certainly before helicopters, flight nurses, paramedics, and life-preserving interventions such as blood volume expanders. In Ontario, for example, the 1930 *Annual Report on the Public Hospitals* reported a tenfold increase in the number of public general hospitals between 1880 and 1930 (to a total of 118).[11] Shimmering new facilities like Sunnybrook Hospital in Toronto, the largest veterans' hospital in the country, were also constructed to welcome injured soldiers after World War II. Many more veterans' hospitals opened across the country; Veterans Affairs Canada operated some 40 facilities at its peak after World War II.[12]

Three types of hospitals evolved in Canada: (a) public hospitals intended to be operated on a not-for-profit basis to treat anyone based on need; (b) private hospitals with conditional (and typically elective) admissions and usually operated for profit; and (c) federal hospitals, which included a range of facilities (including nursing stations and health centres) designed to meet the needs of populations served by the federal government.[13] Public hospitals in Canada today include a mix of general and speciality facilities, the latter including mental health, women's health, and pediatrics.

In her extensive analysis of the history of hospital records, Craig observed that hospitals grew not just in number, but also in "social and medical importance" between 1850 and 1950.[14] Canadians were well aware of the transformational impact of antibiotics and they began to demand access to more procedures (and more complex ones) that, at the time, had to be provided in hospitals. The National Health Grants Program (1948), introduced in Chapter 3, supported the construction of many more hospitals, as well as growth of medical schools and other health science faculties.

It was during this era that the growth of large, urban teaching hospitals really began to take off. It is difficult to tease out the specific policy inputs of the health professions at that time, but it is of interest to note that medical schools—but not nursing schools—and their budgets became increasingly interwoven in complicated ways with the funding of those institutions. The deep connections in medical practice between hands-on clinical care, research, and education became only further entrenched. Physicians in those settings laid down a model whereby they cared for patients, conducted research, and taught the next generation.

At the same time, nursing schools and their faculty were moving steadily away from clinical practice settings. Today most nursing educators and scientists maintain little or no practice in the service areas where the majority of nurses work. Despite the high trust accorded to nurses by the public, herein may lie more of the roots of modern disparities in power, funding, and policy influence between doctors and nurses. The move to strengthen nursing within the academy was an important factor in combating historic gender disparities, especially in research funding. Some of those battles continue today, but certainly nurses have gained a strong foothold in research funding and have established nursing science as a credible source of clinical and health systems evidence. More than two dozen nurses now sit as respected fellows of the Canadian Academy of Health Sciences. The cost of that victory, however, has been the decoupling of nursing science from nursing practice at points of care, and has contributed to the ongoing domination of hospitals and their budgets by physicians.

Growing hospital supply seemingly only fed more demand; as the Canadian Museum of History summarized in its history of medicare, by the 1950s the public thought that "hospitals represented the best that medical science had to offer, because they were now seen as centres of life-saving operations and critical care."[15] The insurance programs that evolved around the growing hospital sector had a similar focus. Despite the push of nurses and organizations such as the Canadian Public Health Association for a range of health care services to come under public insurance, attention never moved much away from acute care hospitals. With the establishment of medicare, hospitals were cemented as the focal point of Canadian health care—and, as Simpson said in his analysis, "to a fault, it remains so today."[16]

Nurses, of course, were not oblivious to shifting trends in health care delivery. It was already clear by the start of World War II that hospitals were growing in size and number, and required a corresponding increase in workforce numbers and skill sets. Short of nurses, hospitals had begun to put in place a variety of auxiliary roles to carry out basic supportive care activities. The shortfall in numbers led CNA to recommend the establishment of a formalized nursing assistant role, and in 1940 CNA published its *Curriculum Guide for Nursing Assistants* to help member jurisdictions struggling with the issue. But while the help surely was needed, the new role almost immediately raised all the issues of boundaries of nursing practice still with us today. As McPherson observed, new roles complicated nursing work in the way they split the attention of registered nurses among direct care, supervision of assistants, and management responsibilities.[17] Fanny Munroe, the first CNA president after World War II, expressed concern about the implications of these divided loyalties and responsibilities, and worried about whether the nursing assistant role could overtake what traditionally had been registered nursing practice.

But in tandem with concerns about the new roles, registered nurses also found bargaining power in the shortages, and began to work more purposefully for improved salaries and other work conditions. Just as hospitals became the focus of health care, they soon became the focus of registered nursing employment. With pressure from professional associations and, later, unions, hospitals began to offer higher salaries than other areas of practice. Over the ensuing decades hospitals became the seat of bargaining power that still drives salary and benefit benchmarks for other categories of workers across the continuum of care today.

Health Care Development After the Canada Health Act: Shifting Perspectives on Population Health

Just as the growth of hospitals across Canada seemed to be reaching its zenith, a report on population health was released by the Honourable Marc Lalonde, a Quebec-born lawyer who served as minister of health from 1972 to 1977 in the government of Pierre Trudeau. Noting that "the demand by the Canadian people for more and better personal health care continues unabated,"[18] Lalonde acknowledged the value of the growing hospital sector but was clearly mindful of its costs; he began to ask explicit questions about its effectiveness.

Lalonde had proposed a conceptual framework for health when he spoke at the Pan American Health Organization meeting in Ottawa in September 1973. With the subsequent endorsement of the provincial health ministers, the framework formed the meat of the report, *A New Perspective on the Health of Canadians*,[19] which began by stating explicitly that health care was only one element leading to good health. Based on an extensive analysis of population health, Lalonde proposed a four-pillar framework of factors contributing to health and illness (for which he credited Laframboise[20])—human biology, the environment, lifestyle, and health care. Today we talk about these pillars as the *determinants of health*.

To reduce risks and improve access to better health, Lalonde proposed that governments should implement five strategies in the areas of health promotion, regulation, research, efficiency in health care (focused on costs, accessibility, and effectiveness), and goal setting for better population health. To accomplish these strategies he offered up 74 recommendations. The report positioned Canada "at the forefront of the public health approach" globally, including its emphasis on the health impacts of social influences and inequalities.[21] This groundbreaking work centred the role of public health in shaping health policy and legislation globally.

The Lalonde report came on the heels of a decade of nation-building legislation under the Pearson and (Pierre) Trudeau governments, and one in which health and social policy were both prominent. Organizationally, the health and social sectors sat within one department, then called Health and Welfare Canada. When Lalonde released his report, Canada's first federal principal nursing officer, Verna Huffman Splane, had served in the role for four years (1968–1972). She was a highly accomplished leader in public health in Canada and globally through her work with the WHO, and she was in the prime of her career by the time she was appointed to the role. When she eventually left the position, Huffman Splane was succeeded by another powerhouse in Canadian nursing, Huguette Labelle, who was a generation younger when she took on the principal nursing officer role (1973–1977). Labelle, meanwhile, continued the charge around public health, primary health care, and public medicare.

In tandem with these strong federal government nurses and their network of allies in provincial and territorial governments, CNA's formidable executive director, Helen Mussallem, had been on the job for a decade by the time the Lalonde report was tabled. She had a reputation for being a tenacious, courageous lobbyist and advocate across a wide range of public policy areas—she rarely felt constrained to nursing directly. E. Louise Miner, who was CNA president from 1970 to 1972, had been director of the Nursing Service Division in the Saskatchewan Department of Public Health during the lead-up to public health insurance under Tommy Douglas. While these nurses certainly did not agree on every issue, together their influence on policy like that laid out in the Lalonde report, through their credibility, experience, and constant input at the most senior levels, was profound. Canada's public health leadership, bolstered by these and many other expert nurses, helped to shape the historic 30th World Health Assembly (1977), where for the first time nursing would be prominent. Mussallem was invited to join the Canadian government's delegation in Geneva—the first time a representative from outside the government was included. With 150 nations present, only two nurses (including Mussallem) were included among the delegations. Of historic interest at this meeting, Canada put forward a resolution on nursing—the first ever at a World Health Assembly—and it was accepted. Importantly, the resolution that became the "Health for All by the Year 2000" global initiative also was tabled and accepted at this meeting. A year later, at the now iconic International Conference on Primary Health Care in Alma-Ata (in what is now Kazakhstan), the 1978

Declaration of Alma-Ata laid out a comprehensive definition of primary health care services and principles, including health as a basic human right.[22]

With these historic documents and charters being developed around the world—and with the esteem in which Canada was held in the wake of the Lalonde report and the global reputation of its doctors, nurses, and health care system—it seemed that Canada might be poised for a change in direction and health system focus. Across the country during the years after universal medicare, the provinces were all considering the issues laid out by Lalonde and tackling health care access, costs, and efficiency in their own jurisdictions. These efforts included reviews of care for specific health issues (e.g., cancer, mental health), health human resources, financing and costs, quality and safety, and full Royal Commissions examining entire systems. At the provincial level nurses led or were appointed to many of the committees, task forces, and commissions. Though the list of initiatives is exhaustive, a few examples from across the country are shown in Table 5.1.

Elected with the largest majority in Canadian history, the Progressive Conservative Government of the Right Honourable Brian Mulroney, who was prime minister from 1984 to 1993, built on the Liberal government's Lalonde report, advancing its thinking around determinants of health and primary health care. In 1986, federal health minister the Honourable Jake Epp tabled *Achieving Health for All: A Framework for Health Promotion*.[23] That report focused on three main challenges: (a) reducing inequities; (b) strengthening disease and injury prevention; and (c) enhancing coping, especially in areas such as chronic disease and mental health. Epp proposed a framework of strategies that included strengthening public participation and community health services, and coordinating health policy to better advantage "mutually-enforcing" health strategies.

Canada would go on to host the first International Conference on Health Promotion in November of that year, organized primarily as "a response to growing expectations for a new public health movement around the world."[24] The Ottawa Charter, tabled at the meeting, laid out principles for action to achieve Health for All by the year 2000—and Canada was again front and centre on the global public health and primary health care stage. Formal nursing policy input in the department at the time was vested in the principal nursing officer, Josephine Flaherty, who served in the role from 1977 to 1994. Flaherty was a prominent public health advocate who had been awarded honourary life membership in the Canadian Public Health Association in 1982 in recognition of the impact of her public health nursing leadership.[25] Nursing input to federal policy again came from an informed and credible health advocate—and Flaherty had the strong support of Ginette Lemire Rodger, who was by then executive director at CNA and a lifelong advocate for the values espoused in the Epp report.

Nearly a decade later, costs were continuing to rise and the system had not been steered away from its treatment focus. Newly elected as prime minister in 1993, Jean Chrétien appointed a National Forum on Health in 1994 "to advise the federal government on innovative ways to improve Canada's health system and

Table 5.1: Examples of Provincial Health Care System Development and Reform Initiatives in the Era of the Canada Health Act, 1980–1999

JURISDICTION	HEALTH SYSTEM DEVELOPMENT AND REFORM INITIATIVES
British Columbia	Royal Commission on Health Care and Costs, 1991
Alberta	Advisory Committee on the Utilization of Medical Services, 1989
	Premier's Commission on Future Health Care for Albertans, 1989
Saskatchewan	*Future Directions for Health Care in Saskatchewan. Report of the Commission on Directions in Health Care*, Murray Commission, 1990
Manitoba	Health Services Review Committee, 1985
Ontario	Task Force to Review Primary Health Care, Final Report (Mustard), 1983
	Health Review Panel, 1987
	Premier's Council on Health Strategy, 1991
	Quality Assurance and Resource Management: The Medical Services Challenges for the 1990s: 1990–1991 Final Report, Task Force on the Use and Provision of Medical Services, 1992
	Devolution of Health and Social Services in Ontario: Refocusing the Debate, Report of the Premier's Health Council on Health, Well-Being and Social Justice, Task Force on Devolution, 1994
Quebec	Comité d'étude sur la promotion de la santé, 1984
	La Commission d'énquête sur les services de santé et les services sociaux, 1988
New Brunswick	Commission on Selected Health Care Programs, 1989
	Health Services Review, 1999
Nova Scotia	Royal Commission on Health Care, 1989
	Leading the Way: Final Report, Task Force on Primary Health Care, 1994
Prince Edward Island	*Health Reform, A Vision for Change: The Report*, Task Force on Health (Cudmore), 1992
Newfoundland and Labrador	Royal Commission on Hospital and Nursing Home Costs, 1984

the health of Canadians."[26] Mr. Chrétien had been elected partly on a promise to strengthen medicare. With the prime minister as chair and minister of health as vice chair, the forum had 24 members and included three nurse leaders: Madeleine Dion Stout, a prominent Aboriginal advocate originally from Alberta, Margaret McDonald from the Northwest Territories, and Judith Ritchie, a past CNA president who was then in Nova Scotia. Based on four pillars of work—values, striking a balance, determinants of health, and evidence-based decision-making—the forum's 1997 report, *Canada Health Action: Building on the Legacy*, recommended action to preserve the health care system by transforming knowledge about health into action, and developing and using stronger evidence to make better decisions.[27] The Canadian Institute for Health Information had been established in 1994, but the forum was strongly focused on scaling up health information, science, and evidence to support health systems and close knowledge gaps. It also recommended nationally insured home care and pharmacare.

With these policy thrusts as a prominent backdrop in the years after the introduction of universal medicare, hospital expenditures as a proportion of total spending did decline, but the costs of hospitals, doctors, and health care overall continued to climb. While Canada has programs to tackle other determinants of health and build services within a broad primary health care framework, these initiatives never caught on at a national level like acute care and treatment did, and recommendations in those areas remained in the background of efforts to improve population health.

21ST CENTURY HEALTH CARE IN CANADA: REFORM AND TRANSFORMATION

Michael Decter suggested in 1994 that the second era of reform might have started with the decision of Saskatchewan's health minister, the Honourable Louise Simard, to convert 50 rural hospitals to health centres, transferring the budget to regional authorities.[28] Saskatchewan had always been home to a lot of hospitals—the quiet comment around policy circles had for some time been that Saskatchewan was a code word for "too many hospitals." Closing or changing the status of any hospital is no small political feat; the public is inevitably up in arms, and nurses and physicians are just as incensed. When she was a member of the National Expert Commission, the Honourable Sharon Carstairs, then a senator, said during deliberations about hospitals versus other care solutions, "Try being the politician who decides to shut down a rural hospital." And the senator may well have been right—Canadians value and cling to their hospitals. Some would prefer to have a hospital close by, even if it doesn't have the best outcomes, rather than see it replaced with a well-functioning health centre. There is something about the big blue square with the white cross that has a deep meaning for Canadians in a way that other sorts of facilities simply do not.

Federal and Pan-Canadian Developments Driving Reform

If the best evidence, climbing costs, and seeming consensus on the need to refocus health care in Canada did not force transformative change, then the harsh financial realities of the mid-1990s certainly did. British nurse leader Tom Keighley says says that in terms of their timing, many policy decisions have one thing in common—"they happen when time runs out"—and in some ways for Canada, time suddenly ran out in 1995.[29]

In his insider look at government, Eddie Goldenberg, who was the prime minister's chief of staff, summarized the Chrétien administration as being coloured by two significant forces: the Quebec referendum issue and a "looming financial crisis" that led the government to make "drastic cuts to programs that had a direct impact on citizens as well as to transfer payments to the provinces."[30] Mr. Chrétien's predecessor (Mulroney) had started to freeze cash transfers to provinces, much as Pierre Trudeau had done before him. By the time Chrétien was elected, health budget cuts had already begun in earnest across the country—with "dramatic cuts" leading to significant job losses in Ontario and Alberta.[31]

When he was elected in 1993, Chrétien inherited a very high national debt and "an alarming annual deficit."[32] Moody's Investors Service had downgraded Canada's debt in 1994, and threatened to do the same in 1995, contributing to already-mounting pressures to cut spending. Abandoning the promises of his government's election platform, reducing the deficit soon became the policy priority. The first major cuts to provincial transfers came in what Goldenberg called the "deficit-slashing budget of February 1995."[33] Through a series of deep cuts to government transfers to provinces and other federal spending, taxes and the federal debt were both reduced significantly, more than $40 billion in deficit was eliminated, and budgets were balanced. By 1998 the federal government tabled the first surplus in a generation[34] and, as the *Canadian Medical Association Journal* put it in 1999, the Right Honourable Paul Martin, Jr., then the minister of finance, "slew Ottawa's deficit dragon."[35] The Canadian government gained global notoriety for its economic prowess, most of it under the leadership of Martin, who succeeded Chrétien as prime minister (2003–2006) after the latter had won three consecutive elections from 1993 to 2003.

Of course, the fallout of the cuts across the country was significant, and health care was no exception. There was a sense of disarray as governments scrambled to reduce costs in response to lost revenue, not surprisingly fuelling discussion of the potential role of more privately delivered (and funded) care and/or the addition of various user fees. The impact on nursing was devastating, and is discussed in more detail in the final section of this chapter and throughout the book.

Riding on its fiscal successes—and it must be said, its popularity among Canadians despite all the cuts—the federal government in 2000 entered into the first of several health accords with the provinces and territories. Reached in part to smooth rocky relationships and growing talk of privatization that was strongly contradictory to the values of the federal Liberal government, the First Ministers' Meeting Communiqué on Health[36] committed to reinvestments in health care that set the stage for a national reform agenda to play out over the ensuing decade. The first ministers agreed to action in eight areas:

1. Access to care
2. Health promotion and wellness
3. Appropriate health care services (primary health care)
4. Supply of doctors, nurses, and other health personnel
5. Home care and community care
6. Pharmaceuticals management
7. Health information and communications technology
8. Health equipment and infrastructure

The first ministers were focused on improvements to primary health care as being "crucial to the renewal of health services," and they also committed to work on multidisciplinary teams. The federal government established an $800 million Primary Health Care Transition Fund (2000–2006) for the use of provinces and territories struggling to reform their primary health care systems. Nurses were prominent in the rollout of a number of the national initiatives flowing from the fund, including *Linking Primary Health Care and Mental Health, Facilitating Inter- and Trans-Disciplinary Work Teams,* and *Linking Chronic Disease Care in the Community and Primary Health Care.* Perhaps the most prominent project led by nurses (and discussed in the final section of this chapter) was the $8.8 million in funding allocated to CNA to lead implementation of nurse practitioners across Canada, known as *Facilitating the Integration of the Role of Nurse Practitioners in the Health System.*

Responding to the earlier recommendations of the National Forum on Health and the 2000 Accord, the Canadian Institutes of Health Research was established in 2000, an arm's-length organization from Parliament, "to create new scientific knowledge and to enable its translation into improved health, more effective health services and products, and a strengthened Canadian health care system."[37]

This agency succeeded the former Medical Research Council of Canada with 13 institutes and some 14,000 researchers. To "accelerate the development, adoption and effective use of digital health solutions across Canada," Canada Health Infoway was established in 2002.[38] It also is governed as an arm's-length agency of Parliament, responsible to the federal minister of health.

The Health of Canadians—The Federal Role (Standing Senate Committee on Social Affairs, Science and Technology, 2002) and Building on Values: The Future of Health Care in Canada (Commission on the Future of Health Care in Canada, 2002)

Provinces and territories had begun reform initiatives in the 1990s and these accelerated early in the new century; examples are shown in Table 5.2. With hints of user fees emerging in some of these—and with legitimate concerns about duplication of effort, a sense of disorder, and the risk of limiting the sharing and uptake of information across the country—the federal government announced in 2000 that it would launch a Royal Commission on the Future of Health Care in Canada, funded at $15 million and to report back in 18 months.

The Long-Grass Strategy of Policy Making

In his opening address to the delegates at the Seventh Annual Workshop of the Canadian Health Services Research Foundation,[40] Philip Davies—then deputy director of the Government Social Research Unit in the United Kingdom Cabinet—warned the audience to be wary of the "long-grass strategy" of policy making. Essentially he advised that when governments don't know what to do, or want to delay making a decision, they might resort to a standard response: fund a pilot study or launch an initiative like a commission. The decision may be seen by the public and even by stakeholders as action because it is visible—the government *did something*. In fact, Davies cautioned, the strategy is more akin to hitting a golf ball off a fairway into the long grass beyond the course. The people who may be lobbying for legitimate policy change will be distracted with the new activity—to continue the metaphor, they will go looking for the ball in the long grass and prolong the game. The result can be that interest groups stop pestering the government temporarily, or even for a significant period of time.

This theory, however, should not be cynically confused with legitimate consultation and study of any given issue. The caution is issued simply to provoke awareness of one political strategy that nurses may encounter.

Table 5.2: Examples of 21st Century Provincial and Territorial Health Systems Reform Initiatives

JURISDICTION	HEALTH SYSTEM DEVELOPMENT AND REFORM INITIATIVES
British Columbia	British Columbia Select Standing Committee on Health (Roddick Committee), 2002
	Conversation on Health, 2007
Alberta	Premier's Advisory Council on Health for Alberta (Mazankowski Council), 2002
	Getting on with Better Health Care: Health Policy Framework, 2006
	Health Action Plan, 2008
	Vision 2020: The Future of Health Care in Alberta, 2008
	Alberta Health Services, *Strategic Direction 2012–2015: Defining Our Focus/Measuring Our Progress*
Saskatchewan	Saskatchewan Commission on Medicare (Fyke Commission), 2001
	Action Plan for Saskatchewan Health Care, 2002
	For Patients' Sake, Patient First Review report, 2009
Manitoba	Health Advisory Network, Task Force on Health Promotion, 2002
	Report of the Manitoba Regional Health Authority External Review Committee, 2008
Ontario	Health Consultation Process, 2002
	Charting a Path to Sustainable Health Care in Ontario (Drummond and Burleton), 2010
	Public Service for Ontarians: A Path to Sustainability and Excellence, Commission on the Reform of Ontario's Public Services, 2012
	Ontario's Action Plan for Health Care, 2012
	Patients First: Action Plan for Health Care, 2015
Quebec	Commission of Study on Health and Social Services (Clair Commission), 2000
	Getting Our Money's Worth: Report of the Task Force on the Funding of the Health System, 2008
	Commissaire à la santé et au bien-être: Rapport d'appréciation de la performance du système de santé et de services sociaux, 2012
New Brunswick	Premier's Health Quality Council, 2002
	Wellness: We Each Have a Role to Play: Individuals, Communities, Stakeholders and Government: Final Report, Legislative Assembly Select Committee on Wellness, 2008

	Transforming New Brunswick's Health Care System: The Provincial Health Plan 2008–2012
	Moving Towards a Planned and Citizen-Centered Publicly-Funded Provincial Health Care System, New Brunswick Health Council, 2011
Nova Scotia	*Changing Nova Scotia's Health Care System: Creating Sustainability through Transformation: System Level Findings and Overall Directions For Change from the Provincial Health Services Operational Review,* 2008
Prince Edward Island	*An Integrated Health System Review in PEI: A Call to Action: A Plan for Change,* 2008
Newfoundland and Labrador	*Strategic Plan 2008–2011,* Department of Health and Community Services, 2008
Nunavut	*Health Integration Initiative, 2011–2014*
Northwest Territories	Minister's Forum on Health and Social Services, 2000
	Northwest Territories Action Plan, 2002
Yukon	*Report of the Yukon Health Care Review Committee,* 2008
	A Clinical Services Plan for Yukon Territory: Final Report, 2014

There was criticism of the government's decision, which some said effectively provided an excuse for it to stay out of health care for nearly two years. The earlier work of the National Forum on Health, another pan-Canadian initiative seen by some as having given the same government breathing room, had largely been set aside in light of the debt and deficit crisis—although aspects of its recommendations were resurrected in the new century. There was also a complicating factor: the Standing Senate Committee on Social Affairs, Science and Technology had begun a systematic study of Canadian health care the year before, under the leadership of the Honourable Senator Michael Kirby, and was set to release an interim report not long after Chrétien announced the new Royal Commission.[39]

Still, the work went ahead. The Royal Commission was led by the Honourable Roy Romanow, former Saskatchewan premier, and is commonly referred to as the Romanow Commission. Mr. Romanow was charged to "review medicare, engage Canadians in a national dialogue on its future, and make recommendations to enhance the system's quality and sustainability."[41] The commission undertook extensive consultations and research across the country, within and beyond governments, and included wide representation of nurses on a variety of topics. In his extensive final report, Romanow provided 47 recommendations intended to make Canadians the healthiest people in the world, with timelines and costs that responded to the following themes revealed by the commission:

- Canadians remain attached to the values at the heart of the system
- Medicare has served Canadians extremely well
- The system is as sustainable as we want it to be
- Canadians want and need a truly national health care system
- Canadians want and need a more comprehensive health care system
- Canadians want and need a more accountable health care system

Both eventually tabled in 2002, Romanow's Royal Commission and Kirby's Senate report were cast by many observers as politically opposed on the left and right, respectively. Kirby's final report[42] did make more references and links to private aspects of care than Romanow's, but it was not as politically right leaning in its tone as some had been predicting. The final report suggested a long list of reform recommendations across its 16 chapters, and some observers were surprised by the calls in both reports for an injection of federal cash. Like Romanow's team, the Senate had undertaken extensive research and cross-Canada consultation, including ongoing discussions with nurses. Given the breadth of consultation and research undertaken by the two national reviews, perhaps it was not surprising that many of their recommendations were similar.

The 2003 and 2004 Health Accords

Extending the accord model used in 2000, the federal government negotiated the First Ministers' Accord on Health Care Renewal in 2003 with the provinces and territories, responding in part to the recommendations of the Royal Commission and the Senate review. The agreement included commitments to action in the following key areas:[43]

- Action on primary health care to ensure home care for Canadians, catastrophic drug coverage, pharmaceuticals management, and improved reporting on progress and outcomes to Canadians
- A diagnostic/medical equipment fund
- Information technology and an electronic health record
- Aboriginal health
- Patient safety
- Health human resources
- Technology assessment
- Innovation and research
- Approaches to improve the health of Canadians

As noted in Chapter 1, Health Canada nurses were instrumental in shaping the 2003 accord, which included $90 million in funding "to strengthen the evidence base for national planning, promote inter-disciplinary provider education, improve recruitment and retention, and ensure the supply of needed health providers (including nurse practitioners, pharmacists and diagnostic technologists)."[44] That work by nurses in a federal policy role followed extensive consultation with nurse colleagues in every province and territory during the preceding years—including professional associations, unions, and so on. Therefore, the policy work carried out by nurses in one role was deeply informed and facilitated by nurses in many other roles; all of them contributed to the final aim of helping to shape policy. In this example we see the dynamic theory, discussed in Chapter 1, in action, with stakeholders (like nurses) outside government exerting an influence on the policy decision-making process.

The same priorities that had been promoted by the federal nursing team in discussions with both Mr. Romanow and Mr. Kirby, and in Health Canada's testimony on nursing human resources to the Romanow Commission led by the office, informed the dialogues inside Health Canada leading up to the accord being signed in September 2003. One of the keys to policy success is consistent and repeated messaging informed by the best available evidence.

To prepare for the 2004 First Ministers' Meeting on Health, CNA collaborated strategically with the Canadian Healthcare Association, Canadian Medical Association, and Canadian Pharmacists Association. Calling themselves informally the G4, the organizations developed common visions and principles for health care around integration, patient-centredness, and affirming and strengthening the Canada Health Act. They agreed to focus on advocacy for reduced wait times for care and treatment, an adequate supply of health human resources, expansion of the insured continuum of care, and the need for predictable, appropriate funding. Again, policy influence was bolstered by consistent, focused messages, in this case spoken by many voices.

On September 16, 2004, Canada's first ministers reached a $41.2 billion, 10-year agreement that was intended to reform and strengthen Canada's stressed health care system. The accord, *A 10-Year Plan to Strengthen Health Care*,[45] responded broadly to the recommendations of the national reviews from 2002 and built on the work started in the 2003 accord. The injection of cash was intended to be a definitive investment in major reforms to health care across the country, including:

- Reducing wait times and improving access
- Increasing the supply of providers through accelerated strategic health human resource action plans

- Providing first dollar coverage by 2006 for a range of home care services
- Primary care reform to improve access, including electronic health records and telehealth
- Improved access to care in the north
- A national pharmaceuticals strategy
- Improvements to disease/injury prevention, health promotion, and public health
- Support for health innovation
- Accountability and reporting to citizens
- In the 2004 accord, Aboriginal health and health care were to be addressed and interwoven. Federal reviews were conducted every three years,[46] the last of which, in 2012, concluded that while there had been some progress, many reform targets had not been met and a great deal of work remained.

Responding to the 2003 accord, the Health Council of Canada was established that same year to monitor and report progress on health systems reform. The Canadian Patient Safety Institute was also established to track and respond to safety and quality issues, and the Public Health Agency of Canada was created in 2004 to strengthen health promotion, wellness, and public health. In 2007, agencies to focus on two key health issues were established—the Canadian Partnership Against Cancer Corporation and the Mental Health Commission of Canada. The Mental Health Commission was a response to the landmark report of the Standing Senate Committee on Social Affairs, Science and Technology in 2006, led once again by Senator Michael Kirby, entitled *Out of the Shadows at Last: Transforming Mental Health, Mental Illness and Addiction Services in Canada*.[47] The Commission released a mental health strategy for Canada in 2012.[48] All of these agencies operate at arm's length from Parliament and report to Health Canada.

There were other important responses to the 2003 and 2004 accords. For example, governments responded to recommendations around improving access with more effective use of nurses. Under a variety of names, telehealth services, largely run by nurses, are one of the most successful innovations responding to Canada's geography and pressing needs for primary care. Telehealth was firmly established over the first decade of the century in British Columbia (2000), Alberta (2003), Saskatchewan (2003), Ontario (2000), Nova Scotia (2009), Newfoundland and Labrador (2006), the Northwest Territories (2004), and the Yukon (2008). Indeed, as noted in the report of the Advisory Panel on Healthcare Innovation, with our "huge landmass and thin population density, as well as our longstanding commitment to telehealth, Canada should lead the world in mobile health and virtual care."[49]

Also tabled in 2006 was the *Final Report of the Federal Advisor on Wait Times.* Led by Brian Postl, who had been appointed in 2005, the initiative was intended "to inquire into the factors contributing to long wait times and to discuss with provinces, territories and stakeholders efforts that could contribute to more timely access to health care services."[50] In 2004, CNA had been a founding partner in the inaugural, pan-Canadian Taming of the Queue Conference, and it participated on behalf of nursing in the following years. Responding to the Postl report, to benchmarks in the 2004 accord, and pressure from the Wait Time Alliance established in 2005, the Patient Wait Times Guarantees Initiative was introduced in 2007 under then federal health minister, the Honourable Tony Clement. To support patient wait times guarantees, which were part of the Conservative election platform in 2006, the new program included "additional support for Canada Health Infoway; the creation of a Wait Times Guarantee Trust; and a Patient Wait Times Guarantee Pilot Fund."[50] Some $612 million was set aside to be used for a guaranteed wait time in one priority area in each of the provinces and territories, and an additional $30 million was available for pilot and project testing. Mindful of the need to contribute meaningfully to a resolution of this issue, CNA published *Registered Nurses: On the Front Lines of Wait Times* in 2009, describing key roles nurses can play in innovative solutions to the wait times challenge.[52] Despite all the effort, outcomes overall have been inconsistent. In a 2013 analysis, Owen Adams—long-standing chief policy advisor at the Canadian Medical Association and a highly respected policy analyst—concluded glumly that "with few exceptions, governments have not expanded benchmarks beyond the initial five areas and in its 2013 report the Wait Time Alliance has reported that in many regions and specialties no substantial or sustained progress has been achieved in recent years."[53]

LIFE AFTER HEALTH ACCORDS

Under Prime Minister Harper, the federal government made a unilateral announcement in December 2011 that it would provide a 6 per cent annual increase in unconditional funding to continue until 2017, after which any further federal increases will be tied to annual GDP growth or 3 per cent per annum, whichever is larger. As a result, with the 10-year accord expired March 31, 2014, and no plan for a new agreement, the Health Council of Canada was shut down.

Mr. Harper would not engage in discussion of a new pan-Canadian agreement on health reform and while he did meet with some premiers individually, he did not take part in the Council of the Federation meetings for a number of years. However, in June 2014 the federal government did launch a new Advisory

Panel on Healthcare Innovation. It was charged to identify "the five most promising areas of innovation in Canada and internationally that have the potential to sustainably reduce growth in health spending while leading to improvements in the quality and accessibility of care."[54] Reporting in July 2015, the panel presented robust evidence in its lengthy report and suggested action in five theme areas:

1. Patient engagement and empowerment
2. Health systems integration with workforce modernization
3. Technological transformation via digital health and precision medicine
4. Better value from procurement, reimbursement, and regulation
5. Industry as an economic driver and innovation catalyst

The panel became the latest in a long line of task forces and commissions to say that a major renovation of the system was overdue, providing plenty of compelling evidence. But in a terse rebuke of Canadian health policy development at the government level, the panel went further, stating in its summary report that its members were "chagrined and puzzled by the inability of Canadian governments—federal, provincial, and territorial—to join forces and take concerted action on recommendations that have been made by many previous commissions, reviews, panels, and experts."[55] The panel concluded in part that

> the lack of integration of healthcare services also reinforces Canada's narrow scope of public coverage, and vice versa. Provinces and territories are justifiably uneasy about the cost implications of adding on more budgetary silos to pay other professionals for needed care or to assume full financial responsibility for covering pharmaceuticals, even though careful spending on these goods and services could more than offset other costs in fully integrated budgets.[56]

A summary of the main pieces of legislation and related federal/pan-Canadian initiatives since the Canada Health Act (1984) are summarized in Table 5.3.

The Council of the Federation and Provincial/Territorial Development and Second-Wave Reform Initiatives

While it is beyond the scope of this discussion to tackle all the provincial and territorial reform initiatives taking place concurrently with the pan-Canadian ones, it is important for nurses across the country to be reminded that they are many and broad in scope. In a 2009 analysis, Lazar observed that a "second wave of

Table 5.3: Prime Ministers, Federal Ministers of Health, and Federal/ Pan-Canadian Reform Initiatives and Legislation Since the Canada Health Act

PRIME MINISTER	DATE	MINISTER OF HEALTH	MAJOR HEALTH LEGISLATION AND INITIATIVES
Pierre Elliott Trudeau (Liberal)	1979– 1984	Monique Bégin	*Canada's National-Provincial Health Program for the 1980s,* report of the Health Services Review, 1980
			Task Force on Federal-Provincial Fiscal Arrangements, 1984
			Canada Health Act, 1984
			Federal Task Force on the Allocation of Health Care Resources, reports 1984
John Napier Turner (Liberal)	1984	Monique Bégin	
Brian Mulroney (Progressive Conservative)	1984– 1993	Jake Epp Perrin Beatty Benoît Bouchard	*Achieving Health for All: A Framework for Health Promotion* (Epp), 1986 The Ottawa Charter for Health Promotion, 1986
Kim Campbell (Progressive Conservative)	1993	Mary Collins	
Jean Chrétien (Liberal)	1993– 2003	Diane Marleau David Dingwall Allan Rock Anne McLellan	Canadian Institute for Health Information established, 1994 *Canada Health Action: Building on the Legacy,* report of the National Forum on Health, 1997 Social Union Framework Agreement, 1999 First Ministers' Communiqué on Health, 2000 Canadian Institutes of Health Research established, 2000 *Building on Values: The Future of Health Care in Canada,* Commission on the Future of Health Care in Canada (Romanow), 2002 *The Health of Canadians—The Federal Role, Volume Six: Recommendations for Reform,* Standing Senate Committee on Social Affairs, Science and Technology (Kirby), 2002 Canada Health Infoway established, 2002

continued

PRIME MINISTER	DATE	MINISTER OF HEALTH	MAJOR HEALTH LEGISLATION AND INITIATIVES
Paul Martin, Jr. (Liberal)	2003–2006	Pierre Pettigrew Ujjal Dosanjh	First Ministers' Accord on Health Care Renewal, 2003
			Health Council of Canada established, 2003
			Canadian Patient Safety Institute established, 2003
			First Ministers' 10-Year Plan to Strengthen Health Care (Health Accord), 2004
			Canada Health and Social Transfer split into Canada Health Transfer and Canada Social Transfer, 2004
			Public Health Agency of Canada established, 2004
Stephen Harper (Conservative)	2006–2015	Tony Clement Leona Aglukkaq Rona Ambrose	*Out of the Shadows at Last: Transforming Mental Health, Mental Illness and Addiction Services in Canada*, report of the Standing Senate Committee on Social Affairs, Science and Technology (Kirby), 2006
			Final Report of the Federal Advisor on Wait Times (Postl), 2006
			Mental Health Commission of Canada established, 2007
			Canadian Partnership Against Cancer Corporation established 2007
			Federal/provincial/territorial Patient Wait Times Guarantees initiative introduced, 2007
			Parliamentary review of the 10-Year Plan to Strengthen Health Care (2004 accord), House of Commons Standing Committee on Health, 2008
			Parliamentary review of the 10-Year Plan to Strengthen Health Care (2004 accord), *Time for Transformative Change: A Review of the 2004 Health Accord*, Standing Senate Committee on Social Affairs, Science and Technology, 2012
			Health Council of Canada closed, 2014
			Unleashing Innovation: Excellent Healthcare for Canada, report of the Advisory Panel on Healthcare Innovation, 2015
Justin Trudeau (Liberal)	2015–	Jane Philpott	New legislation on medical assistance in dying, Cannabis for medical purposes
			Bilateral funding agreements with provinces and territories

... reports was commissioned in the second half of the 1990s and the beginning of the 2000s in the aftermath of the freeze on health spending and with health care by then having become the highest policy priority of Canadians."[57] In many jurisdictions, system support structures similar to the federal and pan-Canadian ones were put in place—including organizations dedicated to safety, quality, research/data, specific diseases and populations, and areas like system performance. For example, formal health quality councils were established in Alberta (2002) and Saskatchewan (2002); British Columbia established its Patient Safety and Quality Council in 2008, the same year New Brunswick created its health council. The pattern continued across the country, and, as noted in Chapter 3, the structure, role, and number of regional health authorities within provinces changed considerably across the country and within jurisdictions in an effort to better manage health care and contain costs.

Established in 2012, the Health Care Innovation Working Group of the Council of the Federation is co-led by two or more premiers and includes the ministers of health as members, with a goal to strengthen shared capacity across health care systems. Priority topics for the working group currently include lowering the costs of pharmaceuticals, appropriateness of care (including team-based delivery models and scope of practice), and prioritizing home care over long-term institutional care for seniors. Significantly, CNA and the Canadian Medical Association have both been included in the innovative work of the group. Examples of leading 21st century health system reports and initiatives at the federal and provincial/territorial levels are summarized in Table 5.4.

SUMMARY AND IMPLICATIONS

The first wave of health systems reform in Canada was focused strongly on creating health care organizations as well as universal access to public health care based on need and not the ability to pay. Over that 45-year period, Canadians built a health care system that in many ways became the envy of the world. But costs steadily grew and sometimes soared, and the link between the dollar inputs and clinical outcomes started to be called into question.

The second wave of reform was characterized by a focus on the areas of improving quality and safety, containing costs sometimes seen to be out of control, and testing and implementing models of care delivery truer to the principles of *right provider*, *right place*, *right care*, and *right time*. Certainly a hallmark of the second wave of reform was its growing focus away from in-patient admissions and traditional institutional walls, moving care closer to the homes and communities of those who need it.

Table 5.4: Summary of 21st Century Federal/Pan-Canadian and Provincial/Territorial Health System Reports and Initiatives

YEAR	FEDERAL/PAN-CANADIAN INITIATIVES	PROVINCIAL/TERRITORIAL INITIATIVES
1999	Social Union Framework Agreement	Health Services Review, New Brunswick
2000	First Ministers' Communiqué on Health	Commission of Study on Health and Social Services (Clair), Quebec
	Canadian Institutes of Health Research established	Minister's Forum on Health and Social Services, Northwest Territories
2001		Saskatchewan Commission on Medicare (Fyke), Saskatchewan
2002	*Building on Values: The Future of Health Care in Canada*, Commission on the Future of Health Care in Canada (Romanow Commission) *The Health of Canadians—The Federal Role, Volume Six: Recommendations for Reform*, Standing Senate Committee on Social Affairs, Science and Technology review (Kirby) Canada Health Infoway established	British Columbia Select Standing Committee on Health (Roddick) Premier's Advisory Council on Health for Alberta (Mazankowski) Action Plan for Saskatchewan Health Care Health Advisory Network. Task Force on Health Promotion, Manitoba Health Consultation Process, Ontario Premier's Health Quality Council, New Brunswick Northwest Territories Action Plan
2003	First Ministers' Accord on Health Care Renewal Health Council of Canada established Canadian Patient Safety Institute established	
2004	First Ministers' 10-Year Plan to Strengthen Health Care (2004 accord) Canada Health and Social Transfer split into Canada Health Transfer and Canada Social Transfer Public Health Agency of Canada established	
2006	*Out of the Shadows at Last: Transforming Mental Health, Mental Illness and Addiction Services in Canada*, report of the Standing Senate Committee on Social Affairs, Science and Technology (Kirby) *Final Report of the Federal Advisor on Wait Times* (Postl report)	Getting On with Better Health Care: Health Policy Framework, Alberta

YEAR	FEDERAL/PAN-CANADIAN INITIATIVES	PROVINCIAL/TERRITORIAL INITIATIVES
2007	Mental Health Commission of Canada established Canadian Partnership Against Cancer Corporation established Federal/provincial/territorial Patient Wait Times Guarantees initiative introduced	Conversation on Health, British Columbia
2008	Parliamentary Review of the 10-Year Plan to Strengthen Health Care (2004 accord), House of Commons Standing Committee on Health	*Vision 2020: The Future of Health Care in Alberta* Health Action Plan, Alberta *Report of the Manitoba Regional Health Authority External Review Committee* *Getting Our Money's Worth. Report of the Task Force on the Funding of the Health System*, Quebec *Wellness: We Each Have a Role to Play: Individuals, Communities, Stakeholders and Government: Final Report*, Legislative Assembly Select Committee on Wellness, New Brunswick Transforming New Brunswick's Health Care System: The Provincial Health Plan 2008–2012 *Changing Nova Scotia's Health Care System: Creating Sustainability Through Transformation: System Level Findings and Overall Directions For Change From the Provincial Health Services Operational Review*, Nova Scotia *An Integrated Health System Review in PEI: A Call to Action: A Plan for Change*, Prince Edward Island Strategic Plan 2008–2011, Department of Health and Community Services, Newfoundland and Labrador *Report of the Yukon Health Care Review Committee*
2009		*For Patients' Sake, Patient First Review*, Saskatchewan
2010		*Charting a Path to Sustainable Health Care in Ontario* (Drummond and Burleton)
2011	Federal government announcement of 6% annual increase in funding (unconditional) to provinces until 2017, then tied to inflation	*Moving Towards a Planned and Citizen-Centered Publicly-Funded Provincial Health Care System*, New Brunswick Health Council Health Integration Initiative, Nunavut

continued

YEAR	FEDERAL/PAN-CANADIAN INITIATIVES	PROVINCIAL/TERRITORIAL INITIATIVES
2012	Parliamentary Review of the 10-Year Plan to Strengthen Health Care (2004 accord), *Time for Transformative Change: A Review of the 2004 Health Accord,* Standing Senate Committee on Social Affairs, Science and Technology	*Strategic Direction 2012–2015: Defining our Focus/Measuring our Progress,* Alberta *Public Service for Ontarians: A Path to Sustainability and Excellence,* Commission on the Reform of Ontario's Public Services Ontario's Action Plan for Health Care *Commissaire à la santé et au bien-être: Rapport d'appréciation de la performance du système de santé et de services sociaux,* Quebec
2013		
2014	Health Council of Canada closed	A Clinical Services Plan for Yukon Territory, Final Report
2015	*Unleashing Innovation: Excellent Healthcare for Canada,* report of the Advisory Panel on Healthcare Innovation	*Patients First: Action Plan for Health Care,* Ontario

And so, the third wave lies ahead. Coming into power in late 2015, Prime Minister Justin Trudeau directed the health minister to focus in several areas:

- "Engage provinces and territories in the development of a new multi-year Health Accord," including a long-term funding agreement and other priorities
- Promote public health in several key areas
- "Work with the Minister of Sport and Persons with Disabilities in increasing funding to the Public Health Agency of Canada to support a national strategy to raise awareness for parents, coaches, and athletes on concussion treatment"
- "Introduce plain packaging requirements for tobacco products"
- "Support the Ministers of Justice and Public Safety and Emergency Preparedness on efforts that will lead to the legalization and regulation of marijuana"
- "Work with the Minister of Indigenous and Northern Affairs to update and expand the Nutrition North program, in consultation with Northern communities"[58]

Initial rounds of negotiations on a health accord were tense, and as of April 2017, most jurisdictions had abandoned the process in favour of bilateral agreements with the federal government. Evidently agreements have been reached that allow them to return to that policy table if more lucrative collective arrangements can be negotiated in the future. Unfortunately there is little evidence that a series of individual agreements will do anything to unlock the gridlock in areas like pharmacare and home care programs recommended in every major reform report since the 1990s and strongly supported by Canadians. The size and spread of the third wave remain to be seen.

DISCUSSION QUESTIONS

1. Why do governments across Canada want to reform health systems?
2. What do Canadians want from and expect of the health system reform agenda?
3. What are the reasons behind the transformation inertia and difficulties inherent in making changes to health systems in Canada?
4. What are the implications of major health system reform policies (e.g., pharmacare, home care, a focus on seniors) for nursing and health care recipients?
5. How effective are health accords in achieving health system reform? Should governments continue to engage in them? What other mechanisms might work?

ADDITIONAL POLICY RESOURCES

INFLUENTIAL PAN-CANADIAN GOVERNMENT HEALTH CARE SYSTEM REFORM DOCUMENTS	
Social Union Framework Agreement (1999)	http://www.scics.gc.ca/ english/conferences. asp?a=viewdocument&id=638_
First Ministers' Communiqué on Health (2000)	http://www.scics.gc.ca/ english/conferences. asp?a=viewdocument&id=1144
Commission on the Future of Health Care in Canada (Romanow, 2002)	http://publications.gc.ca/collections/ Collection/CP32-85-2002E.pdf
The Health of Canadians—The Federal Role, Volume Six: Recommendations for Reform (Kirby, 2002)	http://www.parl.gc.ca/Content/ SEN/Committee/372/soci/rep/ repoct02vol6-e.htm
First Ministers' Accord on Health Care Renewal (2003)	http://healthycanadians.gc.ca/health- system-systeme-sante/cards-cartes/ collaboration/2003-accord-eng.php

A 10-Year Plan to Strengthen Health Care, First Ministers' Meeting on the Future of Health Care (2004)	http://www.hc-sc.gc.ca/hcs-sss/delivery-prestation/fptcollab/2004-fmm-rpm/bg-fi-eng.php
Unleashing Innovation: Excellent Healthcare for Canada, report of the Advisory Panel on Healthcare Innovation (2015)	http://www.healthycanadians.gc.ca/publications/health-system-systeme-sante/summary-innovation-sommaire/index-eng.php

CHAPTER 6

Canadian Nursing Initiatives in the Era of Reform

CHAPTER HIGHLIGHTS

- Introduction
- The Office of Nursing Policy
- Pan-Canadian Government Initiatives to Reform and Strengthen Nursing
- Pan-Canadian Nursing Initiatives Led Outside of Government
- Notes on Nursing Education Reform
- Summary and Implications
- Discussion Questions
- Additional Policy Resources

LEARNING OUTCOMES

1. Describe four pan-Canadian government-led initiatives undertaken to strengthen nursing and facilitate the most effective deployment of nurses across Canada's health systems.
2. Describe five pan-Canadian initiatives undertaken outside of governments to strengthen nursing and facilitate the most effective deployment of nurses across Canada's health systems.
3. Identify major points of change in nursing education over the past 100 years.
4. Discuss the role and value of federal government nursing policy leadership.

Policy Influencer: Dianne Martin

After completing her original practical nursing education in 1979, Dianne Martin, RPN, RN, BScN, MA, went on to complete her BScN and later a master's degree in leadership. She maintains dual registration as a registered practical nurse and registered nurse, and after practicing in clinical care areas she took on leadership roles as a professional practice coordinator in a hospital setting and later as a senior policy analyst with the Nursing Secretariat in the government of Ontario. Martin is the chief executive officer of the Registered Practical Nurses Association of Ontario, a role she has held since 2006, where she has honed her skills as a masterful change agent and collaborator across nursing and health policy spheres. She is especially active in the areas of respectful work environments and removing barriers to optimal scope of practice for all health professionals. Martin is renowned for her steady, innovative, and principled leadership of registered practical nurses and nursing at large in Ontario.

"We need Nightingales for the twenty-first century providing the moral and scientific leadership necessary to advocate for patients using best evidence to deliver effective, safe and compassionate care."

—Sioban Nelson, Vice Provost, Academic Programs, University of Toronto, and Anne-Marie Rafferty, CBE FRCN, Professor of Policy and past Dean, Florence Nightingale School of Nursing and Midwifery, King's College, London[1]

INTRODUCTION

In the years after medicare was first established, nursing organizations across the country undertook a number of reviews focused on aspects of nursing education, development, and practice. For example:

- Royal Commission on Nursing Education, Newfoundland, 1974
- Joint Ministerial Task Force on Nursing Education, Manitoba, 1977
- Department of Health Nurse Practitioner Demonstration Project, Saskatchewan, 1977
- Task Force on Nursing Education, Alberta, 1977
- Commission of Inquiry Concerning the Education and Training of Practical Nurses and Related Hospital Personnel, British Columbia, 1977

Some of this work would inform later policy work at the pan-Canadian level—for example, in the decision to recommend baccalaureate education as the entry-to-practice credential for registered nurses. But nursing was hit hard by the budget cuts that started in the mid-1990s, and the consequences prompted a long roster of more urgent initiatives intended to strengthen—some might say rescue—the nursing workforce. Reflecting the times, provincial government-led initiatives such as Manitoba's Work Life Task Force (2001) and the report of Ontario's Nursing Task Force in 1999, *Good Nursing, Good Health: An Investment for the 21st Century*,[2] were joined by organization-led efforts in the provinces like RNAO's 2002 report, *Tracking the Nursing Task Force (1999): RNs Rate Their Nursing Work Life*.[3]

The number of admissions to first-entry seats in schools for registered nurses dropped roughly 28 per cent, from 12,170 in 1990 to 8,790 in 2000.[4] In the same decade, when the Canadian population grew by 11 per cent, the number of registered nurse graduates dropped by 46 per cent, and registered psychiatric nurse and licensed practical nurse graduates also shrank. As a result of the dramatic drop in graduates, and the fact that the workforce was aging and moving toward retirement, Canada was experiencing a growing RN shortage by the turn of the century and there were concerns that it was set to worsen considerably.

By 1997 CNA had already predicted that, left unchecked, Canada could experience a shortage in the range of 59,000 to 113,000 registered nurses by 2011[5]—prompting the comment by OECD health economists in 2003 that Canada was "galloping just to stand still" in terms of maintaining an adequate nursing workforce. It was in this context that Bob Evans made his comment, cited earlier in this book, that "policy is possible"; dropping the number of nurses in the system quickly and dramatically was precisely what was intended.

Leaders across nursing were increasingly alarmed as realities of the fiscal situation unfolded. In one of the cuts by the Chrétien government, the principal nursing officer role was abolished after Flaherty retired in 1994. Judith Shamian would later reflect with nurses in a policy forum on what the outcomes might have been at those policy tables had strong, credible, and informed nurses been part of the team bringing evidence to bear on the allocation decisions of the mid-1990s. We will never know, of course.

In the lead-up to the 1997 federal election, CNA launched its "1 in 70 Voters is a Registered Nurse" campaign. Nurses made it clear that they were watching the government's actions and were worried about the impacts of cuts on health and health care. Some of the nursing dynamics as examples of policy development are pursued in Chapters 9 and 10. The Chrétien government was re-elected with a small majority in 1997; but the quiet lobbying, public campaigns, and research—such as the Ryten study—were garnering attention. The federal minister of health, Allan Rock, said at the 1998 CNA convention in Ottawa that "no professional group has borne the brunt of health care restructuring more than Canada's nurses."[6] It was at that meeting that the minister announced the establishment of a new, federal nursing policy office, and talk began around the need for a national nursing strategy, a study of the nursing profession, and funding of nursing research.

In 1999, CNA unveiled what it called its "Quiet Crisis" campaign in advance of the federal budget. The association and its members were applying significant pressure on federal, provincial, and territorial governments, pushing for a "reinvestment into quality health care"[7] across the country. The strategy worked: in the 1999 federal budget, a 10-year $25 million Nursing Research Fund was announced and, that spring, Health Canada's new Office of Nursing Policy was opened. Despite the drama of the backstory, there was arguably more political attention to Canadian nursing starting in 1998 than at any point in the history of the profession.

THE OFFICE OF NURSING POLICY

Health Canada's Office of Nursing Policy was positioned strongly in the hierarchy, its executive director reporting to the assistant deputy minister of health policy and communications. Resulting from a confluence of the skills of the leader, the talent recruited to her team, the public positioning of the office, and a wave of support—including similar offices established across the country—the team was able to quickly provide input in a number of key initiatives, partnering in some and leading in others. Table 6.1 provides a list of some key nursing reform initiatives at the federal and pan-Canadian level beginning in 1999.

With the federal office open in 1999, the team immediately connected with the existing group of senior nurses in provincial and territorial governments, where they existed, and the executive director joined the federal/provincial/territorial Advisory Committee on Health Human Resources—an advisory group to the Conference of Deputy Ministers now called the Committee on Health Workforce. A seat at that table, which was made up of some of the most senior health system leaders in governments across the country, was a key point of entry for nursing to networks of policy influence. By 2001, the executive director was appointed vice chair of the committee, solidifying the position of nursing among national health human resources policy decision makers.

To inform its work and priorities, in fall 2000 the Office of Nursing Policy hosted a National Stakeholder Consultation on Nursing and Workplace Health in which nursing stakeholders from all the regulated categories, domains of practice, and regions of the country were brought together.[8] Predictably in such a group, there were areas of agreement and disagreement. For example, participants were cool in their reaction to the idea of adopting aspects of the American Magnet Hospitals program; in January 2015, 15 years later, it was interesting to note the celebration of Mount Sinai Hospital in Toronto becoming the first Canadian organization to achieve Magnet designation. What the participants in that early meeting did have in common was a serious concern about the deleterious effects of system restructuring on the health, safety, and working conditions of nurses. That meeting confirmed the need for the office to focus a pillar of its work on what would become known as Healthy Nurses, Healthy Workplaces. More on that work follows in Chapter 9.

The office also led a number of programs and initiatives to: (a) develop knowledge and evidence, especially as regards health human resources, to support policy decisions; (b) contribute policy advice to advance nursing education and science; and (c) strengthen nursing for Aboriginal Peoples by working with the First Nations and Inuit Health Branch to establish its first national Office of Nursing Services. The team helped in the federal response to the SARS crisis in 2003–2004, and over the same year loaned staff to assist the OECD team in Paris to complete the nursing chapters of the organization's complicated study of the performance of its members' health systems.[9] The office also participated in the federal delegations to World Health Assembly meetings and supported the work of the Chief Nurse Scientist at the WHO. Within its first four years, team members had represented Health Canada at more than 150 domestic and global events and extensively published the nursing policy work of Health Canada, from nursing organization newsletters to peer-reviewed research journals.

The office was well staffed in the years after it was established, and it continued to grow under the leadership of its second executive director, Sandra MacDonald-Rencz. It served as a good example of how nurses positioned in government roles can be highly effective in informing government policy decision-making, and can engage just as effectively with nurses and other providers to explain and seek input on government policy work.

Table 6.1: 21st Century Federal and Pan-Canadian Nursing Reform Initiatives

YEAR	INITIATIVES
1999	• Federal Office of Nursing Policy established, Health Policy Branch, Health Canada
2000	• *The Nursing Strategy for Canada*
	• National Stakeholder Consultation on Nursing and Workplace Health, Office of Nursing Policy

continued

2001	• Federal chief nurse appointed vice chair, federal/provincial/territorial Advisory Committee on Health Human Resources
	• Federal Office of Nursing Services established, First Nations and Inuit Health Branch, Health Canada
	• Dorothy M. Wylie Nursing Leadership Institute established
	• Office of Nursing Policy helps organize Global Nursing Partnerships: Strategies for a Sustainable Nursing Workforce, a meeting including representatives from governments and nursing associations, government chief nursing officers, national and international nursing association leaders, and human resource directors/health planners.
2002	• *Our Health, Our Future: Creating Quality Workplaces for Canadian Nurses*, final report of the Canadian Nursing Advisory Committee
	• Federal/provincial/territorial *Review of Progress of the Nursing Strategy for Canada*
	• World Health Organization/Health Canada Consultation on Imbalances in the Health Workforce
	• Pathfinding for Nursing Science in the 21st Century Think Tank
	• National Nursing Education Think Tank
	• *Planning for the Future: Nursing Human Resource Projections*, CNA, update of 1997 Ryten report
2003	• National Policy Forum on First Ministers' Health Accord, Office of Nursing Policy
	• Executive Training for Research Application (EXTRA) program established, Canadian Health Services Research Foundation
2004	• Inaugural pan-Canadian Taming of the Queue Conference
	• Internationally Educated Nurses National Task Force established under federal/provincial/territorial Advisory Committee on Health Delivery and Human Resources
	• Canadian Health Services Research Foundation grants Canadian Nurses Foundation renewable research funding for the Nursing Care Partnership
2005	• Office of Nursing Policy contributes to development of *Tackling Nursing Shortages in OECD Member Countries* for OECD international health systems performance study
	• *National Survey of the Work and Health of Nurses*
	• *Toward a Pan-Canadian Planning Framework for Health Human Resources: A Green Paper*, CNA and Canadian Medical Association
2006	• *Toward 2020: Visions for Nursing*, CNA
	• *Building the Future: Final Report of the National Occupational/Sector Study of Nursing*
	• *Nurse Practitioners: The Time is Now: A Solution to Improving Access and Reducing Wait Times in Canada*, final report of the Canadian Nurse Practitioner Initiative
	• NurseONE.ca established, CNA national information portal for nurses
	• International Nurses' Forum, *Nurses at the Forefront of HIV/AIDS: Prevention, Care, and Treatment*, International AIDS Conference, CNA

2007	• Office of Nursing Policy leads Health Education Task Force (2007–2013)
	• Canada's first nurse practitioner–led clinic opens (Sudbury)
	• CASN Accreditation Program established
2008	• 100th Anniversary of CNA
	• Canadian Health Outcomes for Better Information and Care initiative established
	• *Advancing Health Through Nursing Science*, CNA, CASN, and Academy of Canadian Executive Nurses
2009	• *Tested Solutions for Eliminating Canada's Registered Nurse Shortage*, CNA update to 1997 and 2002 Ryten reports
	• *Registered Nurses: On the Front Lines of Wait Times*, CNA
	• *Cultural Competence and Cultural Safety in Nursing Education—A Framework for First Nations, Inuit and Métis Nursing*, Aboriginal Nurses Association of Canada, CASN, and CNA
2011	• *Principles to Guide Health Care Transformation in Canada*, Canadian Medical Association and CNA
2012	• *A Nursing Call to Action: The Health of Our Nation—The Future of Our Health System*, final report of the National Expert Commission, CNA
	• *Research to Action: Applied Workplace Solutions for Nurses*, CFNU
	• Office of Nursing Policy is transitioned to Nursing Policy Unit within Health Canada
2013	• *National Nursing Education Summit—Summary Report*, CNA and CASN
	• *Educating Nurses to Address Socio-Cultural, Historical, and Contextual Determinants of Health among Aboriginal Peoples*, CASN
2014	• *National Nursing Education Framework*, CASN
2015	• *Building Our Future: A New, Collaborative Model for Undergraduate Nursing Education in Nova Scotia*, final Report of the Registered Nurse Education Review in Nova Scotia
	• *Framework for Registered Nurse Prescribing in Canada*, CNA

PAN-CANADIAN INITIATIVES TO REFORM AND STRENGTHEN NURSING

Apart from a long roster of nursing reform activities taking place across the individual provinces and territories, three key activities launched in the wake of the 1998–1999 federal funding announcements supporting nursing bear mention: *The Nursing Strategy for Canada*; its offspring, the Canadian Nursing Advisory Committee; and the National Sector/Occupational Study of Nursing. In an ideal world, this third item—the sector study—would have been completed first, providing a broad picture of the nursing sector of the Canadian workforce that would have identified strengths, needs, and gaps on which to build a strategy to renew the profession. But as noted in Chapter 1, the world of policy is rarely ideal or linear, and because the need for action was urgent, the nursing strategy was re-leased years before the findings of the sector study were published. One of the lessons nurses surely have learned from the past two decades is that politicians and policy makers rarely have the luxury of time.

The Nursing Strategy for Canada

The Nursing Strategy for Canada, released in 2000 by the federal/provincial/terri-torial Advisory Committee on Health Human Resources (see Figure 6.1), opened with a clear statement on the level of concern about nursing that had emerged across the country:

> Canada is experiencing a crisis in nursing. This is a view expressed across the country, both in the health system and among the general public. While there are many different perspectives on why this is and what the most prom-ising solutions are, there is significant agreement that the current shortage of nurses is getting worse and that left unchecked, this situation will lead to a deterioration in the quality of the nation's health care system.[10]

Consistent with much of the Advisory Committee's work, the nursing strate-gy was developed to "achieve and maintain an adequate supply of nursing person-nel who are appropriately educated, distributed and deployed to meet the health needs of Canadian residents."[11] The 11 strategies recommended to achieve that goal were organized around (a) unified and coordinated action on nursing issues across the country; (b) improved data, research, and human resource planning; (c) appropriate education; and (d) improved deployment and retention strategies as shown in Table 6.2.

Action on a number of the strategies was relatively swift. A progress report released in 2003[12] revealed that:

- The Canadian Nursing Advisory Committee had been enthusiastically sup-ported, was formed, and completed its work with submission of a final report in 2002. That committee is discussed further in the following section.
- The Canadian Institute for Health Information was expanding its nursing database beyond registered nurses to collect and report on data for all the regulated categories.
- All provinces and territories were taking part in research related to health human resource planning and some were using federal funding to study predictive health human resources modelling.

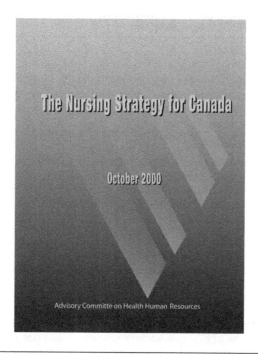

Figure 6.1: Cover of *The Nursing Strategy for Canada*, 2000

Source: Health Canada. (2000). *The nursing strategy for Canada: October 2000.* Ottawa: Health
Canada. Retrieved from http://www.hc-sc.gc.ca/hcs-sss/pubs/nurs-infirm/2000-nurs-infirm-
strateg/index-eng.php.

Table 6.2: Nursing Strategy for Canada Recommendations

THEME	RECOMMENDATION
Unified action	Strategy 1
	The federal government and provincial/territorial governments should immediately establish a multi-stakeholder Canadian Nursing Advisory Committee (CNAC) to address priority issues as identified by the Advisory Committee on Health Human Resources (ACHHR) and the Working Group on Nursing Resources and Unregulated Health Care Workers (WGNR). The key focus for CNAC for 2000 and 2001 will be improving the quality of work life for nurses and providing advice to support the implementation of other strategies of the Nursing Strategy for Canada.
	Strategy 2
	Establish a Nursing Advisory Committee (NAC) (where an equivalent body does not exist) in each province and territory to support the development of strategies for improved nurse human resource planning and management within each jurisdiction.

continued

THEME	RECOMMENDATION
Improved data, research, and human resource planning	Strategy 3 The federal/provincial/territorial governments should encourage the efforts of the Canadian Institute for Health Information (CIHI) and other organizations to develop the information required for effective planning and evaluation of nursing resources.
	Strategy 4 The ACHHR should work with major research funders to identify gaps in current research, profile workforce planning issues for new research funding, and recommend improved mechanisms for the dissemination of these research results to policy makers and managers.
	Strategy 5 The federal government should provide leadership to ensure the development of improved projections for nursing supply/demand requirements to the year 2015.
Appropriate education	Strategy 6 Develop a communications strategy with the goal of increasing the public's awareness of nursing as a positive career choice and increasing the number of qualified applicants to nursing schools.
	Strategy 7 Increase the number of nursing education seats Canada-wide by at least 10% over 1998/1999 levels over the next two years (2000/2002), and base increases in following years upon improved demand projections and provincial/territorial need and capability.
	Strategy 8 Each provincial/territorial NAC or equivalent body should develop a comprehensive strategy to determine what types of nursing human resources are required and for which practice settings, based on an analysis of the needs of the population, the health system as a whole, and the skills and capacities of all types of nurses.
	Strategy 9 Provincial/territorial NACs (or equivalent body) should develop a five-year provincial/territorial Nursing Education Plan based on the comprehensive strategy proposed in Strategy 8.
Improved deployment and retention strategies	Strategy 10 Provincial/territorial NACs (or equivalent body) should identify and support the implementation of retention strategies for their respective workforces that focus on improving the quality of the work lives of nurses.
	Strategy 11 Provincial/territorial NACs (or equivalent body) should examine opportunities to encourage nurses to re-enter the workforce.

- The number of seats in schools for registered nurses in 2001 had increased by some 43 per cent over the 1998/1999 level—a dramatic and rapid turn-around of what had seemed such a desperate situation by 1997.
- Most of the provinces and territories were tackling retention issues and making efforts to recruit nurses back to nursing who had left either by choice or by force during the cuts of the 1990s.[13]

Canadian Nursing Advisory Committee

Establishment of a Canadian Nursing Advisory Committee was the first recommendation of the national nursing strategy, and it was struck in 2001. Made up of expert nurses from the three regulated categories (nurse practitioners were not a regulated category at that time) and representing broad knowledge and interests, the committee commissioned research, accepted submissions, and spoke with stakeholders across the country. Although Quebec had not formally agreed to participate in the committee, a francophone nurse from a Centre local de services communautaires in Quebec was included among the members.

The selection of the chair provides a learning opportunity about policy influence for nurses. While a number of nurse leaders were considered for the committee, after considerable debate and disagreement, it was felt that a prominent Canadian *non*-nurse should be at the helm. Such a leader could help soften an appearance of self-interest in the eventual policy recommendations, and just as important, could provide entry to worlds of policy influencers and decision makers to which nurses might have limited or no access. The selection of these sorts of leaders and allies to head important nursing initiatives is one of the most valuable policy lessons emerging from the policy work by nurses since the turn of the new century.

Michael Decter was selected to lead the Canadian Nursing Advisory Committee with operational support delivered by the federal team. A Harvard-trained economist, Decter was at the helm of a prominent Toronto investment firm, and was (and is) well connected in the world of finance. Importantly, he had served as a cabinet secretary in Manitoba and deputy minister of health in Ontario—the latter during the years of cutbacks that had so drastically affected health care in Ontario. Under then premier Bob Rae, Decter had led negotiations around what was called a *social contract* whereby public servants (including nurses) were forced to take a number of unpaid days off work. The program was one response to the $17 billion deficit that had confronted Mr. Rae when he was elected in 1990—and was very unpopular with nurses.

Decter was well informed about government decision-making, health

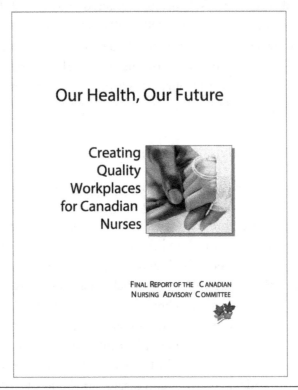

Figure 6.2: Cover of the Final Report of the Canadian Nursing Advisory Committee, 2002

Source: Canadian Nursing Advisory Committee. (2002). *Our health, our future: Creating quality workplaces for Canadian nurses*. Ottawa: Advisory Committee on Health Human Resources. Retrieved from http://www.hc-sc.gc.ca/hcs-sss/pubs/nurs-infirm/2002-cnac-cccsi-final/index-eng.php.

system policy, and structural issues; was concerned about the state of nursing in the wake of the 1990s; and was an unapologetic champion of the potential of nursing to contribute effective responses to emerging population health needs. Decter's leadership of the committee proved to be effective and valuable, and he brought an added benefit of non-nurse neutrality in his approach to including all the regulated categories of nursing during negotiations and in the writing of the final report.

At the end of its one-year mandate, the Canadian Nursing Advisory Committee issued a lengthy report (see Figure 6.2) deeply grounded in evidence and containing 51 recommendations "for policy direction that would improve the quality of nursing work life at the federal, provincial and territorial levels."[14] The recommendations were organized in three pillars as follows:

1. Put in place conditions to resolve operational workforce management issues and maximize the use of available resources.
2. Create professional practice environments that will attract and retain a healthy, committed workforce for the 21st century.
3. Monitor activities and generate and disseminate information to support a responsive, educated, and committed nursing workforce.

All of this work had nurses and policy decision makers talking about nursing and its place in policy across the country, and as chair and champion, Decter helped to move the report to broader health policy and non–health care audiences through his network of contacts and peers.

While the progress report on the national nursing strategy had noted a number of areas still needing action, it should be noted that there was tremendous—probably unprecedented—energy and activity within and around nursing right across the country during this time. Although some activities were sidetracked by the terrorist events of September 11, 2001, and later by the SARS outbreak in 2003–2004, it was a time of a rapid scaling up of nursing participation in health system policy work. Many jurisdictions already had significant activity underway by the time the nursing strategy and other initiatives came to life, and the pan-Canadian work seemed only to add energy to the jurisdictional activities; there was a sense of synergy and movement in those years.

National Sector/Occupational Study of Nursing

To better understand and support policy interventions to strengthen the nursing workforce, in 2001, the Honourable Jane Stewart, minister of human resources development, announced that the Chrétien government would provide $1.8 million (from the Sector Council and Health Canada) over two years for a study of the nursing sector. The nursing profession agreed to contribute a further $2.2 million, for a total $4 million investment.

A sector study typically entails a deep and broad analysis of some sector of the economy and looks at future needs, trends, and conditions related to that sector. The study ultimately took five years to complete, with its final report tabled in May 2006. It took place in two main phases, the first examining the state of the regulated nursing professions, bolstered by 15 technical reports. In the second phase, a pan-Canadian nursing human resource strategy was developed from the findings of the first phase and in consultation with stakeholders from inside and outside government.[15] Initially, the study was been led by co-chairs Mary Ellen Jeans, a past executive director at CNA, and Verna Holgate, then president of the

Canadian Practical Nurses Association. Later in the study the co-chairs changed, with Lisa Little, a nursing and health human resources policy expert then based at CNA, and Annette Osted, the long-serving executive director of the registered psychiatric nurses group from Manitoba and who represented the Registered Psychiatric Nurses of Canada, succeeding Jeans and Holgate.

The study did not unfold entirely smoothly, taking a very long time to get off the ground. As if modelling the difficulty Canada faces in establishing health accords or passing pan-Canadian legislation, many months were spent just to find agreement on terms of reference for the sector study. The initial choice of Jeans and Holgate as co-chairs may have set up the old partisan dynamic of the huge registered nurse group pitted against the practical nurses—and the equally old issue of the registered psychiatric nurses feeling locked out of a position at the head table. The leadership imbalance was exaggerated by Jeans's doctoral preparation and long service as an executive in Health Canada, and before that as the director of the nursing school at McGill University. Early discord between some of the parties around the table only added to the slow start. In retrospect, the lessons of the Canadian Nursing Advisory Committee and National Expert Commission to appoint a neutral chair (and/or co-chair) might have proven valuable in moving the initiative along more quickly and effectively. The final report included 10 main recommendations as part of Phase I, and built on these recommendations by outlining six top-priority strategies for action, summarized as follows:

1. Move away from the language of "scope of practice" and focus on developing management policy to facilitate nurses to practice to their level of competency in various clinical settings.
2. Broaden the nursing human resource planning framework to develop an integrated health human resource strategy.
3. Increase the supply of nurses by increasing the capacity of nursing education programs in Canada.
4. Compile best practices that outline effective workplace strategies that create effective working environments, and maximize nurse and system outcomes.
5. Establish a coordinated pan-Canadian strategy to inform health system managers and policy makers regarding the relationship between workload and quality of patient care and nurse health.
6. Address issues related to workplace health and safety and working environments to ameliorate the effects of overwork and burnout.

The work of the sector study helped to inform health human resources planning activities of federal and provincial/territorial governments over the subsequent years, and an integrated health human resources planning framework was developed as a result.

PAN-CANADIAN NURSING INITIATIVES LED OUTSIDE OF GOVERNMENT

Beyond the pan-Canadian government initiatives described here, there were numerous initiatives at the national level led entirely by nurses, and others funded by governments but led by nursing associations; examples of these follow.

Toward 2020

The Toward 2020 initiative included a suite of projects funded by Health Canada from 2004 to 2006 intended to push nursing forward to imagine new models, new scope, and new directions to contribute to population health trends and demands. The flagship report, *Toward 2020: Visions for Nursing*, which was backed up by a long roster of studies and other work conducted over the term of the funding, suggested

Toward 2020 and the Canadian Nurses Association

Although the Toward 2020 project was carried out with federal funding support and delivered entirely within CNA, the board of directors received but never endorsed the flagship report. That tactic brought with it both advantages and disadvantages. With the report having come from CNA staff, the organization and its board could quite rightly claim it as their own as it suited the situation. When it was criticized (or worse), they could say that the report's conclusions had not been endorsed by the board and were essentially the results of rogue provocation by its authors. In some ways that was a brilliant political strategy. However, remembering that the federal government had asked for a piece of work that would shake things up, CNA's distancing from the report may also cast a revealing light on the risk aversion that characterizes some of its work, and that may have fuelled some of the conflict with RNAO over the years. A decade on, the work still provokes both vigorous criticism and praise, even as some of the scenarios imagined in it seem to be unfolding. Interested readers may view the full report at various sites online.

six scenarios for nursing in the year 2020.[16] The scenarios imagined new models for nursing education, for regulation, and for expanded scopes of nursing practice.

The scenarios were designed to provoke attention and get nurses talking, and provoke they certainly did. Responses across the country were rarely lukewarm; they tended to be white hot or ice cold. Nurse leaders in some sectors—especially education and regulation—seemed particularly incensed, but nurses in direct care generally cheered the work. The study was one of the most popular documents ever released by CNA, with more than 230,000 downloads over its first two years, extensive multi-media news coverage, and presentations to more than 12,000 people in every corner of the country. The work is still studied in a number of nursing programs across Canada.

Canadian Nurse Practitioner Initiative

In 2004, CNA was awarded $8.9 million from Health Canada to advance primary health care renewal with the Canadian Nurse Practitioner Initiative (CNPI). Led by a team of six experts and a national advisory committee, the project had a daunting mandate in its short time. It was expected to "facilitate sustained integration of the nurse practitioner role" across the system and develop the mechanisms and processes to support that massive challenge, including role description, competencies, testing, legislation, and regulations in 13 jurisdictions.[17] The team met its goals and more, delivering:

- Legislative and Regulatory Framework for Nurse Practitioners in Canada
- Practice Framework for Nurse Practitioners in Canada
- Education Framework for Nurse Practitioners in Canada
- health human resources planning recommendations
- change management, social marketing, and strategic communications recommendations
- Canadian Nurse Practitioner Core Competency Framework
- Canadian Nurse Practitioner Examination, Family/All Ages, including blueprint, prep guide, and a guidelines, policies, and procedures manual
- Competence Assessment Framework for Nurse Practitioners in Canada
- Prior Learning Assessment and Recognition Framework for Nurse Practitioner Education and Regulation in Canada
- National NP Education Database and Directory of Educational Programs
- Implementation and Evaluation Toolkit for Nurse Practitioners in Canada
- Health Human Resources Planning Simulation Model for Nurse Practitioners in Primary Health Care.™

After years of ups and downs before 2004, more than 4,300 nurse practitioners now are regulated and deployed in every jurisdiction across Canada.

There were significant challenges in implementing the role, of course, and many remain. The resistance of some physicians has been significant, despite evidence that the role is not a threat to patients or to physician practice or salaries. Nurses too, in some quarters, have not lent their unqualified support. Experience with nurse practitioners seems to correlate with a drop in those barriers.

Messaging from nurse practitioners themselves and from champions like CNA has sometimes been confusing to the public, especially in the language of physician replacement. CNA, other organizations, and some individual nurse leaders have continued to promote nurse practitioners, saying they are not a replacement for doctors, while at the same time saying that the public can see a nurse practitioner instead of a doctor, and that the nurse practitioner is an appropriate primary care provider. For most people, that is "replacement." Canadians have made clear in more than a decade of successive opinion polls that the vast majority of them are happy to see whatever provider is appropriate—they just want access to good care. Whether they are interested in abstract, academic explanations of a nursing model or nursing approach to care is doubtful, and nursing at large needs to find ways to simplify and clarify marketing around the role and its purpose.

The NurseONE Portal

To improve access to information for nurses across the country, CNA received $8.1 million from Health Canada from 2006 to 2012 to develop the first initiative of its kind: an online portal to information for nursing education, research, and clinical decision-making. When NurseONE.ca was launched in 2006, its virtual library offered access to more than 550 e-textbooks, more than 3,700 full-text journals, and 200 continuing education modules. Some functions of the NurseONE portal remain in operation today.

Research to Action: Applied Workplace Solutions for Nurses

The Canadian Federation of Nurses Unions (CFNU) received funding from Human Resources and Skills Development Canada in 2006 to implement pilot projects on critical care and emergency nursing in Cape Breton and mentorship in the Regina Qu'Appelle Health Region in Saskatchewan. These successes pushed the organization to imagine a project of much larger scope, ultimately attracting $4.7 million in funding from Health Canada over three years.[18] Managed by the CFNU with a national steering committee, the initiative, Research to Action:

Applied Workplace Solutions for Nurses, partnered with groups including CNA, the Canadian Healthcare Association, and Dietitians of Canada.

Projects in 10 jurisdictions included "implementation of innovative, research-based strategies to enhance the quality of patient care by addressing staffing issues, to offer support to new nursing graduates and newly hired nurses, and to provide opportunities for education and professional development."[19] Each project was expected to be based in a practice setting and to be developed with partners including employers, unions, governments, and other stakeholders. Results were published in a special issue of the *Canadian Journal of Nursing Leadership*; the projects were successful in involving nurses and others in meaningful changes in a wide range of practice settings. The work successfully promoted awareness of, and a deeper understanding of, the links between nurse characteristics and patient and organizational outcomes.

Cultural Competence and Cultural Safety in First Nations, Inuit, and Métis Nursing Education

From 2008 to 2009, the Aboriginal Nurses Association of Canada (now Canadian Indigenous Nurses Association), CASN, and CNA collaborated to produce an integrated review of literature on cultural competence and cultural safety in First Nations, Inuit, and Métis nursing education. Funded under the Aboriginal Health Human Resource Initiative within the First Nations and Inuit Health Branch at Health Canada, the project was undertaken to understand and address nursing education challenges within and around the three groups. Ultimately, the purpose was to develop a best practice framework to "assist educators to foster cultural competence and safety among students and particularly in relation to First Nations within the Inuit and Métis contexts."[20] The report gave rise to the cultural competence framework published later the same year and still in use today. In 2016, CNA and the Canadian Indigenous Nurses[21] Association entered into a partnership accord, reinforcing "their commitment to collaborate on advancing Indigenous nursing and to address the gap between the health of Indigenous and non-Indigenous Canadians."[22] The Canadian Indigenous Nurses Association office is now housed with CNA House in Ottawa.

The National Expert Commission

By 2010, with an eye to the approaching end of the 2004 to 2014 health accord, CNA leaders had begun to consider the best way to position nursing to be meaningfully involved in whatever negotiations might take place around a succeeding accord or other agreement. After deliberating on a number of topics, it was decided that the association would establish a formal commission to make recommendations on health system reform in ways that maximize the contributions of Canada's nurses. The commission represented one of the most significant personal investments of the nurses of Canada in its generation; the work was funded entirely by members with no outside support.

With lessons such as the success of the Canadian Nursing Advisory Committee in mind, it was decided to establish a governance model that would include two co-chairs—one of which was to be a registered nurse—supported by a team of content experts from a variety of disciplines rather than the usual organizational representatives. Marlene Smadu, then a sitting vice president in the International Council of Nurses, an associate dean of nursing, and past assistant deputy minister and principal nurse advisor in Saskatchewan, agreed to serve as the nurse co-chair. Maureen McTeer, an esteemed author, legal scholar, rights advocate, and policy expert agreed to serve as the non-nurse co-chair. McTeer also brought to the commission many years of direct political experience including being a former candidate for federal parliament. Additionally, as the spouse of Joe Clark, she had spent decades immersed in the lived experience of federal politics and policy from the positions of both leadership and opposition.

Between Smadu and McTeer, the commission was set up with broad connections across health care and beyond. Their reputations made the recruitment of an esteemed panel of commissioners very smooth. The commissioners included:

- Marlene Smadu, RN, EdD, Co-Chair
- Maureen M. McTeer, BA, MA, LLB, LLM, LLD (hons), Co-Chair
- The Honourable Sharon Carstairs, PC, BA, MAT, LLD (hons)
- Thomas d'Aquino, BA, JD, LLD, LLM
- Robert G. Evans, OC, PhD
- Robert Fraser, RN, MN
- Francine Girard, RN, PhD
- Vickie Kaminski, RN, BScN, MBA
- Julie Lys, RN, NP, MN
- Sioban Nelson, RN, PhD, FCAHS
- Charmaine Roye, BSc, MDCM, FRCSC
- Heather Smith, RN
- Rachel Bard, RN, MAEd (ex officio)
- Judith Shamian, RN, PhD, LLD (hon), DSci (hon), FAAN (ex officio)
- Michael Villeneuve, RN, MSc (ex officio, executive lead)

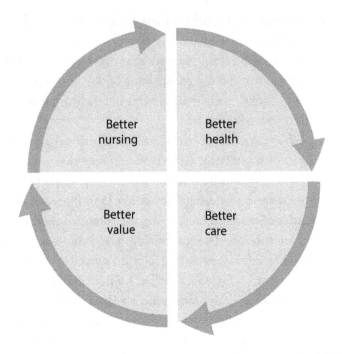

Figure 6.3: Modification of the Triple Aim Model

The commission began its work in June 2011. Although the government announced in December 2011 that there would be no new agreement negotiated to follow the end of the 2004–2014 accord, the work pressed on. In 2011, CNA worked in partnership with the Canadian Medical Association to establish principles to guide the transformation of the health system toward one that is "sustainable and adequately resourced, and provides universal access to quality, patient-centred care delivered along the full continuum of care in a timely and cost-effective manner."[23]

With those principles in mind, and after a year of extensive consultation, research, public polling, and debate, the commission tabled its June 2012 report based on a framework of "better health," "better care," and "better value" after the Institute for Healthcare Improvement's triple aim framework. That framework was developed to describe the key interdependent aims that are considered essential to realizing optimal health system performance.[24] As the Institute describes the "triple aim," the intention is to put forward an integrated approach to:

- improve the patient experience of care (including quality and satisfaction),
- improve the health of populations, and
- reduce the per capita cost of health care.

To those three, a fourth pillar was added in the commission's work: "better nursing," which was intended to refer to the best possible deployment, employment, and engagement of nursing as enabler of the other three elements of the triple aim (see Figure 6.3).

The National Expert Commission offered nine recommendations for action by nurses and about nursing, summarized as follows:[25]

1. Top five in five years
2. Put individuals, families, and communities first
3. Implement primary health care for all
4. Invest strategically in the factors that improve health
5. Pay attention to Canadians at risk of falling behind
6. Think health in all policies
7. Ensure quality and safety in health care
8. Prepare the providers
9. Use technology to its fullest

Within six months, CNA developed 11 project charters to organize responses to the recommendations. The "top five in five" recommendation was intended to

Table 6.3: "Top Five" Goals and Indicators Emerging from National Consensus Meeting, 2013

GOAL	INDICATOR
1. Increase the percentage of primary care practices offering after-hours care.	The percentage of primary care practices having arrangements for after-hours care to see their physician or a nurse.
2. Increase chronic disease case management and navigational capacity in primary care.	The percentage of primary care practices using nurse case managers or navigators for patients with serious chronic conditions.
3. Increase Canadians' access to electronic health information and services.	The percentage of primary care practices offering electronic access for their patients.
4. Reduce hospital admissions for uncontrolled diabetes-related conditions.	All non-maternal hospital discharges (age 15+) with principal diagnosis code for uncontrolled diabetes, without mention of a short-term or long-term complication, in a specified year, per 100,000 population.
5. Reduce the prevalence of childhood obesity.	The percentage of Canadian children between 12 and 17 years of age whose body mass index (BMI) is above a set of age- and sex-specific cut-off points (defined as overweight and obese).

help Canada move toward a top-five ranking among other countries in five health and system outcomes in five years—in time for Canada's 150th birthday in 2017. Commissioners knew well that this was a huge stretch goal, but wanted to push system leaders to rapid, targeted action. In 2013, 32 system experts gathered in a National Consensus Meeting hosted by CNA and, guided by an evidence-driven process, set priorities from among a long roster of possible goals and indicators; they agreed on those shown in Table 6.3.

To follow up other recommendations, CNA held an invitational, pan-Canadian roundtable to lay the groundwork for what would become the *Framework for Registered Nurse Prescribing in Canada*.[26] Another team came together to help develop a screening tool for the Health in All Policies recommendation, which was used during the CNA lobbying day at Parliament Hill in fall 2013. Work focused on safety was led by CFNU, and a national summit co-hosted by CASN and CNA was held to begin the discussion of nursing education reform. Work is ongoing to act on the commission's recommendations.

NOTES ON NURSING EDUCATION REFORM

"In most professions it is taken for granted that better education improves performance but for some strange reason it has been a hard battle to prove this for nurses."

—*Anne-Marie Rafferty, CBE FRCN, Professor of Policy and past Dean, Florence Nightingale School of Nursing and Midwifery, King's College, London*[27]

A few words on reform in nursing education are warranted, since nursing education is, of course, the foundation of everything else nurses do. Without strong, forward-looking nursing education leadership, efforts to strengthen the value, impact, and policy influence of nurses will remain hampered.

Professional registered nursing in Canada evolved after the Nightingale era based on an apprenticeship education model largely housed in hospitals. While many of the programs were able to provide a superb technical training, emphasis was on the *how to* and not always on critical thinking, advocacy, or leadership. In fact, in the earliest days nurses were expected essentially to do the work, stay fairly silent, and not to ask too many questions—especially of physicians or administrators.

The spread of nursing training to so many hospitals, even very small ones, was explained not just by the need for nurses in a growing health care system, but by a growing recognition that student nurses could be deployed to provide so much of the care at little cost—in some cases amounting to indentured labour more than a robust learning experience, as Helen Mussallem observed in a 2008 interview.[28] But that growth in programs came with a cost: beyond the student labour issue, the dubious—or at least uneven—quality and credibility of many programs began to be called into question as early as World War I.

Jean Gunn, who was superintendent of nurses at Toronto General Hospital for over 25 years in the era after Mary Agnes Snively, was already speaking with concern about these issues during her term as president of CNA (1917–1920). Within Ontario she was an important influence on the registration act for nurses, and would go on to be elected first vice president of the International Council of Nurses (1937–1941). Gunn was a lifelong vocal champion of the need for education reform on a global level, believing strongly in the need to separate nursing education from service. Gunn thought then that nursing education should be university based, a position for which she encountered substantial resistance from other nurses.

In part as a result of Gunn's lobbying, Professor G.M. Weir, who was then head of the education department at the University of British Columbia (and later the province's minister of health), was appointed in 1929 to lead a national survey of nursing education. The lead-up to the start of the study was rocky: often ignored (or forgotten) is the fact that the Canadian Medical Association had originally lobbied for the study.[29] This study serves as a glaring example of the pattern in nursing's history of outsiders dominating and developing policy affecting nurses, in this case with almost no nurses involved. Furthermore, difficult relationships between physicians and nurses on a number of fronts were well-known by the mid-1920s—one of which was the perceived creep of nursing into what physicians saw as the exclusive scope of medicine.[30] Thus the involvement of physicians in such a project may not have seemed quite as out of line then as it would now. From our perspective today, it would be unthinkable that nurses, for example, would launch a review of medical education policy and programming in Canada, but the reverse has dogged nursing since its infancy.

Leaders of CNA pushed their way in when the developing nursing education project threatened to proceed without much consultation. Gunn, Mabel Hersey (CNA president, 1928–1930), and other nurse leaders had to insist that nurses be included. In the end, three representatives each from the national medical and nursing associations were appointed under Weir's leadership. Gunn represented nursing along with Jean Browne, from the Canadian Junior Red Cross Society, and Kathleen Russell, a pioneering educator who was then director of the School of Nursing, University of Toronto.

Weir's now famous *Survey of Nursing Education in Canada*—often shortened to the Weir report—was published in 1932 and immediately caused a wave of reaction across the country. It was a damning indictment of the abysmal state of nursing education: in their 2004 review of Canadian nursing education for the National Sector/Occupational Study of Nursing, Pringle, Green, and Johnson summarized Weir as "scathing in his review of practices in many schools at the time, including the practice of admitting students with little if any high school education to schools with no teachers and subsuming any education to the service requirements of the hospitals."[31] Among a host of recommendations, Weir thought nursing should be moved away from hospitals and fully into the education system with the support of government funding. He was unmoved by the protests he'd heard from hospitals, saying that the "training school for nurses provides cheap nursing for the hospital; hence the protests of small, inadequately equipped training schools against closing their schools and staffing them with graduate nurses."[32] Forty years would pass before Weir's vision for nursing education would fully come to life.

By 1936, CNA had generated a proposed curriculum for Canadian nursing schools grounded in Weir's recommendations. But after the initial wave of upset it caused, and the lobbying of visionary nurse leaders who believed in the need to change, in truth there was little uptake of the report given the economic pressures on hospitals and the concomitant need for "respectable" work for women. Cheap labour on the one hand and employment opportunities on the other have been long-standing and powerful forces impeding nursing education reform in Canada.

There were other conferences, meetings, and reports in the decades after the Weir report, and pockets of progress in places like Saskatchewan (so often at the forefront of health system trends), which in 1966 became the first province to transfer authority for hospital schools of nursing from the Department of Public Health to the Department of Education. But the next nurse leader to really take up the education battle with force was Helen Mussallem. She was executive director of CNA from 1963 to 1981, and would become one of Canada's most renowned nurses. Much of her attention from the late 1950s through to the 1970s was focused on nursing education, which she felt had not transformed much, if at all, since the release of the 1932 Weir report. She was relentless in her pursuit of the cause and engendered more than a little irritation along her journey. Mussallem undertook a number of initiatives—often in the face of considerable resistance from nursing practice and education leaders—that culminated in a report on nursing education submitted to the Royal Commission on Health Services in 1965.[33] She had surveyed and studied the nursing programs at 170 hospitals and 16 universities, as well as examining 79 nursing assistant training programs. Building on the Weir work, Mussallem recommended essentially a complete dismantling and revision of existing nursing education such that all hospital programs would be closed and programs would move entirely to colleges and universities.

Introduced in Chapter 3, the Royal Commission on Health Services identified the need to resolve a range of issues including costs, financing, quality of
health care, and the health human resources to support the system. The CNA had
been active throughout the lead-up to and execution of the Commission, with its
past president, Alice Girard, sitting as a member. Girard was a formidable force
in Canadian nursing in her own right. At the time of the Commission she was
the inaugural dean of the first Faculty of Nursing in the country, at Université de
Montréal, where she was also also breaking gender barriers as that university's
first female dean. The brief by CNA made 25 recommendations to improve nursing services in order to strengthen the nation's health care systems. Commission
chair Emmett Hall was in support of CNA's recommendations to steer students
into new, two-year diploma schools to provide more technically focused bedside
nurses, while those who were more academically inclined would be streamed into
university programs aimed at educating nurses equipped to take on leadership
roles in teaching and administration.

In the meantime, Mussallem was ruthless in her condemnation of the inertia
in nursing education, which she felt was not meeting the needs of Canadians, a
problem she thought could have been avoided if the recommendations of Weir
and other studies since its publication had been acted on.[34] But despite alienat-
ing some nurses and other leaders, Mussallem's report and her aggressive lobby
efforts, backed by the Royal Commission on Health Services, would prove to be
transformative. Most Canadian nursing education finally moved—grudgingly in
many cases—out of hospitals and into community colleges and universities across
Canada during the 1960s and early 1970s (although some provinces retained some
hospital programs into the 1990s).

University schools of nursing had existed since the first program in the British
Empire was established at the University of British Columbia in 1919. In 1920,
Dalhousie University established the first Canadian program in public health
nursing, and McGill University started the first Canadian nursing program in
teaching and supervision. But it would be 1933, at the University of Toronto, before a baccalaureate degree in nursing would be offered independently under the
complete control of a university. The first master's degree in nursing was offered at
the University of Western Ontario (1959) and the first nursing PhD program at the
University of Alberta (1991).

For most of the 20th century, only a tiny minority of registered nurses were
university educated. The movement to require a baccalaureate degree to enter registered nurse practice began in earnest during the late 1970s, and with a 1982 decision by the CNA board of directors, the push was on in all provinces (other than
Quebec) to require the degree by the year 2000. Resolutions were tabled at CNA

meetings starting during the 1970s around the degree as a minimal entry to practice, as well as the need to establish master's- and doctoral-level nursing programs
in Canada, and those now are in place across the country. Today, Quebec remains
the only outlier, maintaining a college-level diploma in nursing as the minimal
entry-to-practice requirement.

These evolutions in nursing education were driven in part to position nurses
and their education in line with other leading health professions. But the larger
imperative was the need for nurses to be educated to respond effectively to the
shifting health needs of Canadians, and also to the changing location, pace, complexity, and increasing specialization of health care services. It is disconcerting
that, when resources are tight, some provincial governments still sometimes discuss the option of rolling back registered nurse education to the diploma level, or
shortening the baccalaureate program.

It is now more than 50 years since the last comprehensive review of nursing
education in Canada. Despite the significant social change and upheaval of the past
25 years, recent calls for a comprehensive review of nursing education at the national
level have gone unanswered. The CASN launched a new accreditation program for
schools of nursing in 2007, but the push for more disruptive education leadership has
grown stronger though the years of system reform. Concerns about a number of aspects of nursing education have been expressed in system reviews and reports across
the United Kingdom, the United States, and Canada, including from the National
Expert Commission, which included four senior nursing educators, three of them
university nursing deans, amongst its members.

Change has begun to emerge in small pockets, as it tends to do. The first nurse
leader to respond forcefully to the National Expert Commission's call was Kathleen
MacMillan, then director of the nursing school at Dalhousie University. In the fall
of 2012, she held a small think tank on nursing education and published a report
urging action on reforms discussed by the participants.[35] In 2013, Nova Scotia began a review of undergraduate nursing education across its three schools of nursing
(Dalhousie University, St. Francis Xavier University, and Cape Breton University),
and in 2015, published its plan, *Building Our Future—A New, Collaborative Model
for Undergraduate Nursing Education in Nova Scotia.*[36] In May 2015, the minister
of health and wellness announced $4.7 million in funding for nursing, noting that
"the three Nova Scotia universities that grant nursing degrees will offer a common
curriculum and accelerated programs" as was recommended in the report of the
education review.[37] As one example of action on this strategy, St. Francis Xavier
University and Cape Breton University collaborated "to determine a pathway that
will offer qualified LPNs [licensed practical nurses] block credit for their prior education and work experience and bridging courses that would allow them to apply

to our Accelerated BScN Program."[38] The School of Nursing at St. Francis Xavier University targeted May 2017 for the admission of students to the first offering of the accelerated "LPN to BScN" program.

Scope and Turf Conflict within Nursing

In some ways, nursing is more mired today than ever before in the registered nurse versus licensed practical nurse quandary, distracting nurses from more urgent policy work. Some registered nurses have levelled ongoing accusations of scope creep on the part of licensed nurses (and even sometimes of personal support workers), who they say, based on evidence, are not safe to deliver certain aspects of care. Some have accused government and other health human resources decision makers of deliberately jeopardizing public safety by deploying non-registered nurse staff in the interest of saving money. The intra-nursing battle has attracted negative public and media attention, such as when a Canadian Broadcasting Company (CBC) headline in Saskatchewan blurted "Unhappy nurses vote to turf RN association leaders"[39] after registered nurses there alleged that licensed practical nurses were practicing beyond their scope. The dispute drew significant public attention in the province and more broadly when Steven Lewis put the blame squarely on the Saskatchewan Union of Nurses—whose members also belong to the Saskatchewan Registered Nurses' Association—saying they had been "on the warpath" over scope of practice changes that everyone else knew had occurred.[40] He sided with the practical nurses, accusing the Saskatchewan Union of Nurses of offering up no evidence and engaging in what amounted to "a war over turf and jobs."

Licensed practical nurse leaders have responded to these situations in frustration, pointing to the expanding depth and breadth of practical nurse education, and saying registered nurses are deliberately suppressing the practice of others based on self-interests, not evidence—just as registered nurses and nurse practitioners have accused physicians of doing. Furthermore, they have argued that licensed practical nurses are safe, effective, and cost-efficient providers in many areas across the continuum of health care and ask that evidence, not emotion, guide staffing decisions.

Evidence from the body of research connecting registered nurse entry-to-practice education, experience, expertise, and numbers to outcomes, including morbidity and mortality, is indeed compelling. But the evidence is not all in, and even some of the most robust studies on nurse outcomes have been challenged on certain methodological issues—self-reported data, for example. While it seems increasingly clear that better educated nurses with the right expertise and in the right numbers make a dramatic difference to patient experiences, quality, and safety, the limits of the impact of registered nurses on such outcomes is uncertain. But at least one study has taken on that question: in a retrospective, cross-sectional study looking at hospital data linking educational preparation of nurses with patient mortality published in 2016, the researchers found (like other studies, discussed in Chapters 8 and 12) that baccalaureate nurse education did indeed have an indirect correlation with mortality. However, they also found that above a baccalaureate nurse staffing level of about 70 per cent, there appeared to be "no additional decrease in mortality rates."[41] If these findings are replicated across different countries and settings, they may inform staff mix and optimal staffing levels that could respond to both safety and costs, leaving room for other, less costly providers.

In May 2016, RNAO stirred controversy within the Ontario nursing family with its report, *Mind the Safety Gap in Health System Transformation: Reclaiming the Role of the RN*.[42] Among its recommendations, the association urged Ontario's minister of health and long-term care and the province's Local Health Integration Networks to "issue a moratorium on nursing skill mix changes until a comprehensive interprofessional HHR plan is completed." At the same time, however, the association recommended legislation of an all–registered nurse workforce "within two years for tertiary, quaternary and cancer centres ... and within five years for large community hospitals"[43] and laid out the staff mix expected in long-term care.

Media coverage again revealed the divisive language and tone within nursing.[44] The Registered Practical Nurses Association of Ontario responded, saying that its members are regulated and safe to provide the care they are assigned. Executive Director Dianne Martin went on to say, "Tightening resources and increasing care demands are forcing health-care organizations to take a hard look at what roles each health provider is best suited for as they work to ensure there are enough people to look after patients." She concluded by observing that, "It's in the best interest of every organization and the patients they serve to make sure everyone is using the full extent of their knowledge, skills and judgment."[45] In recorded comments shared through social media, Martin called for collaboration, noting the uncomfortable timing of the report's release during National Nursing Week.[46] She accused RNAO of a "full-out attack on registered practical nurses" and expressed concern with what was perceived as a disingenuous interpretation of some of the data by RNAO. While bemoaning public intra-professional conflicts, Martin eventually responded to the RNAO in a July 2016 *Hospital News* column addressed largely to fellow care providers and sharing the views presented here.[47]

The long-standing divide between the two regulated nursing groups in Ontario, further fuelled by RNAO's choices of language and timing, shows no sign of waning despite calls for collaboration and unity in the interests of patients and nurses. It stands in sharp contrast to the generally collaborative, coalition-building approach that seems to characterize nursing in British Columbia.

SUMMARY AND IMPLICATIONS

Nurses in Canada have been active participants in policy development since Jeanne Mance began her work in the 1600s. The most prominent thread in the public policy work of nurses has been advocacy to achieve what we now call the *triple aim* of better population health, better quality of care, and better value for public dollars. Since the beginning, nurses have been vociferous advocates of the belief that health is a basic human right—and access to health care should be universally based on need and not the ability to pay. Beyond health care, nurses have been effective activists from municipal to national levels in the full range of other determinants of health, including housing and homelessness, food and water, income (e.g., a basic living wage and security in old age), education, and discrimination based on race, culture, and gender. In short, nurses typically have aligned strongly with some of the most vulnerable people in society.

Occasional accusations of self-interest have been levelled at nursing organizations (e.g., more nurses mean more paying members), and unions have perhaps suffered more from that charge than professional associations. However, a growing body of evidence amassed by nurse scientists and other researchers showing the links among nurse education, expertise, staffing patterns, and outcomes will perhaps serve to dampen down that challenge (see Chapter 8). The ongoing high public trust accorded to nurses may suggest that Canadians either don't pay much attention to those allegations or simply don't care about them.

While nursing organizations have informed governments since the earliest days, the public policy work of nursing has escalated considerably in its visibility and sophistication over the past 20 years. The health accords of 2000, 2003, and 2004 were all informed by nursing, and the work of the profession has moved from stand-alone reports to more strategic programs of policy, and even to a formal national commission funded entirely by nurses themselves through their membership in CNA. Collaboration and partnerships are now a normal part of smart policy work by nursing. The decision late in 2015 by CFNU, with CNA as a partner, to draft key elements of a new health accord before the country's ministers of health had their first meeting with a new federal health minister (see Chapter 11) took the policy work of nursing to a new level. The consultative and less centralized stance of the Justin Trudeau government may bode well for nurses' influence on public policy in the course of its mandate.

DISCUSSION QUESTIONS

1. What lessons have we learned from major health systems and nursing

reform reports that could make the best use of nursing across health systems?

2. A generalist baccalaureate degree is required to practice in all Canadian jurisdictions outside Quebec, but most nurses will enter practice directly into specialized settings. How effective is the generalist degree in preparing nurses to enter that practice reality? What areas should be changed or strengthened?

3. Should specialty certification or some other credential be required of all nurses employed in specialty practice settings? Defend your position.

4. What mix of regulated nurses is appropriate for Canadian health care in this century?

5. What should be the key elements of scope(s) of practice regulating nurses and how can we optimize them? How should scopes change, if at all?

6. Should nursing reform include standardized scopes of practice across all jurisdictions? Why or why not?

ADDITIONAL POLICY RESOURCES

NURSING REFORM DOCUMENTS	
Nursing Strategy for Canada	http://www.hc-sc.gc.ca/hcs-sss/pubs/nurs-infirm/2000-nurs-infirm-strateg/index-eng.php
Our Health Our Future: Final Report of the Canadian Nursing Advisory Committee	http://www.hc-sc.gc.ca/hcs-sss/pubs/nurs-infirm/2002-cnac-cccsi-final/index-eng.php
Toward 2020: Visions for Nursing	http://www.cdha.nshealth.ca/system/files/sites/125/documents/towards-2020-visions-nursing-full-document.pdf
Building the Future: An Integrated Strategy for Nursing Human Resources in Canada (Final Report of the National Occupational/Sector Study of Nursing)	https://www.cna-aiic.ca/~/media/cna/page-content/pdf-fr/simulation_analysis_report_e.pdf?la=en
Nurse Practitioners: The Time is Now: A Solution to Improving Access and Reducing Wait Times in Canada	http://www.npnow.ca/docs/tech-report/section1/01_Integrated_Report.pdf
Tested Solutions for Eliminating Canada's Registered Nurse Shortage	https://www.cna-aiic.ca/~/media/cna/page-content/pdf-en/rn_highlights_e.pdf?la=en
Registered Nurses: On the Front Lines of Wait Times	https://www.cna-aiic.ca/~/media/cna/page-content/pdf-en/wait_times_paper_2009_e.pdf?la=en
Principles to Guide Health Care Transformation in Canada	https://www.cna-aiic.ca/~/media/cna/files/en/guiding_principles_hc_e.pdf

A Nursing Call to Action: The Health of Our Nation, The Future of Our Health System (Final Report of the National Expert Commission)	http://www.cna-aiic.ca/expertcommission/
Research to Action: Applied Workplace Solutions for Nurses	http://www.thinknursing.ca/rta
Building Our Future: A New, Collaborative Model for Undergraduate Nursing Education in Nova Scotia	http://novascotia.ca/dhw/nurses/ documents/Registered-Nurse-Education-Review-in-Nova-Scotia-Highlights.pdf
Framework for Registered Nurse Prescribing in Canada	http://www.cna-aiic.ca/~/media/cna/ page-content/pdf-en/cna-rn-prescribing-framework_e.pdf?la=en

NURSING ETHICS

Duncan, S., Thorne, S., & Rodney, P. (2015). Evolving trends in nurse regulation: What are the policy impacts for nursing's social mandate? *Nursing Inquiry, 22*(1), 27–38.

Liaschenko, J., & Peter, E. (2016). Fostering nurses' moral agency and moral identity: The importance of moral communities. *Hastings Center Report, 46*(5), 2–5.

Rodney, P., Buckley, B., Street, A., Serano, E., & Martin, L.A. (2013). The moral climate of nursing practice: Inquiry and action. In J. Storch, P. Rodney, & R. Starzomski (Eds.), *Toward a moral horizon: Nursing ethics in leadership and practice* (2nd ed., pp. 188–214). Don Mills, ON: Pearson Education Canada.

Tronto, J.C. (2010). Creating caring institutions: Politics, plurality, and purpose. *Ethics and Social Welfare, 4*(2), 158–171.

CHAPTER 7

Making Sense of the Dollars: Understanding the Basic Economics of Canadian Health Care

CHAPTER HIGHLIGHTS

- Introduction
- The Flow of Funds to Pay for Health Care
- The Use of Health Care Dollars Nationally
- Health Care Spending in Other Countries
- Summary and Implications
- Discussion Questions
- Additional Policy Resources

LEARNING OUTCOMES

1. Demonstrate a basic knowledge of health system financing and spending by Canadians.
2. Describe key sources of federal, provincial/territorial, and municipal government resources.
3. Describe examples of the main categories of expenditures of federal, provincial/territorial, and municipal governments.
4. Discuss the differences between public and private health care financing, costs, and spending.
5. Discuss the implications of health systems funding, costs, and remuneration for nurses in Canada.

Policy Influencer: Stephen LeClair

Stephen LeClair, BA (Econ), MA (Econ), is an economist originally from the Ottawa Valley who was appointed in March 2015 as Ontario's first financial accountability officer. LeClair's distinguished public service career saw him take on senior roles in the governments of Ontario, Alberta, the Northwest Territories, Yukon, and Canada. Throughout his career his interests and roles have led him to have an impact on health and nursing policy. After serving as the Special Economic and Fiscal Advisor to the deputy minister of finance in the Northwest Territories, LeClair was recruited to the newly minted federal Office of Nursing Policy in 1999 as its first employee and the senior advisor to Canada's chief nurse. In that role he was influential in conducting research and shaping the messaging of the office to place the agenda of nurses' health and wellness firmly at the centre of national health human resources policy development. In a later role with Health Canada, LeClair worked on the 10-Year Plan to Strengthen Health Care and its follow-up reporting. He went on to Alberta, where he assumed the roles of executive director, strategic policy, and for six years during and following the 2008 recession, assistant deputy minister, budget and fiscal policy. In this role, LeClair was responsible for economics, fiscal policy, federal/provincial/territorial relations, and in part for Alberta's budget. In all his positions he has remained a friend of nurses; he keeps engaged and informed about nursing and health care and has brought his extensive experience with and around nurses to bear in the wide-reaching fiscal decisions for which he has been accountable.

"The first lesson of economics is scarcity: there is never enough of anything to fully satisfy all those who want it. The first lesson of politics is to disregard the first lesson of economics."

—*Thomas Sowell, Senior Fellow, The Hoover Institution, Stanford University*

INTRODUCTION

Health care costs and the fiscal sustainability of health systems are perennial topics of angst that support an entire sector of science and policy in Canada. There is good reason for this: as Birch and colleagues said in 2015, independent of changes in the political stripes of different governments, "continued growth in total health care expenditure and the proportion of public spending absorbed by health care strain the capacity of governments to continue funding universal, comprehensive health care."[1]

Economics and the whole fiscal side of health care is an area where nurses and other providers sometimes have dropped the ball in policy work. Health care professionals often can provide compelling emotional arguments for or against any particular policy—and sometimes can also provide solid clinical evidence in support. But while speaking the language of high costs and waste in health care, when a health or finance minister says that a new idea sounds convincing and asks about the cost, timing, and return on investment, then sometimes the answers are less certain. As the discipline and the profession of nursing advance, it is important to build a stronger understanding of economics and how those variables are woven into the development of public policy.

Health Economics

If one speaks of the economics of any given project, typically reference is being made fairly narrowly to cost, sometimes really referring to the resources or revenue, and/or the project budget. However, despite its reputation, the broader concept of the study of economics is not all about mathematics, numbers, or even dollars. In fact, in July 2011, Bob Evans—founding director of the Centre for Health Service Policy and Research at the University of British Columbia—said to delegates during the 8th World Congress on Health Economics in Toronto that "if an economist is giving a speech and puts mathematical equations on a slide, then you know she or he doesn't understand economics."[2] He was deliberately being a bit cheeky, but his underlying message was important: economics is not a purely mathematics or statistical discipline; it's a relationships discipline. Economics is about developing an understanding of the relationships among things, one of which is fiscal costs and how they link to inputs, other resources, allocation decisions, and outcomes in any given market or system.

More formally, Merriam-Webster defines the discipline as "a social science concerned chiefly with description and analysis of the production, distribution, and consumption of goods and services."[3] As implied in the name, *health economics* moves the study to focus on all these variables within or related to health care and health systems. The Centre for Health Services Policy and Research describes health economics as "the study of how scarce resources are allocated among alternative uses for the care of sickness and the promotion, maintenance and improvement of health, including the study of how health care and health-related services, their costs and benefits, and health itself are distributed among individuals and groups in society."[4] This chapter focuses on what Canadians spend on health care, and in Chapter 8 we turn to the returns on those investments.

THE FLOW OF FUNDS TO PAY FOR HEALTH CARE

As introduced earlier in this text, payment for health care in Canada comes from a mix of public and private sector sources. At about 70 per cent and 30 per cent respectively, the national public-private split has been fairly constant over the past 20 years, never varying by more than 1 per cent in either direction (see Figure 7.1). On the public side, Canada operates a single payer system, run by the government in each jurisdiction. Despite criticisms of health care in Canada, our administrative costs are low compared to similarly wealthy nations. As Palmer discussed, "Multi-payer systems are administratively complex and expensive, explaining why the U.S. health insurance industry spends about 18 per cent of its health care dollars on billing and insurance-related administration for its many private plans, compared to just 2 per cent in Canada for our streamlined single payer insurance plans."[5] More urgent than cost, she argued, is the split in equity around access to care—a strong value in the Canadian system, and one of the biggest challenges now facing countries that have adopted multi-payer systems."

For governments to invest in public programs such as health care and public education, of course, they must first generate funds. In Canada, public health care services are funded by a mix of federal, provincial, territorial, and municipal

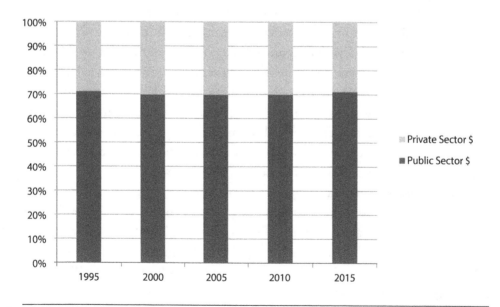

Figure 7.1: Public and Private Health Care Spending in Canada

Source: Canadian Institute for Health Information. (2015). *National health expenditure trends, 1975 to 2015.* Ottawa: CIHI.

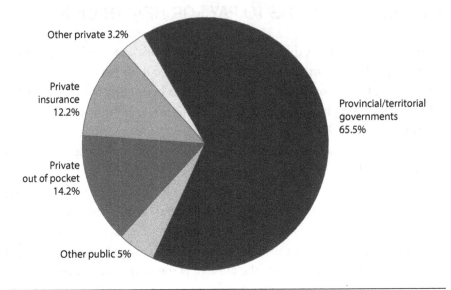

Figure 7.2: Sources of Public and Private Health Care Financing in Canada, 2014

Source: Canadian Institute for Health Information. (2015). National health expenditure trends, 1975 to 2015. Ottawa: CIHI.

governments, so it is important for nurses to develop an understanding of the way monies are collected and spent. Sources of health care financing in Canada are broken down at a high level in Figure 7.2. At 65.5 per cent of total (public plus private) financing, the largest portion of health care costs falls on the public sector side to the provinces and territories. A smaller portion—roughly 5 per cent—is financed by other public sector actors including federal and municipal governments, and through contributions from Social Security Funds. Direct federal contributions in this latter category are outside of and in addition to those made to the provinces and territories through the Canada Health Transfer.

On the private side, payment may be made directly by consumers, out of pocket, for the full costs of any given service, and/or costs may be offset fully or partially through private insurance schemes—a workplace dental or drug plan, for example. Expenses in the "other private" category include costs for non-consumption items that may include capital expenditures for private facilities and health research, for example.[6]

Private, out-of-pocket payment to a dentist or massage therapist, for example, is fairly straightforward. Fees are posted or negotiated, and the client or patient makes a payment. But how that payment relates to costs of the actual hands-on service, payment of other staff (a dental assistant, for example), and to the operation and maintenance of the physical facilities is much less clear. So the flow of dollars paid for services rendered in either of the public or private sectors can be tough to follow. As a result, statistics around the costs of health care can be spun—exasperatingly so at times—to fit a number of storylines. What any given health care service costs, what Canadians actually pay for it, and what it is worth may be three distinctive issues.

Public Sector Financing of Health Care

In a system where health care is often touted to be free, following the trails of public sector costs and spending can be especially perplexing. The task is made even more daunting by the scale of the health systems and number of players involved in funding and delivering care. So before exploring spending patterns further, it is important to understand the sources of revenue that allow governments to fund public health care.

The proportion of spending on the public side of health care breaks down as shown in Table 7.1, based on 2012 data.[7] The various sources of financing are discussed in the ensuing sections.

Federal Government Revenues and Expenditures

Figure 7.3 shows the main sources of federal government revenue as reported by Finance Canada for fiscal year 2013–2014.[8] As the figures reveal, federal income tax remains the greatest source of revenue for the federal government, followed by corporate taxes, the Goods and Services Tax (GST), and other taxes, fees, and duties. Together these sources generated $271.7 billion.

During the fiscal year 2013–2014, the federal government committed to spend $276.8 billion, resulting in a $5.1 billion federal budgetary deficit. Successive

Table 7.1: Public Sector Financing of Health Care in Canada

SOURCE OF FINANCING	$ MILLIONS	%
Provincial/territorial governments	134,655	92.8
Federal government (direct)	6,846.2	4.7
Social Security funds*	2,735.6	1.9
Municipal governments	871.4	0.6
Total	*145,108.2*	*100*

*Social Security funds include Worker's Compensation Boards and Quebec Drug Insurance contributions.

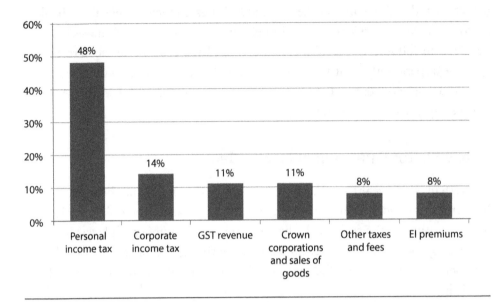

Figure 7.3: Main Sources of Federal Government Revenue, Canada, 2013–2014

Source: Department of Finance Canada. (2014). *Your tax dollar: 2013–2014 fiscal year.* Ottawa: Department of Finance Canada. Retrieved from http://www.fin.gc.ca/tax-impot/2014/html-eng.asp.

budgetary deficits contribute to the cumulative federal debt. Spending in 2013–2014 fell under three categories—transfer payments, program expenses, and public debt—in the proportions shown in Figure 7.4.

Table 7.2 (see page 206) lists examples of programs falling under each category of spending and shows the proportion of spending allocated to various programs. At 29 per cent, the largest category of federal spending is for government operations, including more than 130 departments (ministries), agencies, and other arms of the federal government. After government operations, the largest categories of spending are for direct payments to individuals through programs such as Old Age Security and Employment Insurance (26 per cent), and then transfers to the provinces and territories (22 per cent).

Half of all federal transfers to provinces and territories are targeted to health care (11 per cent of total federal spending). For the sake of comparison, that proportion is the same as the combined total spent by the federal government on national defence (8 per cent, including the Armed Forces) and public safety (3 per cent, including the Royal Canadian Mounted Police, federal prisons, and border security) combined.

The federal government also makes a number of direct transfers to organizations

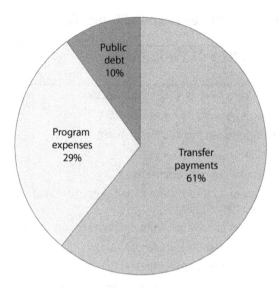

Figure 7.4: Categories of Federal Government Expenditures, Canada, 2013–2014

Source: Department of Finance Canada. (2014). *Your tax dollar: 2013–2014 fiscal year.* Ottawa: Department of Finance Canada. Retrieved from http://www.fin.gc.ca/tax-impot/2014/html-eng.asp.

that support health care. Although it poses no conditions on the provinces, "direct spending in areas of provincial jurisdiction has proven to be somewhat more contentious" than the conditional block transfers.[9] As introduced earlier in this text, direct funding that bypasses provinces but is directed to programs or services they already fund can be problematic. The fiscal value of those direct transfers may be significant: as shown in Table 7.1, they represented 4.7 per cent of public sector health care financing in 2012.[10]

Despite frequent criticism among Canadians about the dollars spent on Parliament—sometimes heightened in the wake of reports of spending irregularities or salary increases—the total operation of Parliament costs less than a quarter of 1 per cent of all spending. Those costs include all salaries (senators, members of Parliament, and staff) and operations of all facilities and services.

A Few Words About the Federal Spending Power

The federal government makes a number of conditional and non-conditional transfers to the provinces and territories. Equalization payments are an example of a non-conditional transfer of federal funds, intended to somewhat level the playing field between more and less affluent provinces—the *have* and *have-not* provinces

Table 7.2: Federal Government Expenditures, Canada, 2013–2014

CATEGORY OF SPENDING	EXAMPLES OF PROGRAMS	PROPORTION OF SPENDING
1. Transfer payments	Cash payments directly to individuals • Old Age Security payments (15%) • Guaranteed Income Supplement • Allowance for Spouses • Employment Insurance (6%) • Canada Child Tax Benefit and Universal Child Care Benefit (5%)	26%
	Transfers to provincial and territorial governments • Canada Health Transfer (11%) • Canada Social Transfer (5%) • Equalization payments and Territorial Formula Financing program (6%)	22%
	Other transfer programs to individuals, governments, and other organizations and groups • First Nations and Aboriginal peoples • Assistance to farmers and other food producers • Foreign aid and other international assistance • Research and development, infrastructure, regional development, and assistance to businesses • Student assistance programs, health research and promotion, the arts, amateur sports, and multiculturalism and bilingualism	13%
2. Program expenses	Operations of government • Government services and programs (26%) • Crown Corporations (3%) • Parliament (less than 0.0025%)	29%
3. Public debt	Interest charges, debt repayment	10%

Source: Department of Finance Canada. (2014). *Your tax dollar: 2013–2014 fiscal year.* Ottawa: Department of Finance Canada. Retrieved from http://www.fin.gc.ca/tax-impot/2014/html-eng.asp.

as they have come to be described. The federal government has intervened in the provincial health care field by using its constitutional spending power, which enables it to make a financial contribution to certain programs under provincial jurisdiction, generally subject to provincial compliance with certain requirements.[11] Federal medicare financing has evolved into block transfers that must meet the conditions of the Canada Health Act, but otherwise are unconditional.[12]

In 2013, the Health Action Lobby joined a chorus of other voices across the country saying that federal government was "steadily distancing itself from dealing with health care challenges and pays insufficient attention to health, although it has considerable responsibility for different aspects of it and the resources, ability and public support to play a role."[13] In its original form, medicare was a 50:50 cost-shared program between federal and provincial/territorial governments. It was under the government of Pierre Trudeau that the retreat from that funding commitment began, replaced in 1977 with the Established Programs Financing Act, the first of a series of block funding models tying increases in conditional grants to GDP.

In his final report, Commissioner Romanow said, "The importance of this change was that after EPF, provincial expenditures on health that exceeded the rate of economic growth and population change were borne exclusively by provincial governments, thus providing the federal government with the predictability it sought in terms of its own expenditures."[14] For the provinces, the program meant more flexibility in use of the funds because they were not targeted just to hospitals and physicians. As the federal government dropped its tax rates, provinces were able to increase theirs. The funding formula provided 50 per cent of the value of the program in the form of a cash transfer, and the remaining half through tax points that were tied to economic growth and equalized to the average across the country.

In 1997, when he was finance minister, Paul Martin, Jr. engineered the Canada Health and Social Transfer, which brought existing federal cash and tax transfers for health care, post-secondary education, and social services and assistance together into a single block transfer.[15] That change led to immediate and significant cuts in transfer payments and a 1 per cent drop in national health spending as a proportion of GDP. As a condition of the 2003 accord, that block-funding mechanism was unbundled in 2004 when Martin was prime minister, becoming the separate Canada Health Transfer and Canada Social Transfer.

The Harper government's announcement in 2011 that the Canada Health Transfer would increase by 6 per cent per annum from 2014 until 2017, after which the formula would be tied to GDP growth, dashed hopes of a renewed health care accord. Combined with a record of distancing itself from health care discussions with the provinces, the decision caused a predictable uproar in most health sectors across Canada. Among nursing organizations, CFNU was especially aggressive in its investigation of the fiscal implications of that policy decision. In a report for CFNU, Mackenzie remarked, "It is easy to get lost in numbers of dollars, in the millions and billions that are difficult to comprehend, and whose significance is difficult to measure against Canadians' direct experience."[16] He concluded that, during the 10 years of the 2004–2014 accord, "federal funding recovered from a low of just over 11 per cent to 23 per cent of provincial and territorial health expenditures." The CFNU has called repeatedly for that funding level to be raised to 25 per cent; in January 2016, in its first meeting with the federal, provincial, and territorial health ministers after the October 2015 federal election, the CFNU pushed the recommendation that federal funding reach 25 per cent by 2025— more on that policy work is cited in Module III.

In an opening message to Mackenzie's report, CFNU president Linda Silas noted that "instead of a shortfall of 36 billion in 10 years, as previously predicted, provinces and territories will lose 43.5 billion in only eight years."[17] Commenting on the study, former Parliamentary Budgetary Officer Kevin Page concluded that "the current arrangements are no longer supporting the Canada Health Act, and Hugh Mackenzie's analysis shows the situation may be even worse than previous studies had predicted."[18] Tholl and his colleagues concluded that the current situation was unsustainable by the provinces. Released in the same month as the CFNU report by Mackenzie, the report of the Advisory Panel on Innovation appointed by the federal government expressed similar concerns about the federal role, concluding that commendable provincial and organizational "efforts to improve healthcare and augment its value are limited in part by a serious shortfall in working capital, and the absence of a cadre of dedicated and expert personnel who can support efforts to initiate and scale-up improvements in healthcare across Canada."[19]

Provincial and Territorial Government Revenues and Expenditures

Provinces and territories generate revenue through taxation, transfers from the federal government (including equalization payments), licenses and fees, and a range of business and non-tax sources that may include, for example, casinos, liquor sales, and public lotteries. In addition to sources of revenue that a province might generate, territorial revenues depend heavily on the federal government. Recall from the earlier discussion of governance that the territories are different from provinces in that they have a direct governance relationship with the federal government and not the Crown. A fiscal transfer program called Territorial Formula Financing helps to provide residents of the three northern territories with a range of public services that the territorial governments could not possibly provide with internal financing. While not entirely comparable to services in large cities in the south, there is at least an attempt to reconcile the geographic isolation through financial injections by the federal government that allow taxation levels of the population to remain bearable.[20]

The breakdown of sources of revenue for Ontario for the interim 2013–2014 fiscal year serves as a good example of provincial revenue categories—see Figure 7.5.

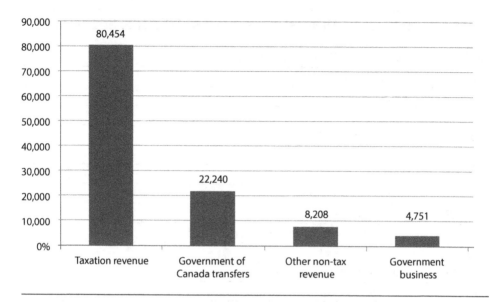

Figure 7.5: Revenue by Source ($ Millions), Government of Ontario, 2013–2014 (interim)

Source: Ontario Ministry of Finance. (2014). *2014 Ontario budget, chapter II: Ontario's economic outlook and fiscal plan.* Toronto: Ontario Ministry of Finance. Retrieved from http://www.fin.gov. on.ca/en/budget/ontariobudgets/2014/ch2f.html.

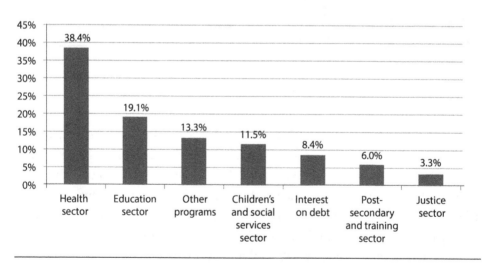

Figure 7.6: Composition of Total Expenses, Government of Ontario, 2014–2015

Source: Ontario Ministry of Finance. (2014). *2014 Ontario budget, chapter II: Ontario's economic outlook and fiscal plan.* Toronto: Ontario Ministry of Finance. Retrieved from http://www.fin.gov. on.ca/en/budget/ontariobudgets/2014/ch2f.html.

Table 7.3: Expenses ($ Millions), Government of Ontario, 2013–2014

EXPENSE	MINISTRY/PROGRAM AREA
48,766.7	Health and Long-Term Care
23,845.7	Education
10,556.0	Interest on debt
10,062.6	Community and Social Services
7,604.7	Training, Colleges and Universities
6,117.1	Other expenses
4,023.0	Children and Youth Services
2,774.3	Transportation
2,347.3	Community Safety and Correctional Services
1,829.5	Attorney General
1,333.5	Tourism, Culture and Sport
947.2	Finance
878.9	Government Services
871.5	Economic Development, Trade and Employment/Research and Innovation
854.3	Agriculture and Food/Rural Affairs
837.3	Municipal Affairs and Housing
757.6	Northern Development and Mines
715.0	Natural Resources
1,829.6	All other ministries and services
126,952	Total expenses ($ millions)

Source: Ontario Ministry of Finance. (2014). *2014 Ontario budget, chapter II: Ontario's economic outlook and fiscal plan.* Toronto: Ontario Ministry of Finance. Retrieved from http://www.fin.gov. on.ca/en/budget/ontariobudgets/2014/ch2f.html

In Ontario's interim budget for that year, total revenue was approximately $115.7 billion. However, the government committed to spend $127 billion, thereby generating a shortfall, or provincial budgetary deficit, of about $11.3 billion. Mirroring the federal situation, that deficit added further to Ontario's cumulative provincial debt. Spending in the budget was allocated in seven categories, shown in Figure 7.6 and expanded in Table 7.3 to show spending for key programs and services.

Notice here that at roughly $48.8 billion, health care was set to consume 38.4 per cent of government spending in Ontario in 2013–2014. As Figure 7.7 shows, provincial and territorial health spending as a proportion of total expenses (projected for 2014) varies considerably across the country. Figures may differ from provincial budget calculations depending on expenses included—for example, whether or not a portion of debt repayment is factored into the costs.

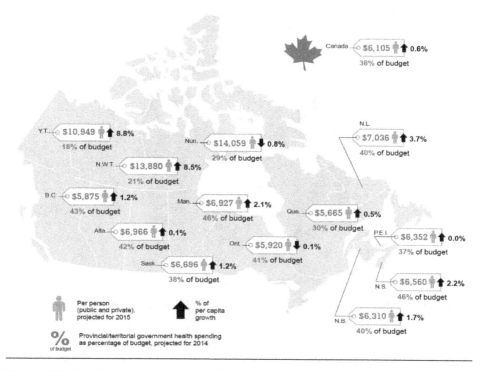

Figure 7.7: Health Spending As a Proportion of Total Provincial/Territorial Government Budgets Projected for 2014

Source: Canadian Institute for Health Information. (2015). *National health expenditure trends, 1975 to 2015.* Ottawa: CIHI, p. 17.

Municipal Governments

Municipal sources of revenue and their program expenses vary considerably within and across provinces and territories. Compounded by differing definitions of those categories of expenses, direct comparisons are difficult. And since funds may be received from provincial and federal governments to support various aspects of programs and services (including public health), caution must be exercised to avoid double-counting health care costs and financing sources.

Because Ontario government revenue and expenditures were cited as examples in this chapter, revenue and expenses for the City of Toronto, Ontario (population 2.6 million in 2011), are cited here as an example. Figure 7.8 shows revenue sources for Toronto, which combined to a total of $9.6 billion.

Main expenditures for the City of Toronto are listed in Table 7.4 in descending order of cost. With expenses totalling $9.6 billion, the budget for 2014 was balanced. While aspects of health care may be buried in other categories when one takes into account broader determinants of health (e.g., housing, children's services), the city

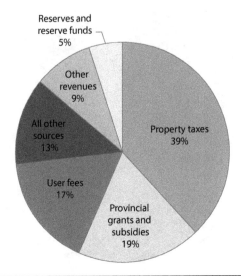

Figure 7.8: Sources of Revenue, City of Toronto Operating Budget, 2014

Source: Adapted from City of Toronto. (2014). *Toronto 2014 budget.* Toronto: City of Toronto.
    Retrieved from http://www1.toronto.ca/City%20of%20Toronto/Strategic%20Communications/
    City%20Budget/2014/PDFs/About%20the%20budget/2014BudgetAtAGlance_Report_S0.pdf.

explicitly spends 7 per cent of its total budget (or $672 million) on health care ser-
vices that include Toronto Public Health (2.6 per cent), long-term care homes and
services (2.4 per cent), and emergency medical services (2 per cent).

Like Vancouver, Montreal, and other larger cities and metropolitan areas,
Toronto's revenues and expenses are significantly out of proportion with the scale
and needs of the medium-sized and smaller cities and towns that make up most of
Canada; for example, Toronto's budget is about the same as the entire provincial
budget for Nova Scotia.

While direct comparisons are problematic, for the sake of illuminating the
different situations in Canadian municipalities of different sizes, sources of revenue and expenditures for the cities of Calgary, Alberta (population 1.1 million in
2011), Moncton, New Brunswick (population 138,644 in 2011), and Thompson,
Manitoba (population 13,123 in 2011), are shown in Tables 7.5 and 7.6. Note that
category figures do not necessarily add to a total of 100 per cent; they are high-
lighted strictly for the purpose of comparing similar revenues and expenses across
the three cities.

It is difficult to find directly comparable data, but look, for example, at expenses on transportation—more than 5 times greater in Moncton than Thompson;
and protective services spending—nearly 10 times higher in Thompson than

Table 7.4: Composition of Total Expenses, City of Toronto Operating Budget, 2014

EXPENSE	MINISTRY/PROGRAM AREA
17.8%	Toronto Transit Commission
12.2%	Toronto employment and social services
11.3%	Toronto Police Service
9.8%	All other services
7.4%	Governance and internal services
6.9%	Other expenses
6.7%	Shelter, support, and housing administration
4.5%	Debt charges
4.4%	Toronto Fire Services
4.3%	Parks, Forestry and Recreation
4.2%	Toronto Children's Services
3.5%	Transportation services
2.6%	Toronto Public Health
2.4%	Long-term care homes and services
2.0%	Emergency medical services
$9.6 billion	*Total expenses*

Source: Ontario Ministry of Finance. (2014). *2014 Ontario budget, chapter II: Ontario's economic outlook and fiscal plan.* Toronto: Ontario Ministry of Finance. Retrieved from http://www.fin.gov. on.ca/en/budget/ontariobudgets/2014/ch2f.html

Moncton. Given the widely varying differences in spending patterns, nurses in these settings would expect that nursing practice and health care programs could vary just as widely. Other determinants of health may drive the sorts of programs that are needed or that can be afforded (e.g., public health programs). If significant funds are allocated to criminal justice, then less may be available to support programs that might prevent crime (e.g., housing, food security, safe injection sites). As such, the sorts of programs offered at the municipal level across Canada typically vary widely.

The Flow of Funds from Governments to Organizations

We will not pursue a lengthy discussion of the models by which individual organizations receive their funding from provinces, territories, and/or municipal governments; the number and range of models across the country is exhaustive and frequently changes. Nurses would be better served to seek the most current

Table 7.5: Comparison of Sources of Revenue for Calgary, Moncton, and Thompson, 2015

SOURCES OF REVENUE	CALGARY	MONCTON	THOMPSON
Property taxes	43%	87%	35%
Other municipal revenue sources		9.3%	3%
Unconditional grants		3.7%	
Grant in lieu			21%
Provincial/federal grants			16%
Sale of goods and services	31%		14%
Transfers			11%
Total	$3.5 billion	$144.3 million	$28.2 million

Sources: City of Calgary. (2015). *Action plan 2015–2018*; City of Moncton. (2015). *Your municipal tax dollars at work*; City of Thompson. (2015). *2015 financial plan*.

Table 7.6: Comparison of Composition of Selected Total Expenses for Calgary, Moncton, and Thompson, 2015

MINISTRY/PROGRAM AREA	CALGARY	MONCTON	THOMPSON
Transportation	17%	76.4%	14%
Recreation and culture		16.6%	13%
Protective services	13%	3.5%	33%
General government		3.5%	8%
Environmental health services			4%
Public health and welfare			1%

Sources: City of Calgary. (2015). *Action plan 2015–2018*; City of Moncton. (2015). *Your municipal tax dollars at work*; City of Thompson. (2015). *2015 financial plan*.

information from each jurisdiction. Most physicians across Canada bill public insurance systems directly in a fairly straightforward fee-for-service (or fee-for-visit) basis. But the funding trail for health care organizations is, of course, more complex. Across the country, various models of regionalization (mentioned in Chapter 3) have established the structures through which funding flows between ministries of health and organizations such as hospitals. Funding may be tied to population size, health needs, the sorts of services/procedures provided

The Fee-for-Service Model

The fee-for-service model has been the source of considerable debate throughout its history, and was a key sticking point in the Saskatchewan doctors' strike in 1962. While historically the majority of physicians have favoured it, there is some evidence that attitudes may be changing. In a British Columbia survey of newly graduating physicians reported in 2016, more than two-thirds (70 per cent) did not want to work in a fee-for-service model, preferring instead alternative models, including blended payment or even full salary. The College of Family Physicians of Canada, which conducted the survey, cited earlier work of Wranik and Durier-Copp in concluding that "salaries can be a useful tool for recruiting and retaining physicians in rural and remote areas. Incomes in an FFS system would be less useful in attracting physicians to these low-density areas. Instead, salaries offer a stable, predictable, and sufficient income for those working in areas with a low population density."[21] Interest in fee-for-service payment may have peaked with the baby boomer generation, and if the study can be replicated, the findings may hold promise for recruiting physicians to rural, remote, and other hard-to-staff settings, as well as for exploring alternate remuneration models.

(and their efficiency and costs per case), and in some cases to performance. For example, a hospital chief executive officer may have some portion of salary held back if certain performance criteria are not met.

THE USE OF HEALTH CARE DOLLARS NATIONALLY

How Much Are Canadians Spending on Health Care?

Having looked at a high level at the public-private spending split, and examples of government revenues and expenditures, it is important now to look at the larger picture of what Canadians are spending nationally for different health care programs and services. Health care spending in Canada, both per capita and as a proportion of GDP, has grown steadily in the medicare era beginning in the late 1960s. Concern has especially grown when health care costs outpace inflation. Health care is a tremendously pricy investment for Canadians—with expenditures consuming an estimated 41.5 per cent of aggregate revenues in all provinces and territories in 2010–2011, up nine percentage points from 2000–2001.

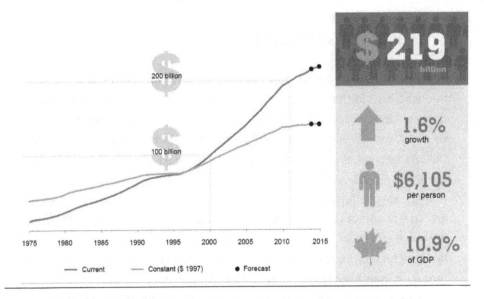

Figure 7.9: Canadian Health Care Expenditure Trends, 1975–2014

Source: Canadian Institute for Health Information. (2015). *National health expenditure trends, 1975 to 2015.* Ottawa: CIHI, p. 6.

National health expenditures grew rapidly during the 1970s and into the 1980s, levelled off when Chrétien reined in federal spending during the mid-1990s (discussed in Chapter 4), and then began to grow again over the first 15 years of the new century.[22] As depicted in Figure 7.9, the rate of growth has begun to slow, but total expenditures nonetheless continue to rise, growing by some 2.1 per cent between 2013 and 2014.

Canadians spent about $219 billion on health care in 2015—more than at any other point in our history. For the sake of comparison, Table 7.7 highlights total health expenditures in Canada for 1975 and 2014 by source and distribution of financing. As a proportion of GDP, total health expenditures have risen by 57 per cent during that 40-year period. Combined provincial and territorial spending (bolstered by federal transfers) in 2014 had increased by more than 16 times over the 1975 spending. However, while the raw dollars have increased, the proportion overall falling to the provinces and territories decreased from 71.4 per cent to 65.5 per cent. Public sector spending as a proportion of total expenditures dropped from 76.3 to 70.5 per cent, while private sector spending grew from 23.8 to 29.5 per cent (see Figure 7.10). As the proportion of spending for hospitals has been reduced and people move more quickly out of hospitals after procedures (if they are admitted at all), more and more financial responsibility is falling to individuals—and that is reflected in the rising proportion of private sector spending.

Table 7.7: Total Health Expenditures, Canada, 1975 and 2014

TOTAL HEALTH EXPENDITURES	1975	2014
Total health expenditures in current dollars ($ millions)	12,199.4	214,907.0
Per capita health expenditures ($)	527.1	6,045.2
Total health expenditures as a % of GDP	7.0	11.0
TOTAL HEALTH EXPENDITURES BY SOURCE OF FINANCING ($ MILLIONS)		
Provincial governments	8,709.3	140,772.4
Federal government direct	398.3	6,916.8
Municipal governments	71.6	821.8
Social Security Funds	121.1	2,982.7
Total public sector (total of the above four sources)	9,300.3	151,493.7
Total private sector	2,899.2	63,413.6
DISTRIBUTION OF TOTAL HEALTH EXPENDITURES BY SOURCE OF FINANCING (%)		
Provincial governments	71.4	65.5
Federal government direct	3.3	3.2
Municipal governments	0.6	0.4
Social Security Funds	1.0	1.4
Total public sector (total of the above four sources)	76.3	70.5
Total private sector	23.8	29.5

Source: Canadian Institute for Health Information. (2014). *National Health Expenditure Trends, 1975 to 2014*. Ottawa: CIHI.

Figure 7.11 breaks down total health expenditures as a proportion of GDP by province and territory for 1981 (the first year for which comparative data were available) and 2014. Expenditures as a proportion in relation to GDP rose in every jurisdiction except Newfoundland and Labrador, where they dropped from 11.9 to 7.9 per cent. Growth was sharp in several jurisdictions, and compared to the Canadian average of 11 per cent in 2014, nine jurisdictions exceeded this level, the most dramatic being Nunavut, where health expenditures account for more than 19 per cent of GDP. Health expenditures as a portion of GDP grew by more than 50 per cent in British Columbia, Alberta, Manitoba, Ontario, and Nova Scotia; the highest growth was in the Yukon, where expenditures more than doubled to 12.7 per cent.

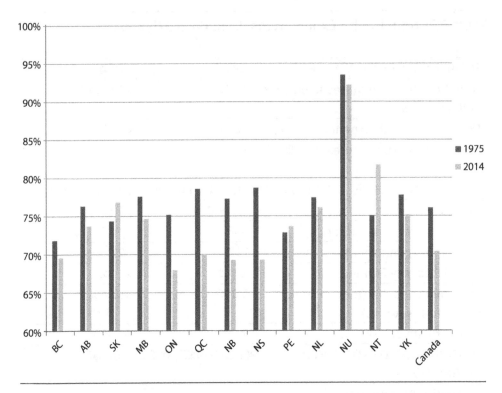

Figure 7.10: Public Sector Portion of Total Provincial/Territorial Health Expenditure, Canada, 1975 and 2014

Source: Canadian Institute for Health Information. (2014). *National health expenditure trends, 1975 to 2014.* Ottawa: CIHI.

How Are Canadians Paying for Health Care?

The public-private financing split across the country also changed between 1975 and 2014, with the public sector proportion of total expenditures dropping nationally by 5.7 per cent and dropping in every jurisdiction other than Saskatchewan, Prince Edward Island, and the Northwest Territories (see Table 7.8). Increases in public sector financing of health care grew most in the Northwest Territories, where the change was 6.6 per cent, and decreased most in Nova Scotia, where it dropped by 9.3 per cent. While decreases in public sector spending dropped in all the other jurisdictions, the changes were greatest in Ontario (7.2 per cent), Quebec (8.2 per cent), and New Brunswick (8 per cent). In 2014 the highest provincial public sector financing as a proportion of GDP was in Saskatchewan (77 per cent) and the highest private sector financing was in Ontario (31.9 per cent). Only three other jurisdictions outside Ontario (British Columbia, New Brunswick, and Nova Scotia) have private sector funding exceeding 30 per cent.

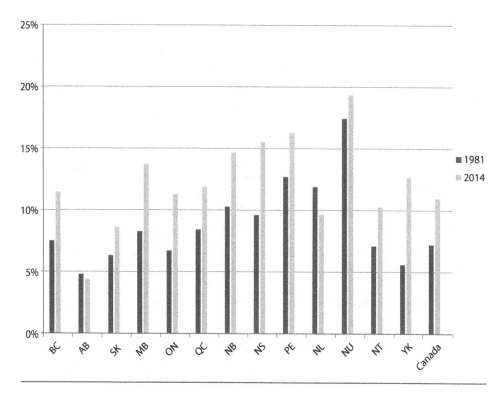

**Figure 7.11: Total Health Expenditure as a Percentage of Provincial/
Territorial GDP, Canada, 1981 and 2014**

Source: Canadian Institute for Health Information. (2014). National health expenditure trends,
1975 to 2014. Ottawa: CIHI.

**Table 7.8: Total Provincial/Territorial Health Expenditure in Public and
Private Sectors, Canada, 1975 and 2014**

TOTAL PROVINCIAL/TERRITORIAL HEALTH EXPENDITURE IN PUBLIC AND PRIVATE SECTORS		1975 (%)	2014 (%)
Canada (average)	Public	76.2	70.5
	Private	23.8	29.5
British Columbia	Public	71.9	69.7
	Private	28.1	30.3
Alberta	Public	76.4	73.9
	Private	23.6	26.1
Saskatchewan	Public	74.5	77.0
	Private	25.5	23.0

continued

Manitoba	Public	77.7	74.8
	Private	22.3	25.2
Ontario	Public	75.3	68.1
	Private	24.7	31.9
Quebec	Public	78.8	70.6
	Private	21.2	29.4
New Brunswick	Public	77.4	69.4
	Private	22.6	30.6
Nova Scotia	Public	78.8	69.5
	Private	21.2	30.5
Prince Edward Island	Public	73.0	73.8
	Private	27.0	26.2
Newfoundland and Labrador	Public	77.6	76.3
	Private	22.4	23.7
Nunavut (first column figure is for 1999)	Public	93.6	92.3
	Private	6.4	7.7
Northwest Territories	Public	75.2	81.8
	Private	24.8	18.2
Yukon Territory	Public	77.9	75.4
	Private	22.1	24.6

Source: Canadian Institute for Health Information. (2014). *National health expenditure trends, 1975 to 2014.* Ottawa: CIHI.

What Health Care Services Are Canadians Purchasing?

Health spending has for some time been heavily concentrated in services that fall broadly under the umbrella of acute and treatment care—especially to physicians, drugs, hospitals, and other institutions that together account for 70 per cent of all health care spending. Costs are rising steadily in the first three of those categories, as illustrated in Figure 7.12, with physician costs significantly outpacing the others.

Table 7.9 offers a comparison of the distribution of health expenditures for selected health care services in 1975 and 2014. Most striking in these statistics are changes in hospital and drug expenses. The portion of expenditures for hospitals has dropped by a third since 1975—reflecting our journey away from the bed, and toward a "portable, more mobile era of health care" as Porter-O'Grady said in 1998.[23] He noted that, in the United States, inpatient operating room services had dropped from 86 per cent of cases in 1978 to a near

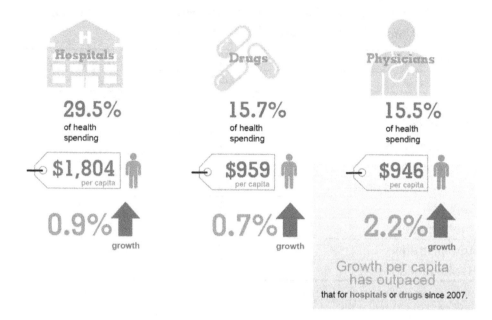

Figure 7.12: Health Spending on Hospitals, Drugs, and Physicians in Canada, 2015

Source: Canadian Institute for Health Information. (2015). *National health expenditure trends, 1975 to 2015.* Ottawa: CIHI, p. 13.

total flip 20 years later in 1998, when some 80 per cent of the same services were provided as outpatients; of course, Canada has been on the same journey. Prescribed drug expenditures have increased by more than 100 per cent to 13.4 per cent of total expenses.

Public and private spending on hospitals have both decreased over 40 years, while spending on both sides for pharmaceuticals has increased—see Table 7.10. Spending for physicians continues to rise on the public side but has dropped slightly on the private side; the costs of nursing are buried largely in the categories of hospitals, other non-hospital institutions, and public health, and steadily rising nursing salaries and benefits contribute to the rising costs in those categories.

As Browne and colleagues pointed out in work done for the National Expert Commission, significant resources are focused on a relatively small number of health care consumers.[24] They cite statistics from the collaborative 2010 study conducted by the Ontario Association of Community Care Access Centres, Ontario Hospital Association, and Ontario Federation of Community Mental Health and

Table 7.9: Examples of Distribution of Total Health Expenditures by Use of Funds, Canada, 1975 and 2014

EXPENDITURES	1975 (%)	2014 (%)
Hospitals	44.7	29.6
Other institutions	9.2	10.3
Physicians	15.1	15.5
Dental services	6.1	6.1
Prescribed drugs	6.3	13.4
Non-prescribed drugs	2.5	2.4
Capital	4.4	4.1
Public health	3.3	5.3
Administration	2.8	3.1
Health research	0.8	1.6

Source: Canadian Institute for Health Information. (2014). National health expenditure trends, 1975 to 2014. Ottawa: CIHI.

Addiction Programs,[25] which concluded that in Ontario, just 1 per cent of system users account for 49 per cent of combined annual hospital and home care costs, and 5 per cent account for 84 per cent of costs. Frequently having complex and multiple co-morbid conditions, these users tend to require more care, including hospital emergency room and inpatient readmissions.

The Canadian Institute for Health Information similarly found that in the category of public spending on pharmaceuticals at the national level, a relatively small proportion of Canadians were responsible for significant spending. In 2015, more than half of beneficiaries accounted for 5.6 per cent of total program spending (less than $500 per beneficiary), while 13.9 per cent of beneficiaries accounted for 67.3 per cent of spending ($2,500 or more per beneficiary). In that latter group, just 2.1 per cent of beneficiaries were associated with a third of all drug spending.[26]

As health system policy is developed going forward, nurses and other decision makers need to constantly return to data like these to inform effective decision-making around cost control. Ontario, for example, has responded to this quandary with its Community Health Links program, designed to better coordinate care for such patients among the patients and their families and friends, hospitals, family doctors, long-term care facilities, and community organizations.[27] There may be little merit in massive, system-level reform if tackling a discrete group of users could achieve significant results.

Table 7.10: Total Health Expenditure by Use of Funds in Public and
Private Sectors, Canada, 1975 and 2014

EXPENDITURES		1975 (% DISTRIBUTION OF FUNDS)	2014 (% DISTRIBUTION OF FUNDS)
Hospitals	Public	55.2	37.9
	Private	11	9.6
Other Institutions	Public	8.6	10.4
	Private	11.3	10.1
Physicians	Public	19.5	21.6
	Private	0.9	0.8
Dental services	Public	0.6	0.5
	Private	23.6	19.6
Vision care	Public	0.4	0.3
	Private	6.6	5.9
Other professionals	Public	0.5	0.6
	Private	2.8	5.7
Prescribed and non-prescribed drugs	Public	1.7	8.0
	Private	31.7	34.4
Capital	Public	4.0	4.4
	Private	5.5	3.4
Public health	Public	4.4	7.6
	Private	0	0
Administration	Public	2.9	1.8
	Private	2.5	6.2
Health research	Public	0.8	1.5
	Private	0.8	2.1
Other spending	Public	1.4	5.3
	Private	3.3	2.4

Source: Canadian Institute for Health Information. (2014). National health expenditure trends, 1975 to 2014. Ottawa: CIHI.

What Is the Cost of Nursing?

Teasing out spending on nursing is no small task. Beyond physicians, health human resources costs are typically rolled up in larger categories such as *hospitals* or *other institutions*. Because they make up so much of the staff in hospitals, it is often assumed that nurses make up the majority of costs. A closer examination calls that assertion into question.

For the purposes of this text, an attempt was made to determine a gross estimate of the costs of registered nurses (RNs), licensed practical nurses (LPNs), and
registered psychiatric nurses (RPNs) on a national scale. Nurse practitioner costs
were not included. The calculation was based on the following assumptions for the
sake of the exercise:

1. The average, full-time 2015 registered nurse salary estimate of $77,773 by
   CFNU is representative of the country.
2. Average full-time registered psychiatric nurse salaries are equal to average
   full-time registered nurse salaries.
3. Average licensed practical nurse salaries were calculated to be 74 per cent
   of average registered nurse salaries based on scales from the Manitoba
   Nurses Union (where licensed practical nurse salary is approximately 74
   per cent of registered nurse salary) and Nova Scotia Nurses Union (where
   licensed practical nurse salary is approximately 73.4 per cent of registered
   nurse salary). It was assumed for this exercise that this salary is representative of the country.
4. All part-time staff (PTE) in all categories work 0.5 of a full-time equivalent (FTE), meaning that they all work half time.
5. Benefits in all categories and all employment statuses (full- or part-time)
   equate to 20 per cent.
6. Data provided by the Canadian Institute for Information on the number
   of regulated nurses in each category and the numbers working full- and
   part-time were used to calculate the total estimated costs per category—
   see Table 7.11.

Based on this gross estimate, the costs of all regulated nurses in all categories (n=402,851 in 2014) other than nurse practitioners across Canada add up
to roughly $27.4 billion, or 12.5 per cent of $219 billion total annual spending.
By comparison, there were 77,674 physicians in Canada in 2013 according
to CIHI, accounting for 15 per cent of total annual health spending. Since
nurses are spread across so many settings, not just hospitals, if this estimate
of total national nursing costs is valid, then the notion that nurses make up
the majority of hospital costs should be abandoned. A closer examination may
indeed reveal that nursing accounts for the largest portion of the health human
resources costs in nurse-intensive settings (e.g., emergency rooms, critical care
units, acute medical and surgical inpatient units, and labour/delivery/post-par-
tum care units in hospitals), and if that is the argument being made it should
be clarified as such.

Table 7.11: Gross Estimate of Annual Cost of Nursing in Canada, 2014

CATEGORY	TOTAL NUMBER, FULL-TIME (FT) AND PART-TIME (PT)		SALARY	COSTS PER CATEGORY
RN	289,239		$77,773/FTE	
	FT 58.5%	169,205	77,773 x 169,205 FTE	$13,159,580,465
	PT 41.5%	120,034	77,773 x 120,034 FTE x 0.5	$4,667,702,141
Total RN: $17,827,282,606				
LPN	107,923		$77,773 x 0.74 = $57,552/FTE	
	FT 48.5%	52,343	57,552 x 52,343 FTE	$3,012,444,336
	PT 51.5%	55,580	57,552 x 55,580 FTE x 0.5	$1,599,370,080
Total LPN: $4,611,814,416				
RPN	5,689		$77,773/FTE	
	FT 62%	3,527	77,773 x 3,527 FTE	$274,305,371
	PT 38%	2,162	77,773 x 2,162 FTE x 0.5	$84,072,613
Total RPN: $358,377, 984				
Sub-total				$22,797,475,006
+20% benefits				$4,559,495,001.20
Total				$27,356,970,007

Notes: Canadian Institute for Health Information. (2015). *Regulated nurses, 2014*. Ottawa: CIHI; Assumptions: (a) CFNU estimate $77,773 per full-time registered nurse is representative of the country; (b) registered psychiatric nurse salary is equal to registered nurse salary; (c) licensed practical nurse salary—calculated at 74% of registered nurse salary based on Manitoba Nurses Union (74% of RN salary) and Nova Scotia Nurses Union (73.4% of RN salary)—is representative of the country; and (d) part-time staff in all categories work 0.5 of full-time.

HEALTH SPENDING IN OTHER COUNTRIES

In an ongoing effort to understand and improve Canada's health systems, health expenditures and system outcomes are regularly compared to counterparts, usually other OECD members. As shown in Figure 7.13, Canada ranked eighth in spending on health as a proportion of GDP using 2012 data—the last year for which all country data were available.[28] Note that Canada's current spending has risen since the 10.2 per cent figure recorded by OECD 2012 data.

Canada spends significantly more on health care per capita and relative to GDP than the OECD average of 8.9 per cent. Setting aside the outlier of the

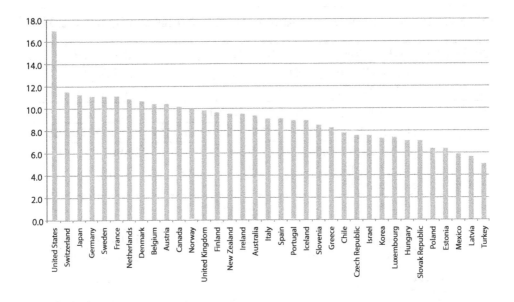

Figure 7.13: Total Health Expenditures as a Percentage of GDP, OECD Members, 2015

Source: Organisation for Economic Co-operation and Development. (2015). Health expenditure and financing. Retrieved from http://stats.oecd.org/index.aspx?DataSetCode=HEALTH_STAT#

United States, Canada's closest company—the group of nations spending 9 to 11 per cent of GDP on health—includes Austria, Belgium, Denmark, Germany, Greece, Hungary, Korea, New Zealand, Norway, Slovakia, and Switzerland. The public-private spending split based on total health expenditures of these nations is shown in Figure 7.14[29] and system performance based on these investments in explored in Chapter 8.

SUMMARY AND IMPLICATIONS

After discussing the structure and reform of Canada's health systems in the past two chapters, Chapter 7 has laid out the landscape of health care spending in Canada today. The public-private spending divide has remained relatively constant over the past 20 years, hovering around a ratio of 70:30 per cent. Proportionate spending on hospitals has declined over the past half century, but hospital, doctor, and drug costs continue to account for 60.7 per cent of health spending. Other institutions use up 10 per cent of spending, leaving less than 30 per cent for all other health and health care services needed across Canada.

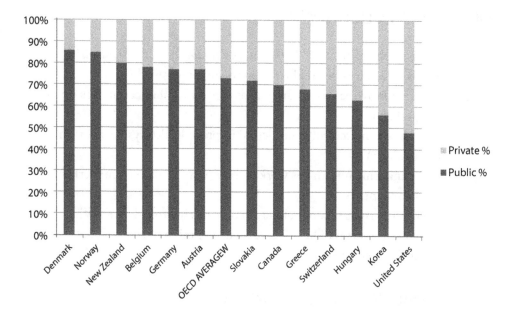

Figure 7.14: Private–Public Spending as Proportions of Total Health Expenditures in 2012, Select OECD Nations

Source: Organisation for Economic Co-operation and Development. (2015). *OECD health statistics 2015.* Paris: OECD.

As efforts to rein in costs continue, in part by moving services outside of traditional hospital settings, Canadians are being forced to pay for more services out of pocket (more on this in Chapter 12). As more and more services shift away from institutions like hospitals, Peter argues that the Canada Health Act "is becoming increasingly incapable of protecting the health needs of Canadians"— and she lays the blame for this shift squarely at the feet of spreading neoliberal political ideology.[30] Desperate attempts to simply save money may imply a less sinister, or at least less well thought-out, explanation for some policy choices. However, Rodney and her colleagues are critical of that thinking, calling out efficiency trumping quality as a result of the "widely held assumption that actions to save money in health care and other social services are inherently justifiable."[31] Given the prickly ethical issues at play, nurses undertaking policy work should be well informed about the categories of revenue and spending discussed here, as well as some notion of relative costs of programs and services, and the implications for Canadians of shifting spending patterns.

DISCUSSION QUESTIONS

1. What is the difference between *sustainability* and *affordability*? How should these ideas be employed in nursing policy work?
2. We often hear that "costs are out of control." What can nurses do about that problem?
3. What financing reform is needed to improve health systems performance in Canada? Why?
4. What financing reform has worked to improve health system performance in other countries?
5. What is the right mix of publicly and privately funded care? Why?
6. What other sources of health care financing might be tapped that have not already been considered?

ADDITIONAL POLICY RESOURCES

INTERNATIONAL ECONOMICS ORGANIZATIONS	
International Labour Organization	http://www.ilo.org
International Monetary Fund	http://www.imf.org
Organisation for Economic Co-operation and Development	http://www.oecd.org
United Nations	http://www.un.org
World Bank	http://www.worldbank.org
World Economic Forum	https://www.weforum.org

CHAPTER 8

Effects and Outcomes of Health Policy: Population Health Status and the Performance of Canada's Health Systems

CHAPTER HIGHLIGHTS

- Introduction
- "Are We Getting the Results that Matter?" How Healthy Are Canadians?
- "Are We Doing the Right Things to Make an Impact on the Health of the Populations We Are Serving?" The Performance of Health Systems in Canada
- What Is the Return on Investment in Nursing Services?
- Summary and Implications
- Discussion Questions
- Additional Policy Resources

LEARNING OUTCOMES

1. Identify leading population health outcomes in Canada.
2. Describe key measures of population health status.
3. Demonstrate an understanding of the range of factors that determine the health of Canadians.
4. Describe four key social, economic, environmental, or Aboriginal factors that have a significant impact on health.
5. Demonstrate knowledge of the performance of Canada's health systems based on key health system performance metrics, indicators, and outcomes, and in the context of international comparisons.
6. State five examples of evidence pointing to the performance, effectiveness, and/or return on investments in the nursing workforce.

Policy Influencer: Gina Browne

Dr. Gina Browne, RN, BScN, MS, MEd, PhD, Hon LLD, FCAHS, recently retired from her role as a professor in the School of Nursing at McMaster University in Hamilton, Ontario. At McMaster University she also served as an associate member of the Department of Clinical Epidemiology and Biostatistics and she was the founder and director of the Health and Social Service Utilization Research Unit. Beyond her teaching, research, and administrative duties, Browne has maintained a clinical practice as a family therapist since 1978. In her scientist role, she led and developed a decades-long program of research linking broad determinants of health with service utilization, with a particular focus on clients having a range of challenges leading them to simultaneously use services in both the health and social sectors. Her work shed light on the high costs to the quality of life of the individuals affected and the high fiscal costs for health and social systems. In 2012, she led development of a landmark report that shaped the recommendations of the National Expert Commission.[1] Famous for her humorous delivery of complex information, it is often said that "Gina thinks the unthinkable, says the unsayable, and does the undoable!"

"The consequence of the traditional view is that most direct expenditures on health are physician-centered, including medical care, hospital care, laboratory tests and prescription drugs. When one adds dental care and the services of such other professions as optometrists and chiropractors, one finds that close to seven billion dollars a year are spent on a personal health care system which is mainly oriented to treating existing illness."

—*The Honourable Marc Lalonde, 1974*[2]

INTRODUCTION

To this point, a basic history of the development, governance, and reform of Canada's health systems has been explored and a picture of public and private spending on health systems laid out. Nurses undertaking policy analysis also need to think about the returns on investments of time, energy, and dollars. This final chapter of Module II responds to the "so what?" questions, that is, the impact of all that spending and hard work on the health of Canadians, and what sorts of system performance outcomes are being achieved as a result of policy choices.

When she was interviewed about taking office as the new director general of the WHO in 2007, Margaret Chan said, "We must stay in our core business.... What is important to me is, are we getting the results that matter? Are we doing the right things to make an impact on the health of the populations that we are serving? These questions have to be asked."[3] Those are good questions to ask about any health system. And in addition to those, we must be mindful of the realities of what outcomes matter most to governments, the public, and providers such as nurses; they might all be different. It is in the spirit of exploring these fundamental questions that this chapter is organized.

"ARE WE GETTING THE RESULTS THAT MATTER?" HOW HEALTHY ARE CANADIANS?

"We hope that the nurse, with her knowledge of hygiene and sanitation and the care of the body in health and illness, will be an educator, and we lay much stress upon this."

—*Lillian Wald, American nurse pioneer and founder, Henry Street Settlement*[4]

As discussed in Chapter 5, Canadians have gained 20 years of lifespan, on average, over the past 100 years—"a good indicator of overall health" in any country, the Conference Board of Canada argues.[5] Canadians today live a decade longer than the global average and our life expectancy is near the top of the 194 nations reported by the WHO (see Figure 8.1). During their lives, Canadians certainly are healthier in many ways than they were in 1916, and healthier than people in many other countries today. Sexually transmitted infections continue to be problematic, but a great deal of communicable disease has otherwise been beaten down thanks to better hygiene, vaccines to fight traditional diseases like polio, and disease-prevention measures driven by public health campaigns as in the case of newer diseases like HIV/AIDS. Canadians have access to infection-fighting antimicrobials that continue to be life-saving and life-prolonging supports in the worlds of multiple trauma, general surgery, and infectious diseases for which there are no vaccines.

By comparison with many areas of the world, the health status of Canadians is immeasurably better. But comparing Canada to global averages is not very helpful. It is when looking to similarly wealthy, politically stable fellow OECD nations with democratically elected governments and similarly advanced health care and social systems that population health status becomes more worrisome—especially when set against Canada's high spending on health care. As the Conference Board of Canada concluded about our health status, relative to our peer countries, "Canada's performance is weak on key indicators."[6] And while Canada has indeed gained the upper hand in the fight against many infectious and communicable diseases, a growing body of evidence shows that our longer lives are increasingly likely to be lived in the company of one or more non-communicable (or chronic) diseases.

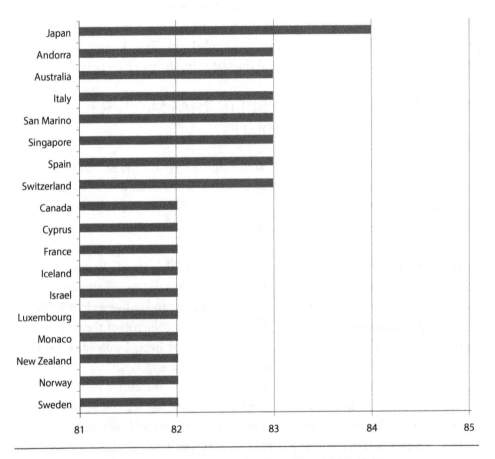

Figure 8.1: Average Life Expectancy for Top 18 of 194 Nations

Source: World Health Organization. (2014). *Global health observatory repository: Life expectancy: Data by country.* Geneva: WHO.

Health Status of Your Region

To learn more about population health status where you live, go to the following link and explore: http://www12.statcan.gc.ca/health-sante/82-228/index.cfm.

Measures of Population Health Status

Based on selected health indicators (including perceived health, body mass index, and rates of disease) Statistics Canada reports that Canadians are "generally healthy" and population health status remained fairly stable from 2003 to 2008.[7] The department reports that Canadian men are more likely than women to be overweight or to have diabetes, and they die younger (as they do in all Western nations), but in general they rate their personal health as better than women rate theirs.

Based on 11 leading population health indicators, the Conference Board of Canada's Report Card accorded Canada a B grade for its tenth-place ranking among 17 OECD nations.[8] There is good news in the finding that fewer Canadians die today from a number of the causes that led to deaths during the 1960s and 1970s. So "progress is being made," with Canada doing best in self-reported health status, premature mortality, and mortality due to circulatory diseases—the latter of which has finally begun to decline in some groups (see Table 8.1).[9] The second tier of health outcomes, given B grades, included life expectancy, mortality due to respiratory diseases, mental disorders, and medical misadventures. The other four indicators all achieved a C grade.

While progress in some areas is noted, the Conference Board of Canada's conclusion that Canada is sliding back in some areas is a concern; overall, the country has dropped from its fifth-place ranking during the 1990s to tenth today. As nurses and others consider health policy options, Table 8.2 may help shed light on areas where priority action may be required. Particular concern arises in the areas of respiratory diseases, diabetes, musculoskeletal diseases, infant mortality, and medical misadventure. There have been some criticisms of the methodology and data used in the large cross-border comparisons and the scoring, but other studies and outcomes seem to support them for the most part. For example, concern is expressed about respiratory diseases, and they continue to account for a significant number of emergency room visits; medical misadventure is a worry, and Canada's health system safety has been found to be a serious concern.[10] Across the country, concerns about diabetes rates have emerged in nearly every jurisdiction and population sector.

Population Health Indicators

To explore each of the Conference Board of Canada population health indicators, visit the following webpage, then click on individual indicators: http://www.conferenceboard.ca/hcp/details/health.aspx.

Table 8.1: Ranking of Population Health Indicators, Canada, 2015

GRADE	POPULATION HEALTH INDICATOR
A	Self-reported health status
	Premature mortality
	Mortality due to circulatory diseases
B	Life expectancy
	Mortality due to respiratory diseases
	Mortality due to mental disorders
	Mortality due to and medical misadventure
C	Mortality due to cancer
	Mortality due to diabetes
	Mortality due to musculoskeletal system diseases
	Infant mortality

Source: Conference Board of Canada. (2015). *Canada health ranking.* Ottawa: Conference Board of Canada. Retrieved from http://www.conferenceboard.ca/hcp/details/health.aspx.

Table 8.2: Population Health Indicator Rankings, Canada, 1960s to 2000s

INDICATOR	1960s	1970s	1980s	1990s	2000s
Life expectancy	B	B	B	B	B
Self-reported health status	n/a	n/a	n/a	A	A
Premature mortality	C	C	C	B	B
Mortality due to cancer	B	B	C	B	B
Mortality due to circulatory diseases	C	B	B	B	B
Mortality due to respiratory diseases	A	A	A	B	A
Mortality due to diabetes	C	C	B	C	D
Mortality due to musculoskeletal system diseases	n/a	B	A	B	C
Mortality due to mental disorders	A	B	B	B	B
Infant mortality	B	B	B	C	C
Mortality due to and medical misadventure	n/a	n/a	B	A	B

Source: Conference Board of Canada. *Health: Canada benchmarked against 15 countries.* Ottawa: Conference Board of Canada. Retrieved from http://www.conferenceboard.ca/hcp/details/health.aspx.

Table 8.3 shows provincial and territorial rankings on selected indicators, and Table 8.4 shows overall rankings of countries and Canadian provinces and territories. Together these may point to potential policy solutions in other jurisdictions. Within Canada, British Columbia and Ontario achieved the highest overall scores in the Conference Board Report Card, while the lowest scores fell to Newfoundland and Labrador and the three territories, each of which were ranked below the lowest international comparator, the United States.

Table 8.3: Conference Board of Canada Report Card Scores for Select Population Health Indicator Rankings, Canadian Provinces and Territories

INDICATOR	CA	BC	AB	SK	MB	ON	QC	NB	NS	PE	NL	NU	NT	YT
Life expectancy	B	A	B	D	C	A	B	B	C	C	C	D-	D-	D-
Premature mortality	A	A	B	D	D	A	A	B	B	B	B	D-	D-	D-
Infant mortality	B	B	D	D-	D-	C	C	B	C	B	D	D-	D-	D-
Self-reported health	B	A	A+	A	A+	A+	A+	A	A	A	A	A	A+	A+
Self-reported mental health	B	B	A	A	A	A	A	B	B	B	A	D	B	B
Cancer	A	A	A	B	C	C	C	C	D	C	D	D-	D-	D-
Heart disease/ stroke	D	B	C	B	B	B	A	B	B	C	C	A	C	B
Respiratory	C	B	B	B	B	B	B	C	C	C	C	D-	D	D
Diabetes	B	C	B	D	D	D	B	C	C	B	D-	A+	A	D-
Nervous system	C	B	B	B	B	B	B	B	B	B	B	A	A	B
Suicide	B	B	B	C	B	B	B	B	B	A	B	D-	C	A

Table 8.4: Conference Board of Canada Country and Province/Territory Report Card Scores on 11 Population Health Indicators

	REPORT CARD GRADE				
Jurisdiction	A	B	C	D	D-
Country	ITALY	AUSTRALIA	AUSTRIA	DENMARK	
	JAPAN	CANADA	BELGIUM	IRELAND	
	SWITZERLAND	FINLAND	NETHERLANDS	UNITED STATES	
		FRANCE	UNITED KINGDOM		
		GERMANY			
		NORWAY			
		SWEDEN			

continued

Province/ Territory	BRITISH COLUMBIA	ALBERTA	NEW BRUNSWICK	MANITOBA	NEWFOUNDLAND AND LABRADOR
		ONTARIO		NOVA SCOTIA	
		PRINCE EDWARD ISLAND			NORTHWEST TERRITORIES
					NUNAVUT
		QUEBEC			YUKON TERRITORY

The Challenges of Chronic Disease and Aging

"Improvements in managing seniors with chronic conditions can lead to the prevention of complications and comorbidities as well as improved effectiveness and cost-efficiency of healthcare for seniors."

—*Canadian Institute for Health Information, 2011*[11]

In a Canadian Academy of Health Sciences study, more than 4 in 10 Canadian adults reported suffering from one of seven common non-communicable diseases—arthritis, cancer, emphysema or chronic obstructive pulmonary disease, diabetes, heart disease, high blood pressure, and mood disorders (not including depression).[12] From among these, cancer, diabetes, cardiovascular disease, and chronic respiratory disease are associated with lifestyle factors that could be modified by healthy public policy fully in the domain of nursing practice. Risk factors for all four include "physical inactivity, unhealthy eating, smoking and the harmful use of alcohol."[13] In addition, risk factors include a broad spectrum of other determinants including (but not limited to) the environment, income, education, and stress levels. In turn, the Alzheimer Society of Canada[14] cites research finding that "a healthy diet, regular exercise, maintaining an active social life, and engaging in intellectually stimulating activities can reduce the chances of developing Alzheimer's disease or related dementia, and can slow its advancement once it has begun."[15]

While communicable and non-communicable diseases and injuries are spread across all age groups, central in the health status of Canadians in this century is the aging of the population. That variable is inextricably linked to health—so barring a transformative change in the health status of that aging population, aging also will be a predictable driver of health services utilization over the coming generation.

Different studies have found that many seniors report their health as quite good, even when they appear to outsiders to have various health and social challenges. However, the Public Agency of Canada noted that "the percentages with overall good health, good functional health and independence in activities of daily living declines sharply with age."[16] Also, the more chronic conditions present, the less likely seniors are to self-report good health.

As presented in background work prepared for the National Expert Commission,[17] major health challenges among Canadian seniors include:

- rising rates of cancers between 2000 and 2009;
- rising rates of diabetes;
- increased number of falls and increasing severity of injury from falls correlated with age;
- high and growing rates of dementia (estimated at 1 in 11 Canadian seniors);
- depression rates estimated at 10 to 15 per cent; and
- seniors may suffer from all the other illnesses and injuries affecting Canadians, including heart disease and stroke, lung diseases, and kidney disease, and they account for more of the morbidity and mortality related to the leading diseases than younger Canadians.

Seniors who are healthy don't use a lot more health services simply by virtue of their age; utilization is correlated with chronic disease.[18] The longer Canadians live, the more likely they are to accumulate non-communicable diseases, and the more of those they have, the more medications they take and more health services they use. Three-quarters of Canadians aged 65 and over report having one chronic condition and about one-quarter have three or more. Not surprisingly, those seniors use more health care services: the Canadian Institute for Health Information reports that seniors having more than two non-communicable conditions "report poorer health, take more prescription medications and have the highest rate of health care visits among seniors with chronic conditions."[19]

Ramlo and Berlin calculated that in British Columbia, per capita health spending almost doubles every decade after the age of 65, reaching $8,425 at age 75 and $16,821 at age 85.[20] They also found that the number of those older people is rising disproportionately—266 per cent growth in numbers in the 85–89 age cohort over the 30 years from 1979 to 2009, for example. This dynamic poses a critical policy conundrum: a lot more health expenditures for older people having non-communicable health conditions coupled with a rapidly growing number of those seniors, especially the group sometimes called the *old* old. Well ahead of Canada in its aging curve, Japan in 2016 already had more than 61,000 citizens over the age of 100, bringing huge implications for health and social systems. The related Canadian health expense spending trends are shown in Figure 8.2.

End-of-Life Costs

Most people who die in Canada are older, and a number of studies over the past decade have made clear that, for many of us, our highest health care utilization

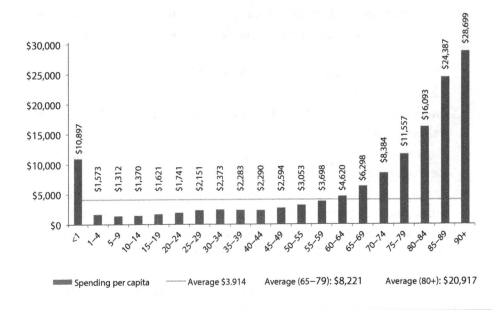

Figure 8.2: Total Provincial/Territorial Health Spending per Capita by Age Group, 2013

Source: Canadian Institute for Health Information. (2015). *National health expenditure trends, 1975 to 2015.* Ottawa: CIHI.

and costs will arise during the final year of life. That presents a fiscal problem when the number of deaths in Canada is set to double over the next 20 years.

A 2007 study of deaths in Western Canada found that 62 per cent of those who eventually died had been admitted to hospital at least once during the year before dying, and 58 per cent of the deaths happened in a hospital.[21] In their 2013 review of the issue, Fowler and Hammer cited evidence that the numbers were even higher, finding that "hospitals remain the provider of end-of-life care for 70% of Canadians" and that up to 15 per cent are admitted to critical care units during their final hospital admission.[22]

Studying some 265,000 deaths in Ontario, Tanusepturo and his colleagues found average costs of $53,662 during the final year of life, accounting for a total bill of $4.7 billion—roughly 10 per cent of all government spending on health care.[23] At 42.9 per cent, the highest portion of the total cost arose from acute care, which was used by three-quarters of those who eventually died. About a quarter of subjects had used long-term care and 6 in 10 used home care. Overall costs "rose sharply" during the final three months of life, largely driven by inpatient care.[24]

"ARE WE DOING THE RIGHT THINGS TO MAKE AN IMPACT ON THE HEALTH OF THE POPULATIONS WE ARE SERVING?" THE PERFORMANCE OF HEALTH SYSTEMS IN CANADA

"Where you live does matter. Access to high-quality care still varies across the country. And disparities in health status remain."

—*Health Council of Canada*[25]

Rising gross health care costs have been fuelled in part by the roughly 50 per cent increase in the Canadian population over the 40 years since the mid-1970s; assuming other factors stay constant, more people mean greater demand for care, including nursing services. That growth accounted for a 1 per cent increase in health expenditures per year over the decade 1998 to 2008.[26] Despite the fear about growing numbers of seniors in the population, during the same period "population aging contributed an annual average growth of only about 0.8%."[27] However, raw numbers are only part of the story of cost drivers. Individually, Canadians use more health care services than they did during the 1970s: per capita health expenditures have multiplied by a factor of nearly 12 times above the 1975 level. Some of those costs reflect raw demand, but they also reflect dramatically higher health human resources costs (including a doubling of physician fees between 1998 and 2008), myriad new diagnostic and treatment techniques, the ubiquitous use of expensive technology, more drug use and higher drug costs, and health care inflation costs exceeding general inflation.

What Is the Link between Health and Health Care?

Canadians are spending a lot more on health care, and living longer, but as discussed in the previous section of this chapter, the country is achieving some middle-of-the-pack rankings for population health status and has slipped in rankings on key outcomes. What is the message? Is there a disconnect in those findings about health status and health care? Consider some key outcomes:

- Canada spends more on health care per capita and as a proportion of GDP than the OECD average.
- The hospital proportion of national health expenditures has decreased significantly over 40 years; currently there are roughly 73,000 hospital beds in operation across the country.[28]

- Spending on drugs and physicians has increased, and Canadians pay more for doctors, and a lot more for pharmaceuticals, than the OECD average.
- Compared to other OECD nations Canada has significantly fewer hospitals, fewer physicians (but higher physician costs) and fewer nurses.
- Canada's average hospital stays are longer than the OECD average, which may reflect sicker patients (given poorer population health scores), high numbers of alternate-level-of-care beds, and/or some combination of these and other factors.
- Canadians pay more than similar countries for hospitals, although hospital-level costs are not terribly out of line with OECD comparators. Procedure costs in hospitals often are higher than when they are provided in other settings.
- Approximately 1 million Canadians are receiving home care at any given time.[29]
- Private spending has crept up over the years, more in some provinces and territories than others. As patients are discharged from hospitals, or avoid admission altogether, some costs that used to be covered by public medicare (because they fell under publicly insured hospital costs) have been moved to the private side, driving up out-of-pocket costs for individual Canadians.

The Commonwealth Fund's 2014 ranking of 11 national health systems offers up some revealing findings that point starkly to the importance of making the distinction between health and health care as policy decisions are made. Criticism has been levelled against these sorts of survey-based rankings, but they attract significant attention from decision makers, media, and the public. Also, as noted in the previous sections, the findings seem to be validated in other country-level studies and reports of patient experiences—and given their repetition over many years, they do offer one view of possible trends.

As shown in Figure 8.3, ranking first place in 8 of the 11 categories measured, the country with the highest health system ranking overall was the United Kingdom. The United Kingdom spends less on health per capita and by proportion of GDP than any of the 10 other countries—and it also has second-lowest ranking for healthy lives (see Table 8.5). The country was given a C grade for population health in the Conference Board of Canada rankings. France, on the other hand, was ranked ninth overall by the Commonwealth Fund—including having the lowest or second-lowest scores for patient-centredness and access issues—but is ranked first for healthy lives and was given a B score by the Conference Board.

These outcomes present something of a conundrum; despite spending less, one nation appears to have a first class health system but poor health—and the other has mediocre scores for its system performance and has the highest rating for healthy lives.

Canada again ranked second-last overall (as it has in earlier rankings by the Commonwealth Fund), having the lowest or second-lowest rankings in the areas of safety, timeliness, and efficiency of care, placing ninth overall for quality and eighth for healthy lives. The Canadian Adverse Events Study in 2004 found an error incidence rate in adult general hospitals sampled of 7.5 per cent, of which more than a third were considered highly preventable. What is more, at the time of that study, Canadians spent more than a million extra days in hospitals due to complications in their care every year, and it was estimated that between 9,250 and 23,750 deaths from adverse events could have been prevented.[30] In addition, safety concerns persist: a 2016 study by the Canadian Institute for Health Information and the Canadian Patient Safety Institute found that patients are harmed in 1 out of every 18 hospitalizations and that

COUNTRY RANKINGS

Top 2
Middle
Bottom 2

	AUS	CAN	FRA	GER	NETH	NZ	NOR	SWE	SWIZ	UK	US
OVERALL RANKING (2013)	4	10	9	5	5	7	7	3	2	1	11
Quality Care	2	9	8	7	5	4	11	10	3	1	5
Effective Care	4	7	9	6	5	2	11	10	8	1	3
Safe Care	3	10	2	6	7	9	11	5	4	1	7
Coordinated Care	4	8	9	10	5	2	7	11	3	1	6
Patient-Centered Care	5	8	10	7	3	6	11	9	2	1	4
Access	8	9	11	2	4	7	6	4	2	1	9
Cost-Related Problem	9	5	10	4	8	6	3	1	7	1	11
Timeliness of Care	6	11	10	4	2	7	8	9	1	3	5
Efficiency	4	10	8	9	7	3	4	2	6	1	11
Equity	5	9	7	4	8	10	6	1	2	2	11
Healthy Lives	4	8	1	7	5	9	6	2	3	10	11
Health Expenditures/Capita, 2011	$3,800	$4,522	$4,118	$4,495	$5,099	$3,182	$5,669	$3,925	$5,643	$3,405	$8,508

Figure 8.3: Overall Rankings of Health Systems, Commonwealth Fund, 2014

Source: Davis, K., Stremikis, K., Squires, D., & Schoen, C. (2014, June). *Mirror, mirror on the wall: How the performance of the U.S. health care system compares internationally.* New York: The Commonwealth Fund. Retrieved from http://www.commonwealthfund.org/publications/fund-reports/2014/jun/mirror-mirror.

Table 8.5: Commonwealth Fund Ranking of Health Systems, Spending on Health Care, and Healthy Lives Rankings

COUNTRIES LISTED BY COMMONWEALTH FUND RANKING (2014)	HEALTH SPENDING PER CAPITA, $US	% GDP SPENT ON HEALTH CARE (2012)	PUBLIC % GDP (2012)	PRIVATE % GDP (2012)	HEALTHY LIVES SCORE
1. United Kingdom	3,405	8.5	83	17	10
2. Switzerland	5,643	11.0	66	34	3
3. Sweden	3,925	10.8	85	15	2
4. Australia	3,800	8.8	68	32	4
5. Germany	4,495	10.8	77	23	7
5. Netherlands	5,099	11.0	87	13	5
7. New Zealand	3,182	9.8	80	20	9
7. Norway	5,669	8.8	85	15	6
9. France	4,118	10.8	79	21	1
10. Canada	4,522	10.2	70	30	8
11. United States	8,508	16.4	48	52	11

Source: Davis, K., Stremikis, K., Squires, D., & Schoen, C. (2014, June). *Mirror, mirror on the wall: How the performance of the U.S. health care system compares internationally.* New York: The Commonwealth Fund. Retrieved from http://www.commonwealthfund.org/publications/fund-reports/2014/jun/mirror-mirror.

"about 20% involve more than 1 occurrence of harm."[31] Beyond the human suffering, that rate translates to significant costs, with more than 1,600 hospital beds every day occupied by patients harmed during their care and requiring a longer hospital stay. Even more alarming, Chris Power, chief executive officer of the institute, reports that one Canadian dies every 17 minutes related to an adverse event suffered during the course of care

Spending nearly 100 per cent more as a proportion of GDP than the top-ranked United Kingdom (and 150 per cent more per capita), the United States again placed last overall. It has the lowest proportion of public spending and lowest ranking for healthy lives.

The countries with the closest match between health system rankings and healthy lives are Switzerland, Sweden, and Australia—they all ranked in second to fourth positions in both categories. At 85 per cent, Sweden spends significantly more on the public contribution to health expenditures than Switzerland (66 per cent) or Australia (68 per cent), and has the highest score for healthy lives of the three.

Social, Economic, Environmental, and Aboriginal Determinants of Health

"Politics is the most important determinant of health."

—*Ritika Goel, MD, family physician, Toronto*

Many international health systems do well in managing health crises that improve individual health; certainly that is rarely truer than in the case of well-educated, insured, wealthy, heterosexual, male, Caucasian Americans who live in large urban areas and have access to rescue services and acute care that are unparalleled in the world. However, the Commonwealth Fund findings seem to support the notion that the link of those acute treatment services to broader population health is much less clear. While one should not infer cause and effect, of course, these sorts of findings shed an interesting light on other evidence driving the question of how much health care is linked to population health.

In his *Report on the State of Public Health in Canada 2008*, Chief Public Health Officer David Butler-Jones noted, "The origins of public health in this country can be traced back to traditional Aboriginal teachings that highlight the importance of maintaining and restoring balanced health through social and environmental sensitivity."[32] In this decade, hard scientific evidence tells a similar tale: Browne, Birch, and Thebane argued that the balance between social and health spending is more important to better health outcomes than raw dollars spent on health care alone.[33] However, Canada and some other nations seem to have wandered from that balanced approach to what actually creates good health in favour of treatment of disease and injury.

Canada's health system is the eighth most expensive in the world. Canadians have made a collective decision to invest a lot of dollars in formal health care as the route to better health. But in leading a Senate review of determinants of health, the Honourable Senators Wilbur Keon and Lucie Pépin—a physician and a nurse, incidentally—concluded that three-quarters of health is attributable to

Explore Your Health System

The Canadian Institute for Health Information offers a digital tool to explore the health of Canadians and the health system. Go to the following link to search by hospital, long-term care organization, city, health region, province, or territory: http://yourhealthsystem.cihi.ca/hsp/indepth.

factors beyond health care and that "fully 50% of the health of the population can be explained by socio-economic factors."[34] These factors include income, education, housing, access to healthy food and water, and issues such as perceived social standing and social support. Of course, genetics, gender, race, and discrimination also all play important roles.

The places we live—the small towns and huge cities around us—also exert many influences on our health. Cities have been described as "complex systems, with urban health outcomes dependent on many interactions and feedback loops."[35] Far beyond nursing and health care, "modification of the physical fabric" may require good urban planning to improve health. This is a special challenge in places like Toronto, where trends since the 1970s are reversing and the inner city core is growing faster than suburbs.[36] The OECD argued for the value of *resilient cities*, which it defined as being "characterised by adaptive capacity, robustness, redundancy, flexibility, resourcefulness, inclusiveness and integration."[37] Importantly for nursing policy work, OECD identified "addressing the issues of social inequality" as a major policy lever to build resilience—adding that doing so "requires inputs from diverse policy sectors, ranging from labour, economy and housing to health, education and social services."[38]

In our country, Aboriginal status is a strong determinant of health—some might say it is the most important determinant of poorer health outcomes. During meetings of the National Expert Commission, representatives of First Nations, Métis, and Inuit asked that nurses explicitly acknowledge the term "Indigenous determinants of health" going forward. The data cited in this chapter could hardly make the case plainer. Where there are concentrations of wealth, education, and privilege—British Columbia and Ontario, for example—the population health rankings are highest. And where the concentrations of Aboriginal Peoples are highest—Manitoba, Saskatchewan, and all three territories, for example—the outcomes are the worst. In a commentary on the long-standing and "shamefully apparent" health inequities between Indigenous and non-Indigenous Canadians, Alika Lafontaine, president of the Indigenous Physicians Association of Canada, worried that "these disparities have become normalized and accepted."[39]

In their synthesis for the National Expert Commission,[40] Muntaner, Ng, and

The Social Determinants of Health

For an excellent primer on the determinants of health in Canada, check out *Social Determinants of Health: The Canadian Facts*, by Juha Mikkonen and Dennis Raphael: http://www.thecanadianfacts.org/

Chung "confirmed the findings of the leading research on determinants of health: there is a clear and direct association between income and health. Low-income Canadians have the highest rates of death, illness and health-care use, while middle-income individuals and families have worse health outcomes than the highest-income groups ... regardless of whether income is measured at individual, household, or neighbourhood levels."[41] They concluded that income, housing, food insecurity, and social exclusion are especially important determinants that drive and sustain health inequalities over the life course. These issues have been long-standing, prominent policy issues in large urban settings like Vancouver and Toronto. They continue to receive attention from media through constant advocacy by nurses and social care providers such as social workers. Many physicians have stepped up to the plate too; some have even prescribed money or an income as the required treatment. And around the housing issue, physicians like Raza and Goel in Toronto have shared articulate messages with the media, saying, for example, that "experts in health are often trained to focus on the provision of health care services, often sending patients back into the social and economic conditions that made them sick. Nowhere is this more evident than in the case of individuals experiencing homelessness or living in unsafe, precarious housing."[42]

The Conference Board of Canada concluded in 2012 that "most top-performing countries have achieved better health outcomes through actions on the broader determinants of health" and that leading countries place a strong focus on health drivers such as education, early childhood development, income, and social status to improve health outcomes.[43] More recently, in an analysis of 16 indicators (determinants) of health, the Canadian Institute for Health Information concluded that inequalities persist and that in over 15 years "little or no progress has been made in reducing inequalities in health by income level in Canada."[44]

WHAT IS THE RETURN ON INVESTMENT IN NURSING SERVICES?

One of the clever mantras that evolved in Canadian nursing during the mid-2000s—"nurses have more face time with the public than any other profession"—built on the notion that nurses are everywhere in health systems across Canada and that they provide more care in the system than any other provider. If this refrain is true, then what is the return for Canadians on their significant investment in nursing? If nurses are absent, patients and populations get sicker and even die; but what happens when they are present? What does some $27.4 billion—an estimate of the cost of Canadian nursing (not including nurse practitioners) cited earlier—actually purchase in return for all that face time?

Performance of the Nursing Workforce

A compelling body of evidence makes clear that when they are effectively deployed, employed, rewarded, and engaged, nurses exert massive impacts on population health, health care, system quality, safety, and overall value for dollars invested. Importantly, and often not given due emphasis, nurses exert equally significant impacts on physical and emotional healing. Nurses sometimes have been reluctant to claim *cure* in favour of *care*. Both matter, of course, and as the data reveal, both are part of excellent nursing practice.

Our understanding of the effects of nurses and nursing care on individual, organizational, and system outcomes has grown dramatically over the past 20 years. The collection of nurse-sensitive inputs and outcomes data is increasing across the system. Some of the push has come from researchers, who, apart from conducting individual studies on the topic, have supported initiatives such as the Canadian Health Outcomes for Better Information and Care (C-HOBIC) project. This initiative was launched to introduce "a systematic, structured language to admission and discharge assessments of patients receiving in acute care, complex continuing care, long-term care or home care."[45] Pressure for information also has come from decision makers in organizations and governments to inform their allocation decisions. The results of C-HOBIC are improving identification of indicators that support collection and analysis of comparable data—in short, to enable the comparison of apples to apples and not oranges. The Canadian Institute for Health Information supports analysis of nursing outcomes by collecting and providing syntheses of the composition and employment patterns of regulated nurses (and other providers) across Canada. Under the leadership of nursing informactics leaders Lynn Nagle and Peggy White, a symposium to further advance pan-Canadian nursing data standards in Canada was held in Toronto in April 2016. A second symposium was held in April 2017, attracting more than 100 participants from every Canadian jurisdiction and resulting in an action plan with targeted milestones and outputs to move this agenda.

The body of nursing outcomes research is vast, and while much of it is focused on hospitals, there is information emerging from other areas of practice as well. In the following sections, consider just a few examples of the impacts of nursing entry-to-practice education, nursing expertise (a reflection of years of experience, professional development, and specialty certification), and staffing numbers on individual, organization, and system outcomes.

The Impact of Entry-to-Practice Nursing Education on Individual, Organization, and System Outcomes

- Studying the impact of education on mortality and failure to rescue, Kendall-Gallagher and colleagues found that in hospitals, a 10 per cent increase in the proportion of baccalaureate-prepared nurses reduced the odds of adjusted 30-day mortality and failure to rescue by 6 per cent.[46]
- In a nine-country European study (420,000 patients in 300 hospitals) each 10 per cent increase in the number of baccalaureate nurses in the staff mix was associated with a 7 per cent decrease in the likelihood of death within 30 days of admission. Furthermore, the mortality rate dropped by 30 per cent where there were more baccalaureate-educated nurses (60 per cent) and their patient assignments were lower (six patients each) than those having lower numbers of baccalaureate nurses (30 per cent) and caring for more patients (eight patients each).[47]

The Impact of Nursing Expertise on Individual, Organization, and System Outcomes

- In the study by Kendall-Gallagher and colleagues cited above, when baccalaureate-educated nurses had additional specialty certification, the odds of 30-day mortality and failure to rescue were reduced by an additional 2 per cent.[48]
- In rehabilitation settings, it was found that a 6 per cent increase in the proportion of registered nurses with specialty certification in rehabilitation was associated with a one-day drop in average length of stay.[49]
- As years of registered nurse experience rise, fall rates among patients drop, as do hospital-acquired pressure ulcer rates.[50]

The Impact of Nurse Staffing on Individual, Organization, and System Outcomes

- We have known since early in the 2000s that as the number of patients per nurse climbs in hospital surgical settings so do risk-adjusted 30-day mortality and failure-to-rescue rates—and those "nurses are more likely to experience burnout and job dissatisfaction."[51]
- Lower proportions of professional nurses in hospital units are associated with higher medication errors and higher wound infections.[52]
- In a landmark Canadian study in 2006, the Tourangeau Research group at the University of Toronto found lower 30-day hospital mortality rates

in association with a number of variables, including higher proportions of registered nurses and baccalaureate-educated nurses, better staffing and resources, a higher use of tools such as care maps to help guide the care, and higher quality reported by the nurses. Their study revealed that a "10% increase in the proportion of Registered Nurses was associated with six fewer deaths for every 1000 discharged patients."[53]

- Higher numbers of hours provided by regulated staff improve outcomes and reduce length of stay, while lower regulated nursing hours are correlated with more medication errors and wound infections. In other words, vigilant, well-educated eyes on patients is what cures them. Buhlman concluded in 2016 that "the link between more bedside nurses and a better patient experience isn't surprising. That the correlations stretch across all experience domains—not just those that examine quality and frequency of nurse-patient interactions—is eye-opening."[54] More eyes lead to better outcomes, and as Mitchell observed, "having fewer patients per nurse or more direct nursing care hours per patient day is associated with fewer adverse outcomes, in particular mortality, failure to rescue and some specific adverse events, particularly among surgical patients." Summarizing these relationships, she said conclusively, "This association is no longer in dispute."[55] Convinced by the evidence, Jack Needleman—a University of California, Los Angeles non-nurse scientist of global repute in this area of research—said in November 2015 that whether or not nurse staffing should be strengthened depends on one thing only: the value patients, providers, and funders assign to avoided complications and deaths.[56]

- In magnet hospitals in the United States, where there are "significantly better work environments and higher proportions of nurses with bachelor's degrees and specialty certification," patients faced 14 per cent lower probability of mortality and 12 per cent lower probability of failure to rescue.[57]

- In a 2009 analysis of the economic value of professional nursing, the research team led by Dall in the United States examined the relationship between staffing levels of registered nurses in acute care hospitals and nursing-sensitive patient outcomes.[58] They concluded that each additional registered nurse employed in hospitals would generate more than $60,000 in reduced medical costs and improved national productivity annually. Their analysis suggests that adding 133,000 full-time registered nurses to the hospital workforce would (a) save 5,900 lives per year; (b) save at least $1.3 billion in productivity value of averted deaths—nearly $10,000 per registered nurse; and (c) decrease hospital days by some 3.6 million. They estimated the national productivity value of nurse-influenced shorter stays to be (conservatively) $231 million, or $1,700 per additional registered nurse per year.

- In the Massachusetts public school system, a one-year trial of school nurses found that the program generated a net benefit of $98.2 million back to society—a gain of $2.20 for every dollar invested. The researchers concluded that the study "demonstrated that school nursing services ... were a cost-beneficial investment of public money, warranting careful consideration by policy makers and decision makers when resource allocation decisions are made about school nursing positions."[59]

- Early measures of the registered nurse prescribing initiative in the United Kingdom have revealed high levels of patient satisfaction and confidence, no significant differences in prescribing patterns between doctors and the nurse prescribers in hospitals, a better utilization of skill sets on hospital wards, improved access to care for patients, minimal errors by the nurses, and the whole project has allowed physicians to focus more on patients needing their level of diagnosis and care.[60]

- In a study of nurse practitioners in collaborative practice with physicians in rural British Columbia, patients had more time with each visit, the job satisfaction of physicians and other team members improved, access to care was enhanced in the community (especially for harder-to-serve populations), emergency room visits and hospital admissions dropped, and physicians' intentions to remain in the work environment increased.[61]

- Finally, in their review of evidence conducted for the National Expert Commission, Browne and team analyzed 27 high-quality reviews that met their criteria from among an original compilation of more than 4,000 papers focused on comparative models of nursing care for people with chronic conditions. For the work, they classified nursing intervention studies where at least 50 per cent of the intervention was provided by nurses. Some of these involved nurse replacement (for physician) models and, in others, nurses were used to supplement the usual care, either alone or as part of a multidisciplinary team. As a result, they found that "models of proactive, targeted nurse led care that focus on preventive patient self-management for people with chronic disease are either more effective and equally or less costly, or are equally effective and less costly than the usual model of care."[62] Specifically, they found that: 13 models were more effective and less costly; 2 models were more effective for the same cost; 7 models were equally effective and less cost; and 5 models were equally effective for the same cost.

In study after study, the impact of nursing care—especially registered nurse and nurse practitioner care, which have been studied most often—has revealed significantly positive returns on investments: fewer deaths and fewer complications, fewer admissions and readmissions to institutions, faster healing and shorter lengths of stay in hospitals, more satisfied patients and happier team members, and lower costs for those footing the bill. And despite the strategic, ongoing lobbying and marketing of physicians calling for more doctors and more doctor care, there are cracks in some of that narrative as well. Analyzing American physician workforce data and outcomes in 2007, for example, Weiner argued that "above a certain threshold, more is not better. As use of services increases, quality and health related outcomes (at least to the degree we can currently measure it) do not improve." There is value in more generalist physicians delivering primary care, but Weiner cited studies showing that "as the supply of specialists per population increases, indicators of quality of care decrease, costs increase, and population mortality does not change."[63]

Adding advanced practice nurses to the mix only makes things better. In a 2010 synthesis for the Canadian Health Services Research Foundation, DiCenso and Bryant-Lukosius found a "striking consistency in findings across studies and the consolidation of these findings in a number of systematic reviews" showing that "advanced practice nurses are effective, safe practitioners who can positively influence patient, provider and health system outcomes."[64] For nurse practitioners in primary care settings, findings included higher satisfaction and better quality care than physicians, and no differences in measures such as number of prescriptions, return visits, or health outcomes. In addition, in hospitals there either were no differences or an improvement in outcomes such as mortality, morbidity, complications, and length of hospital stay. Outcomes for clinical nurse specialists were similarly positive.

The findings of Browne and colleagues have especially profound implications in a system clamouring for better quality while containing costs: they showed that for chronic disease management, an area of growing demand in Canada, nursing care is as effective as or more effective than traditional models for the same or less cost—no small assertion in a system plagued with long wait times and too few physicians interested in working with this population. What is more, care for chronic diseases aligns well with the existing scope of nursing practice. The policy implications of these findings are discussed in the closing chapter.

SUMMARY AND IMPLICATIONS

Material in this module has explored evidence that Canadians live longer lives than the citizens of most other countries, and over the past century our growing investments in health care have helped defeat many communicable

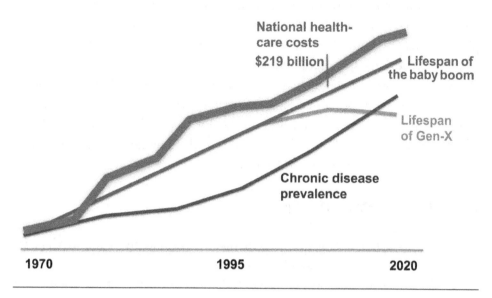

Figure 8.4: Trends in Canadian Health Care Costs, Life Expectancy and Disease Burden

Note: These are trend lines only.

diseases and mitigate the impacts of non-communicable illnesses and injuries. Paradoxically, however, the evidence tells us that, left unchecked, those longer lives are likely to be lived in the troubling and costly company of chronic health problems that tend to grow in number and severity in old age. And, for the first time, some analysts have predicted that the generations after the baby boomers could live shorter, sicker lives than their parents. Figure 8.4 depicts these troubling trends.

If the assertion of the National Expert Commission that the ability of episodic, acute care to have an impact on population health is limited is true, then our collective and constant fuelling of acute care, treatment, and cure is an increasingly questionable investment. Certainly the system can do a quick and effective job rescuing individual health, and for those who suffer a heart attack or are injured in a car crash, they will be grateful for its effectiveness. However, in a country with a growing number of seniors, growing rates of chronic disease, a growing number of deaths (related to the high number of seniors), a small sector the population using a lot of services, and whole groups of citizens whose health problems seem to be driven by determinants not amenable to acute care, then the proportion of resources allotted to doctors, drugs, hospitals, and other institutions is worrying. The system rallies well to sudden illness or injury, but that seems to be the only way it knows how to rally. While it is fit for purpose around rescue, it is a poor choice of care and use of funds to help frail older people, those having multiple co-morbid health problems, or Canadians who need compassionate end-of-life care options.

Knowing some of these challenges, we turn in Module III to think about how to take on the tasks of making policy change. How can nurses act to change things to create a better match between health care and emerging population health needs? How are those policy decisions made, how can nurses be involved, and what challenges lie on the road ahead?

DISCUSSION QUESTIONS

1. What is the role of the state in shaping population health in Canada? How could and should it be reformed?
2. What could Canada's governments do differently to use their resources to improve population health?
3. What should be the role of nurses in improving population health?
4. What actions could nurses and nursing organizations take toward reconciliation with Aboriginal Peoples by addressing population health outcome disparities?
5. What are the links among determinants of health, population health, nursing, and public policy?
6. How should nursing be reformed to improve population health, quality and safety of care, and return on investments in health care?
7. How should nursing respond to improve the health of Canada's growing population of seniors?

ADDITIONAL POLICY RESOURCES

HEALTH SYSTEMS DATA AND RESEARCH

Canadian Academy of Health Sciences	http://www.cahs-acss.cav
Canadian Institute for Advanced Research	http://www.cifar.ca
Canadian Institute for Health Information	http://www.cihi.ca
Evidence Network of Canadian Health Policy	http://umanitoba.ca/outreach/ evidencenetwork
Health Council of Canada	http://www.healthcouncilcanada.ca
McMaster Health Forum	http://www.mcmasterhealthforum.org

HEALTH SYSTEMS SAFETY, QUALITY, AND PERFORMANCE

Accreditation Canada	https://www.accreditation.ca
Canada Health Infoway	http://www.betterhealthtogether.ca
Canadian Foundation for Healthcare Improvement (formerly Canadian Health Services Research Foundation)	http://www.cfhi-fcass.ca/Splash.aspx
Canadian Patient Safety Institute	http://www.patientsafetyinstitute.ca
Institute for Healthcare Improvement (United States)	http://www.ihi.org

MODULE III

From Ideas to Legislation: How Are Health Policy Decisions Made?

Building on knowledge about the governance, structures, functioning, and funding of health systems developed in the first two modules, Module III explores conceptual models and practical examples of the ways policy happens. Thinking back to an example in Module I, how is it that there is mandatory seat belt legislation across Canada today when there were no seat belts in cars 50 years ago? Why is it unacceptable to smoke cigarettes in most public places in Canada when people in many other countries smoke everywhere? Public policy drove the legislation of these behaviours. Public policy also tells us where and when Canadians are allowed to sell, buy, and consume alcohol depending on the province in which they live, how child-care services are funded and delivered, at what times of the year hunters may hunt and fishers may fish, and who may access home care at what cost. Policy is everywhere in our lives every day.

Public policy, of course, does not simply appear. It is the result of work by real people, often over years and even generations. And while it is a complex and complicated endeavour, as was introduced in Chapter 1, there are models that can help to understand how policy gets done. This module presents theoretical steps in the policy process and discusses examples of tools commonly used by nurses and others in policy development, including lobbying, briefing notes, position papers, royal commissions by governments, and pro-fession-led initiatives such as the National Expert Commission.[1]

Public policy is dependent on difficult, often politically risky, decision-making; there are very few public policies that do not provide some outcome that accords an advantage to one group while denying something to another. The questions of who gets what public services and why are thorny ones indeed. They depend on priority setting and the subsequent allocation of resources. The ways those decisions are made are no less muddy. They may be driven by scientific evidence, for example, or by ethical principles, by eco-nomic considerations, or by emergency situations that threaten human lives. In most major pieces of legislation, aspects of many dynamics may come into play as public and health policy decisions are made.

What might overrule the most rigorous decision-making process is the complicating factor of politics. That may mean the personal preference, be-liefs, or even desire for power of a decision maker, or the ideology of a po-litical party. It may bring into play constituencies such as supporters of the decision maker (e.g., voters), the opinions of the public at large, and, as in all things, timing. This module examines these spheres of influence in policy in-cluding the public, noted above, but also forces such as the media. The public and members of the media may have interests in any number of public policy issues, but also may be cast as interest groups in the policy-making process. Similarly, nurses have many interests in public policy development; nursing organizations are interest groups in the world of health policy. Also introduced here are what are sometimes called the "I" forces—ideas and ideology, inno-vation, institutions, interests and interest groups, and intuition—with an eye to understanding how these forces may act to shape health policy. Examples of actions, roles, and effectiveness of individual nurses, and of the nursing profession in influencing public policy and health system transformation, are introduced.

The final chapter of Module III closes this introductory exploration of policy for nurses by looking forward to the system-level challenges lying ahead, and to ways nurses and nursing might engage in policy solutions to resolve them. The First Ministers' 10-Year Plan to Strengthen Health Care—more commonly known as the 2004 Health Accord—certainly had an impact on some of its in-tended outcomes, but left many of them unresolved. Much work remains and nurses should hold the reins on some of these. Among the most urgent prob-lems are the immediate health care needs of Canadians, including strategies to support the affordable, healthy aging of a huge cohort of older Canadians, and to prevent and manage chronic disease. Important to addressing both of those challenges are the unresolved issues of access to affordable pharmaceuticals and to insured home- and other community-based care. The public discourse on ethical challenges, including globalism, medical tourism, end-of-life care, palliative care, medical assistance in death, and futile care, has been dominated by physicians even when so much—in some cases nearly all—of the care is managed and delivered by nurses.

CHAPTER 9

Models of Policy Development

CHAPTER HIGHLIGHTS

- How Does Policy Happen? Frameworks and Models
- An Evolving Conceptual Model of Policy Development for Nursing
- Summary and Implications
- Discussion Questions
- Additional Policy Resources

LEARNING OUTCOMES

1. Discuss different approaches and models that have been developed to explain and predict the policy development process.
2. Describe the key elements of policy development in a theoretical *policy cycle* model.
3. Describe how problems are identified and moved to the public policy agenda, and state three nursing examples of the same.

Policy Influencer: Madeleine Meilleur

Madeleine Meilleur, RN, LLB, is a nurse who was also educated as a lawyer with a specialty in labour and employment law. Beyond her roles with health-related boards and organizations, and after serving as a city councillor in Ottawa (2001–2003), she went on to be elected as a (Liberal) member of Ontario's provincial parliament in four consecutive elections beginning in 2003. She brought her nursing and legal knowledge to various portfolios in cabinet, serving as minister of culture, community and social services, community safety and correctional services, francophone affairs, and finally as the attorney general of Ontario.[1] Reflecting on her policy successes at the time of her resignation in June 2016, she cited having "led the passage of laws promoting the social inclusion of persons with developmental disabilities, spearheaded efforts to introduce a new and strengthened Ontario Heritage Act, made sprinklers mandatory in retirement homes and vulnerable care occupancies, and undertaken a number of initiatives that have furthered access to justice across Ontario."[2] Her leadership also was pivotal in saving Ottawa's Hôpital Montfort—the only French-speaking hospital in Ontario—when its closure was recommended by the Ontario Health Services Restructuring Commission in 1997.

"Enduring progress is forged in a cauldron of both principle and compromise."

—*William J. Clinton, former president, United States*

HOW DOES POLICY HAPPEN? FRAMEWORKS AND MODELS

Up to this point, the discussion has focused on the types of history, information, and dynamics nurses need to be equipped to understand and engage effectively in the worlds of nursing and health policy in Canada. However, while examples of nursing influence on policy have been introduced, this module attempts to respond to the more fundamental question, "How do you do the actual work of policy development? How does it happen?" The tools and strategies in this module come from a mix of sources, including policy publications and lessons emerging from the practical experiences of nurses in policy roles over the past 20 years.

While the process of policy development can quickly look daunting at a systems level, it is useful to take a step back and be reminded of the basic stages

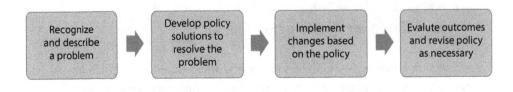

Figure 9.1: Basic Steps of Policy Development

underlying most models of policy making and change depicted in Figure 9.1. Except in the most basic circumstances, the process is rarely this straightforward or linear, and that is especially so in areas as complex as health and social policy.

A model for public policy development suggested by the University of Texas at Austin is more inclusive of the complexity of public policy development, including six overlapping stages in a circular cycle model as shown in Figure 9.2. Notice here the introduction of a fiscal component—cost is almost always a central issue in public policy deliberation. The process in this model is described as including "additional mini stages in a process that never ends."[3]

Circular conceptual models can help portray a sense of flow and also emphasize the ongoing nature of policy development, as mentioned in the University of Texas description. The idea of a process that never ends underscores the notion that, once developed and adopted, the evidence, content, and impact of policy

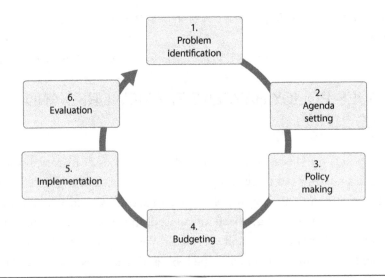

Figure 9.2: Theoretical Public Policy Process, University of Texas at Austin

Source: Liberal Arts Instructional Technology Services. (2015). *The public policy process.* Austin, TX: University of Texas at Austin. Retrieved from http://www.laits.utexas.edu/gov310/PEP/policy.

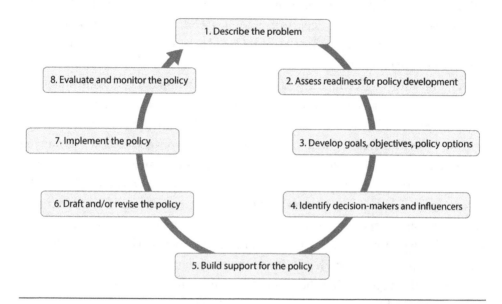

Figure 9.3: Eight Steps to Developing a Healthy Public Policy, Public Health Ontario

Source: Public Health Ontario. (2013). *At a glance: The eight steps to developing a healthy public policy.* Toronto: Public Health Ontario.

should be monitored, revised as necessary, or abolished when it is no longer relevant. One of the collective failings in the world of public policy, including nursing policy, is that it is sometimes left to stagnate, often exerting its influence long after its relevance has passed.

Closer to home, Public Health Ontario offered up a helpful, eight-stage model in 2013 that includes and builds on some of the elements and principles of the University of Texas model (see Figure 9.3).[4] While the Texas model describes stages, the Public Health Ontario model is prescriptive, laying out very helpful actions, steps within the major stages, and practical suggestions to support the development of public policy. Each of these models helped to inform the model discussed in the following section.

AN EVOLVING CONCEPTUAL MODEL OF POLICY DEVELOPMENT FOR NURSING

When it opened in 1999, the federal Office of Nursing Policy was an entirely new unit within Health Canada, staffed and structured to position nursing more prominently than had been the case in the preceding generation. The policy office titling also signalled an explicit focus, which included its mandate to "bring the perspectives of nurses to the department's policy work and decision-making"[5] and, in the reverse, to take the work of Health Canada out to the world of nursing and health care more broadly.

The breadth and complexity of the issues that immediately confronted the team made clear that some sort of tool was required to organize them, understand their contexts, and help set priorities. Consider the earlier example of the high nursing absenteeism rate, which began to come up in conversations across nursing in the late 1990s. Confronted with that issue, the team immediately needed to understand where the information was coming from, who knew about this issue, who was doing work in this area across the country, what evidence had been developed, and what policy responses, if any, had been implemented and tested. In short, to inform the department's policy work, intelligence gathering was necessary to fully identify the problem, position it in the context of other related issues, and help the team think through whether they should engage with it and how.

A number of different models of policy development were examined by the team over the first year of the office's operation, including the previous work of Kingdon[6] and Milstead.[7] But transformative conceptual help came at the Annual Couchiching Conference in August 2000. Focused on the conference theme, The Future of Health Care in Canada, the opening keynote panel included Fraser Mustard, Sir Michael Marmot, and Alvin Tarlov—from Canada, the United Kingdom, and the United States, respectively. At the time, Tarlov was director of the multi-university program in society and population health in Houston, professor at the School of Public Health at University of Texas, Houston, and a senior fellow in health policy at Rice University. In his presentation, he outlined what he called a "simple, logical framework with which to formulate policies to improve population health."[8] For those in the audience struggling with ways to categorize policy issues and organize related work, he was encouraging: "I want you to feel confident that a common-sense methodology and a simplified conceptual framework will get you there and that you will make a lot of good sense out of it."[9]

Tarlov had published his framework in 1999, describing it in eight steps over two stages as follows:

> The initial phase, in which public consensus builds and an authorizing environment evolves, progresses from values and culture to identification of the problem, knowledge development from research and experience, the unfolding of public awareness, and the setting of a national agenda. The later phase, taking policy action, begins with political engagement and progresses to interest group activation, public policy deliberation and adoption, and ultimately regulation and revision.[10]

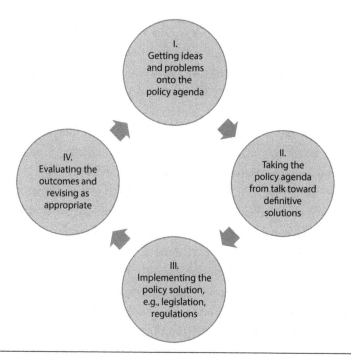

Figure 9.4: Stages of Public Policy Development, Implementation, and Evaluation

He laid out a useful way of breaking down and thinking through the steps in a cycle of policy development, from idea to legislation and/or regulation. Once policy is formalized through legislation or regulation, there still remain the important stages of implementation and evaluation. In the case of health policy, for example, implementation may mean changes in funding mechanisms for regional health authorities, in the operation of a community health clinic, or in the scope of practice of nurses.

A policy being formalized is, of course, a long way from the change(s) in behaviour the policy is designed to bring about—think of the decades-long challenges around public smoking mentioned earlier. Therefore, to be most helpful to nurses, a more comprehensive model of policy development must include the concepts in Tarlov's policy cycle in addition to stages of implementation and then evaluation of the impact of the policy as it plays out in reality. Those four stages, discussed in more detail in this chapter, are depicted in Figure 9.4. Notice the similarity here to the very basic four stages of policy development described at the beginning of this chapter.

The happenstance of the Couchiching event would prove to be a game changer for the Office of Nursing Policy, not just for organizing and monitoring its own work going forward, but in how it enabled the team to explain its work and communicate its policy development process. The framework described by Tarlov was broad and sophisticated enough to be useful in categorizing and analyzing complex rosters of issues. But importantly, the model also was compelling because it was straightforward and fairly easy to understand within the team and to communicate to others; practicality in these matters is important. Always with full credit to Tarlov's foundational influence on the work, Health Canada nurses adapted some of the language to suit their work, considered other published frameworks, and developed a tool to understand and organize activities.

The evolution of that tool for use by nurses (and others) continues and some of the terms have changed over time as a result of experience and new thinking. However, the underlying principles and flow have remained quite solid for the past 15 years. It has proven to be a useful model to teach, understand, and operate within the sphere of public policy development—if one subscribes to a pluralist view of policy making that assumes forces outside governments have a role. When analyzing the state of any policy issue, this tool is helpful in thinking about its context and dynamic, what work has been done, and what work lies ahead.

Earlier publications referred to the first two stages of the conceptual model simply as the *Policy Cycle*.[11] The first phase of ramping up knowledge, options, and awareness around a problem or issue, is summarized as "Getting to the Policy Agenda." The second phase, "Moving into Action," includes taking evidence, experience, and awareness into the action of political engagement, consultation, policy development, and on to legislation and/or regulation. For this text, the model is expanded in Figure 9.5

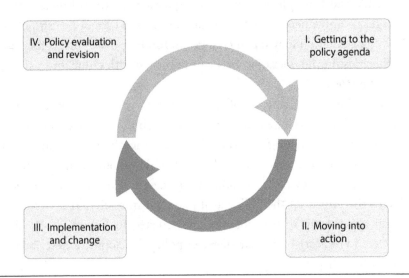

Figure 9.5: Four Main Stages of the Policy Cycle

to show those two stages, as well as the phases of implementing policy and then evaluating outcomes and revising the policy as necessary. Examples of the federal Office of Nursing Policy's work in the area of the health of nurses are threaded throughout this chapter to illustrate ways the team attempted to intervene to influence policy development at different stages.

Phase I: Getting to the Policy Agenda

The first phase of policy development includes the four steps depicted in Figure 9.6 and discussed in the following pages. Examples of nursing policy work are used in discussions of the various steps.

Step 1: Values and Beliefs

All stages and steps in any policy development depend on the existence of some underlying set of values and beliefs. In Canada, good and practical examples can be found in our Constitution Act (1867) and its Charter of Rights and Freedoms. At the opening of the Charter are the words that lay out a basic set of values and beliefs across Canadian society: "Everyone has the following fundamental freedoms: (a) freedom of conscience and religion; (b) freedom of thought, belief, opinion and expression, including freedom of the press and other media of communication; (c) freedom of peaceful assembly; and (d) freedom of association."[12] Those are clear belief or value statements about expectations in Canadian society. In the American Declaration of Independence of July 4, 1776, a similar underlying value set is set down in the words, "We hold these truths

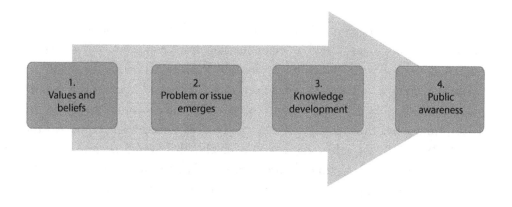

Figure 9.6: Phase I Steps in Policy Development:
Getting to the Policy Agenda

to be self-evident, that all men are created equal, that they are endowed by their creator with certain unalienable rights, that among these are life, liberty and the pursuit of happiness."[13] These sorts of founding ideas lay out the landscape of a nation and the value sets with which its citizens will be treated—and with which it is expected they will conduct themselves in public.

Both countries are members of the United Nations, and have signed on to uphold the Universal Declaration of Human Rights.[14] Among the 30 articles in the declaration are values that have profound social and health implications in our own country. Consider Articles 25 and 26, for example, which state that:

Article 25

a. Everyone has the right to a standard of living adequate for the health and well-being of himself and of his family, including food, clothing, housing and medical care and necessary social services, and the right to security in the event of unemployment, sickness, disability, widowhood, old age or other lack of livelihood in circumstances beyond his control.

b. Motherhood and childhood are entitled to special care and assistance. All children, whether born in or out of wedlock, shall enjoy the same social protection.

Article 26

c. Everyone has the right to education. Education shall be free, at least in the elementary and fundamental stages. Elementary education shall be compulsory. Technical and professional education shall be made generally available and higher education shall be equally accessible to all on the basis of merit.

Note that Canada vowed to uphold the values of this declaration—including the important conditions related to secure housing, food, education, and a range of health and social services—when it was tabled by the member nations in 1948.

Beyond being a signatory to the Universal Declaration of Human Rights, and in the years after the Lalonde report positioned Canada so prominently on the global primary health care stage, the Pierre Trudeau government supported the WHO's 1977 "call for achieving a level of health that would permit everyone to lead a socially and economically productive life" by the year 2000.[15] Over the next year, Canada helped its WHO fellow members to develop the Declaration of Alma-Ata, which it then vigorously promoted and signed in 1978. The opening statement of that declaration "strongly reaffirms that health, which is a state of complete physical, mental and social wellbeing, and not merely the absence of disease or infirmity, is a fundamental human right and that the attainment of the highest possible level of health is a most important world-wide social goal whose realization requires the action of many other social and economic sectors in addition to the health sector."[16]

When we think about the first phase of a health policy development model, these various beliefs and values—enshrined in the constitution and in the global declarations about health and social rights that Canada has agreed to uphold—provide a strong base on which to ground thinking and decisions about outcomes and progress. Therefore, as a starting point, one value that has emerged in Canada is the importance of health care as a public good. Helm and Mayer pointed to public health and education as important examples of societal infrastructure that form "the sub-structure of an economy on which other structures, systems and activities are built."[17] They included public health among innovations that "have laid the foundations for economic activity around the world in every sector, in most cases over several centuries."[18] Health care fits their definition of infrastructure that, along with other kinds of services, has laid the foundations for economic activity around the world in every sector, in most cases over several centuries. Canadians might add to that the example of the traditional postal service, Canada Post, which some have argued is a public good that, like health care, should be treated as a not-for-profit entity—one that comes with fiscal costs that drive other benefits—and not one whose value should be measured through fiscal profit.

Related to the idea of not-for-profit public good, an important and specific value of Canadians around health care is found in their unwavering support of the Canada Health Act. Another is that the presence of a safe, well educated, regulated, and healthy nursing workforce is important to the delivery of programs that respond to all our other beliefs and values about health and health care.

Step 2: Problem or Issue Emerges

There is particular value in remembering the elements of a robust primary health care system outlined in the Alma-Ata declaration, which Canada agreed should minimally include:

- education concerning prevailing health problems and methods of preventing and controlling them;
- promotion of food supply and proper nutrition;
- an adequate supply of safe water and basic sanitation;
- maternal and child health care, including family planning;
- immunization against the major infectious diseases;
- prevention and control of locally endemic diseases;
- appropriate treatment of common diseases and injuries; and
- provision of essential drugs.

Problems in the health sector typically emerge when one of these values is not being met, or not met fully—think of the E. coli outbreak in the drinking water in Walkerton, Ontario, in 2000,[20] the SARS outbreak in 2003, the H1N1 outbreak in 2009, or the inability of so many Canadians to afford prescribed (or even over-the-counter) medications today. These examples represent problems meeting our underlying values about safe water, spread of endemic disease, and provision of essential drugs. Within these values, we see the roots of policy work related to social problems that impact health, such as inadequate housing and its tie to the reality of the Canadian climate—for example, that life-threatening inner-city heat in the summer and freezing cold in winter are both significant threats to the homeless and those with inadequate housing.

Nurses and nursing have featured prominently in many policy initiatives over the past century. Sometimes it is a lack of nurses that prompts a policy response: a news story about a child requiring transfer to a different facility due to a lack of

Values in Policy Development

With regard to the place of values in policy development, students of the topic may wish to read the report by Giacomini and colleagues. They offer lessons for consideration:

- "Values are like atoms. Values seem to be everywhere, like atoms—all pervasive, extremely important, yet often invisible.
- Values are not just preferences.
- Values are not just individuals' deep-rooted beliefs.
- Individual and collective values are made of different, incommensurable substances.
- Weighing values tells us little about what to do with them.
- And values are also like onions. Studying policy values critically leads the policy analyst through layers of reasoning that is definitional ... as well as instrumental ...
- Strive for the big picture and critique its parts. Values can be found in many actors and may take many forms.
- Reading between the lines is necessary and difficult.
- Evidence is not value free."
- From platitudes to policies—our relationship with values involves developmental philosophical and discursive aspects.[19]

available nurses to provide intra-operative or post-operative care usually provokes a rapid response, freeing up funds for more nurses or to open closed hospital beds. The problem in that example emerges from a failure to meet the values that (a) appropriate treatment of common diseases and injuries should be accessible, (b) nurses are important to the treatment equation, and (c) having a qualified nursing workforce in place to meet the access to health care is imperative.

In the wake of provincial and territorial efforts to contain costs during the 1990s, and especially after the austerity budget of the Chrétien government in 1995, many regulated nurses were removed from the system through early retirements, shutting down seats in nursing schools, and other measures. While some money was saved in the short term by having fewer nurses in the system, there were long-term costs from which, arguably, nursing and health systems have yet to recover. Understandably, the uncertainty of that time provoked tremendous anxiety across the profession. One of the impacts of unionization—a mix of both beneficial and detrimental effects, depending on one's place in the chain of events—was the movement of nurses within institutions across program areas based on seniority. A consequence of nurses being fired was that many nurses who survived the cuts were moved from their areas of clinical specialty and/or personal preference—assuming that an experienced nurse wants to be and/or can be easily or safely moved to other sectors of clinical practice. This sort of policy would be considered ridiculous in most professions and utterly unacceptable in nursing's closest counterpart, medicine. Other nurses were coaxed to take early retirement packages and still others were let go altogether. The mess created, including the amount of care being left undone, meant that some of those same nurses who had been urged to take early retirement packages were nearly immediately hired back—creating a whole new policy problem.

There was less formal measurement in the 1990s of outcomes such as job satisfaction and turnover than exists today. However, nurses and others in management and leadership positions across the provinces and territories certainly had a sense that nurses were unhappy, and, not surprisingly, that the workforce was in a general state of upset. By 1999, nurses doing policy work were beginning to hear concerns from across the country about staffing problems and difficulties managing budgets, due to problems such as high use of overtime staff and external agency nurses. Some of the feedback was verbal, but publications also were beginning to emerge pointing to concerns about shortages of nurses, an aging nursing workforce, and the interaction among nurses, their workplaces, and patient outcomes. Unhappy nurses drove up staff turnover, later found to be near 20 per cent per year in Canada (higher in critical care areas), and costing organizations roughly $25,000 per nurse.[21]

During that period (1998–2001) scattered comments grew into what seemed like a chorus across the country, and evidence began to grow, with nurse managers and others increasingly commenting that it seemed like there was a lot of absenteeism due to illness. At the same time there was growing concern about the impact of the whole situation on quality of care. Could this emerging constellation of problems be a symptom, and/or a cause, of the perceived chaos across health systems, particularly in costly hospital and institutional settings? The pursuit of more information in this area led to establishment of a key pillar of work over the first decade of the new century that included definitive interventions and programs that remain a legacy of the Office of Nursing Policy and its partners within and beyond Health Canada.

Step 3: Knowledge Development

Knowledge development to inform policy decision-making may entail a wide range of activities, from computer-based literature searches (which may be called environmental, landscape, or horizon scans depending on the task at hand) to in-person meetings, stakeholder consultations, surveys, and formal research that may include extensive, random-controlled trials. Usually some combination of tools and techniques are employed, and examples of the main ones are described in Chapter 10.

Urgent in the early work of the Office of Nursing Policy was the need to quantify the talk being heard across the country and synthesize the available evidence. To be concrete, the office assumed a four-tiered approach to the research steps of its knowledge development:

1. Constant scanning with a nursing and health systems lens.
2. Commissioning formal research and/or promoting studies underway.
3. Participation of team members as lead or co-investigators in new research.
4. Interpretation and dissemination of research.

The Nursing Health Services Research Unit

The Nursing Health Services Research Unit based at the University of Toronto and McMaster University has now wrapped up its work, having functioned for 25 years (1991–2016). To learn more about the work of the Nursing Health Services Research Unit, go to http://nhsru.com.

To learn more about the current work of the Center for Health Outcomes and Policy Research at the University of Pennsylvania, go to http://www.nursing.upenn.edu/chopr.

Data from Canada's Labour Force Survey proved to be illuminating when it was found that the absenteeism of nurses exceeded all other occupations, including jobs such as heavy equipment operators and construction workers.[22] By 2001, registered nurse absenteeism was 311,364 hours per week—the equivalent of 8,956 full-time positions. Perhaps not surprisingly, overtime being worked by registered nurses climbed—someone still had to provide care in the absence of other nurses—exceeding 240,000 hours per week or more than 7,000 full-time positions. Most of that was paid overtime at premium costs.[23] It is a concern that, more than 15 years later, the absenteeism and overtime problems remain significant, as discussed in Chapter 12.

The impact on quality of care from having fewer registered nurses across the system became increasingly clear and worrying as a growing body of science confirmed the hunches of real providers whose eyes were on the outcomes. It was not long before significant pieces of research, mostly from Canada and the United States, began to correlate the number, education level, and specialty certification status of nurses in the mix of staff with patient experiences, costs, and outcomes such as morbidity and mortality. Health Canada nurses were actively involved in supporting the funding, execution, and dissemination of a number of those studies, many of which were conducted under the leadership or structure of the Nursing Effectiveness, Utilization and Outcomes Research Unit based at the University of Toronto and McMaster University under the leadership of Drs. Linda O'Brien-Pallas and Andrea Baumann, respectively. That research unit had a wide reach through its relationships with leading researchers across the country. In the United States, the Health Canada team worked extensively with the International Hospital Outcomes Research Consortium led by Linda Aiken and her team in the Center for Health Outcomes and Policy Research at the University of Pennsylvania School of Nursing.

Typical of studies at the time, a 1998–1999 study of more than 8,000 Ontario registered nurses, led by the Ontario arm of the International Hospital Outcomes Research Consortium, found that more than 50 per cent of nurses who provided narrative comments "voiced strong concerns about the intensification of workloads" that were the result of a toxic combination of dwindling numbers of nurses, the same number or more patients per nurse, sharply higher acuity, policies "favouring reduced length of stay," and more non-nursing responsibilities—all leading to a more complex and exhausting work environment.[24] As discussed in Chapter 8, those sorts of nursing outcomes played out across the following decade and continue today.

Step 4: Public Awareness

Decision makers may be highly influenced by the voting public and public opinion. Surveys about public attitudes and beliefs can be valuable tools for influencing policy change, and being recognized and respected by the public, as nurses generally are, is a key asset in the policy game. Canadians place very high trust in nurses, as was noted earlier in this text, so they pay attention to stories about nurses and health care.

Creating public awareness may be a very direct, hands-on strategy undertaken by individual nurses. For example, in July 2016, Cathy Crowe and other social justice advocates blasted the Canadian National Exhibition in social and traditional media for its decision to stop offering free admission to people with disabilities. Their eyes are always on the broad determinants of health, including income and who can access what services and privileges across society. The free pass to the exhibition had been a long-standing, small offering to help people with disabilities (many of whom have fixed, low incomes) enjoy a public activity with fellow citizens. Within 48 hours the organization bowed to the outcry and reversed the decision—although its language was decidedly more nuanced than those who protested: "Over the last couple of days, CNE customers and members of the broader community have shown considerable interest in, and provided valuable feedback regarding the proposed changes to the admissions policy."[25]

Two weeks later, during a growing heat wave in Toronto, Crowe whipped up public attention and support again, this time to urge Toronto officials to open cooling centres, with Facebook messages like, "#Humidex40 is trending. Come on City of Toronto and open the cooling centres. Upgrade the heat warning!" And she posted very clear messages in social media providing technical information that other advocates could use in snowballing support. For example, using her Facebook page, she said:

> Last week when I was at City Hall I learned that most councilors did not realize that when a heat alert is called by the Medical Officer of Health it doesn't mean the cooling centres are open. They only open when the alert is elevated to 'extended'. So just to be clear, as of approximately 2 p.m. today with temperatures predicted this afternoon to be 37C and feeling like 45C with humidity, the alert has not been elevated. The cooling centres for vulnerable people (homeless, poor seniors, people in rooming houses and others without air conditioning) ARE NOT OPEN.

Crowe went on to name the mayor and Board of Health chair, telling people how to contact and pressure them. Furthermore, pulling all the social determinants together, she spoke articulately through social media about the reality for people living on limited/fixed incomes: by mid-month they might not have fiscal resources left to get to the cooling centres. Crowe similarly targets city officials in very public ways in the winter by pushing the public to demand more shelter beds for homeless people during cold spells.

Also in Toronto, Leigh Chapman posted similar messages during 2016 about the issue of safe injection sites, effectively increasing public and media awareness by drawing attention to the "not in my backyard" stances of some Toronto neighbourhoods. (Crowe lashed out in a rabble.ca column on the same issue, mincing no words in calling it a "vile form of speaking and acting fuelled by ignorance, fear and hate."[26]) Speaking candidly about the death of her brother, who had become homeless and suffered from addictions, Chapman's dramatic testimony to a city committee prompted a lengthy newspaper article focused on Ontario's homeless population.[27] These sorts of examples bring to life the recommendations of the University College London Lancet Commission (introduced in Chapter 1) that "city governments should work with a wide range of stakeholders to build a political alliance for urban health. In particular, urban planners and those responsible for public health should be in communication with each other."[28] Chapman's strategy worked, and policy was developed directly as a result of strategic nursing input in alliance with other advocates.[29]

Returning to the Office of Nursing Policy work back in 2000, when the office turned dry absenteeism data into the phrase "nurses are the sickest workers in the country," the tide of public awareness turned. It was pushed in interviews and in articles in professional publications[30] and it soon began to appear in popular media stories, including newspapers. The nurses' stories rang true with the public, who had begun to notice that wait times for many services were growing and who were scrutinizing every aspect of health care. With a few exceptions, far from being critical of nurses, Canadians who had experienced the health care system often commented that "the nurses all seemed to be running all day." So the situation escalated to the point that concerned Canadians—and public interest in health care—became so intense that health care is rarely out of the top two or three public policy concerns. Through all the years of reform, nurses have maintained their position at or near the top of the professions most trusted by Canadians—firefighters, emergency medical technicians, nurses, pharmacists, and physicians, according to a 2012 Ipsos-Reid survey conducted for Postmedia News and Global Television.[31]

Phase II: Moving into Action

Nurses have often been quite effective in bringing issues forward, and getting them into the policy agenda. However, as happens across all sectors of society, the ball sometimes gets dropped before the rest of the policy work is done. Fatigue may be a factor by that point, and/or it may be that once an issue begins to attract public attention, we believe other reasonable people will somehow carry it forward to a sensible resolution. That, of course, is not always the case, and the larger process is better understood today. There is a great deal more to be done after a policy agenda begins to achieve public awareness in order to nail down real solutions and see them implemented. This second major phase of policy development in the model also includes four main steps, as shown in Figure 9.7.

Step 5: Political Engagement

Essential in policy development is understanding and engaging stakeholders, and being clear about one's target audiences. Nurses learning about policy development typically may be urged to think about three categories of target audiences, noting that the categories may overlap: (1) stakeholders who may be influenced by the eventual policy or legislation; (2) stakeholders who could be allies in helping to advance the policy work; and (3) stakeholders who might be likely to resist or obstruct the eventual policy or legislation. Obviously one hopes to activate those most likely to be helpful to the cause, but it is just as important to engage with or at least monitor those against the cause. Both sides may have powerful influence, for better or worse, and can bolster or sink the work; better to know up front who sits on each side and engage, or at least inform, them as early as possible. Where feasible, it is of value to leverage support from those on your side, and minimize resistance from those opposing—or at least mitigate the damage they could do.

For a lot of nursing policy and health system work on the public side, audiences typically include stakeholders at one or all of the levels shown in Table 9.1.

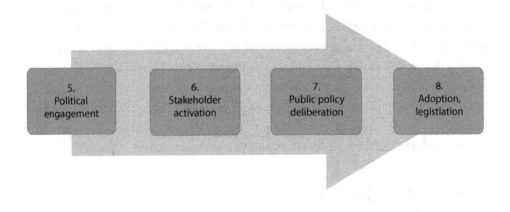

Figure 9.7: Phase II Steps in Policy Development: Moving into Action

Some groups outside these categories also may have a role—for example, clinical and health services researchers, the health science education sector, accreditors, and the constant pressure (sometimes competition) from the private sector.

Political decision makers are, of course, critical players in the development of health policy and must be engaged early and often. Political engagement in this case normally refers to engaging formal political decision makers—the elected and appointed officials in various levels of governments who make the macro- and meso-level allocation decisions about funding and services; this level of engagement is especially critical where the ultimate objective is legislation. Without the support and, ultimately, leadership of politicians it is not likely that ideas will move beyond concern to action. The other audiences listed in Table 9.1 are discussed in the next section.

Remembering the governance structures discussed in Chapter 2, working with the right political leaders is critical. Depending on the objective, one might need to approach and engage a cabinet minister in the executive branch—for example, the minister of health or other ministers whose mandates are related to the topic. For other purposes, it might be more effective to engage with a well-placed backbencher (a non–cabinet member of the governing party in the legislative branch) who may be persuaded to introduce a private member's bill. Overall, it is valuable to play the cards judiciously and with transparency, engaging with

Table 9.1: Typical Stakeholders in the Development of Nursing and Health Policy

	TARGET AUDIENCE	ROLE
Macro-level Decision Makers	Federal, provincial, and territorial government officials	Direct the funding of health systems and services at national, provincial, or territorial levels
Meso-level Decision Makers	Municipal government, Aboriginal government, and regional health authority officials	Direct the funding and monitor outcomes of health organizations within regions or communities
Micro-level Decision Makers	Executives, managers, and other organizational decision makers	Direct the funding of health programs and manage care and human resources within organizations
Providers, Regulators, Unions	Health professionals and support staff	Implement allocation decisions and deliver health services
Voters, Taxpayers, Users	The Canadian public	Pay for and use publicly funded health services

opposition parties so they are aware of key issues, but all the while making efforts to support the minister(s) and governments who will be responsible for tabling bills and legislation. At the federal level, knowing which senators could support a bill toward legislation is important, since this group gives final approval to every bill. At any one time there are normally nurses and other health professionals sitting as senators, for example, who might prove to be helpful allies or worrying foes; it is important to identify them and know where they stand on issues. The same holds true for band councillors in First Nations, municipal councillors, and other officials at the city and town level—and for all the people in the governance structures in health care at regional and organizational levels.

For nurses and others in the business of policy development at a formal level involving government legislation—whether at the federal, provincial/territorial, Aboriginal, or municipal level—it is helpful to learn the mechanics of the process by which ideas are tabled for discussion and ultimately how they work their way to laws and/or regulations. There are multiple points at which one could and should intervene with political regimes during that long process. A multi-pronged approach could include private meetings with political leaders and their staffs, direct personal engagement with the legislative committee that will lead the study of the bill after second reading in the legislature, and brief, professional presentations during formal hearings or other consultations called by any level of government. At the federal level, once a bill has passed through the House of Commons, a very similar process is repeated in the Senate, where, again, there are similar opportunities for points of intervention.

National nursing associations like CFNU and CNA have resources to support some formal activities during which they can engage with political decision makers. The CFNU, for example, hosts regular "Breakfast on the Hill" sessions where elected and appointed officials are invited to breakfast, which usually includes a short presentation on a salient policy issue and allows plenty of time for networking and talking. They have become increasingly popular and well attended over the years, and they allow an opportunity to inform, cajole, and remind leaders of issues important to the organization and/or to nursing at large. During Nursing Week 2016, CFNU developed a compelling, easily understood presentation on the impact of nurses on patient, organizational, and system outcomes to help inform policy decisions, and distributed it for use by its members in Nursing Week meetings with politicians across the country. In its May 2016 Breakfast on the Hill, the topic was pharmacare, picking up on the presentation made to federal, provincial, and territorial health ministers in January 2016—an ongoing reminder of the work left to do.

To continue the street nurse examples from Toronto cited earlier, Cathy Crowe has lived and breathed a social justice value set throughout her professional life. She is well-known among city officials and stays on top of all the relevant meetings, votes, and consultation opportunities. While she certainly creates awareness of links to the same issues happening at the provincial and national levels, she has mastered political engagement in Toronto by doing the hard work of sustaining a decades-long effort that has paid off in her access to decision makers and power to influence policy from the outside. Newer to the task, Leigh Chapman, mentioned earlier, has achieved early successes in her articulate appearances before city committees that have helped sway votes in favour of establishing a homeless shelter and a safe injection site, despite vociferous opposition.

Nurses should be aware of engagement opportunities that may include formal meetings with ministers, deputy ministers, assistant deputy ministers, and teams within governments working in the area of policy interest; formal presentations to parliamentary, Senate, legislature, and municipal committee hearings; and consultation opportunities that arise frequently. Formal and off-the-record personal meetings can help to nourish rich networks that help support policy work across a career, and not just within one setting.

As a result of efforts by the Office of Nursing Policy team to connect with political leaders at many levels, the nursing agenda and the federal team became well-known within federal, provincial, and territorial governments across the country. However, political engagement is a very much a political game, and that reputation came with both political benefits and risks. Borrowing from the Goldilocks metaphor, the leadership style of Judith Shamian, the office's executive director, was too aggressive and chaotic for some, not forceful enough for others, and "just about right" for those falling in the middle of the policy bell curve. Personality was especially an

How a Bill Becomes a Law

For an excellent graphic walk-through of the process at the federal level, visit http://www.parl.gc.ca/About/Parliament/SenatorEugeneForsey/inside_view/follow_bill-e.html.

The provinces and territories also have websites describing the process—see, for example, Nova Scotia (http://nslegislature.ca/index.php/proceedings/how-a-bill-becomes-law), Quebec (http://www.assnat.qc.ca/en/abc-assemblee/projets-loi.html), and Alberta (https://justice.alberta.ca/programs_services/law/Common_Questions_Library_Law/HowAreAlbertasLawsPassed.aspx/DispForm.aspx). Look up your province or territory and learn the process before you wade into the world of policy development.

issue in 1999, when Health Canada was described as coming out of a period of demoralization, and when the people working there were "groping for a role in the face of controversies, cutbacks and criticism."[32] As a result, the fit of a new person, imported from outside into a senior role and not always obedient around government roles and processes—set against a large, long-standing, rules-laden bureaucracy— was an unhappy one for some. Reflecting on her own style, Shamian said she has "no difficulty in setting high standards and expecting people to achieve them. There is no point in aiming too low, and I do not deal well with mediocrity. I push my staff hard to accomplish a lot, and I am impatient with poor performers."[33] But with insight into some of the costs of the style that has driven her success, Shamian noted that her approach to work "can at times be overwhelming and my enthusiasm and high standards can be intimidating. When this happens, if my antennae aren't well tuned, I may miss the cues, leaving people feeling frustrated or 'at sea.'"[34]

As a result of the successes of the Office of Nursing Policy and its networks around the country, a proposal was floated initially during the tenure of minister of health Allan Rock for a program that could recharge and strengthen the nursing workforce over a decade. Elements of the proposal included funding to support undergraduate nursing education, an expansion of graduate school funding and seats to help renew the nursing education workforce (at the time, faculty were much older on average than the workforce itself), and a program to ramp up nurse practitioners. There was a great sense of political engagement, energy, and move-ment toward something new for the national nursing workforce in the interest of better care—until the sunny Tuesday morning of September 11, 2001, when the nursing agenda was derailed along with so many others. Many of the problems that the renewal program was designed to alleviate persist today, and in some ways the momentum for nursing in those heady days was never recovered.

Step 6: Stakeholder Activation

Once political engagement has begun (or at the same time it is beginning), it is just as important to look more broadly to other potential audiences—essentially made up of (a) the employment sector where nurses work and health services are delivered, (b) the people who provide and support health care services, and (c) Canadians at large, including individuals, associations, and interest groups, who make the most fundamental allocation decisions with their votes and who both pay for and use health systems. Political engagement from the inside is import-ant, but the influence of outside actors can be just as powerful, if not more so. Politicians do respond to public opinion and effective lobbies.

At the national level, CNA has a long history of identifying allies and building partnerships to help support and accelerate its work. Some are one-on-one activities, including a close historic association with the Canadian Medical Association. The two groups tend to keep one another informed of unfolding policy issues and often come together on key issues of mutual interest, for example, in *Principles to Guide Health Care Transformation in Canada*, developed and published by the two organizations in 2011.[35] Of course, organized medicine is a powerful lobby, so the two organizations benefit from affiliation with one another in the long term.

Other policy work may demand a more time-limited stakeholder engagement strategy. When the Nursing Research Fund established by the federal government in 1999 was set to expire in 2009, for example, the CASN, CNA, and the Academy of Canadian Executive Nurses came together to propose new funding to the federal government. Together they informed other leading nursing groups of the need for a renewed research fund and gained support from unions and other groups. Acknowledging that they were operating in a very different political climate from 1998–1999, *Advancing Health through Nursing Science*, a proposal for some $80 million in funding to support capacity building in nursing science, was presented twice to the federal finance committee in the lead-up to annual budgets, but was not successful in securing any further funding. In retrospect, the due diligence around early and ongoing political engagement may have been inadequate, but in reality, signals were becoming very clear that the Harper government was pulling away from those sorts of initiatives, especially when they related to health care and health human resources.

Other stakeholder engagement can be cemented in partnerships that are formalized and long-standing; in March 1991, nurses helped establish the Health Action Lobby, a coalition that has grown from 7 to 41 health care associations representing more than 500,000 providers and consumers of health care.[36] The group originally came together in response to the potential for a significant drop in federal funding under then Prime Minister Mulroney.[37] The executive directors of the Canadian Hospital Association and CNA served as co-chairs. The work within and across these stakeholder groups continues today with a focus on strengthening and sustaining public medicare, including funding concerns. Coalitions of health providers like these can be very influential because the providers tend to be valued and respected by the public.

The National Expert Commission engaged in extensive stakeholder consultations across the country, holding formal meetings with representatives of the public, governments, health professionals, and business sectors in 19 cities. Dozens of private, one-on-one meetings with government and health system officials, journalists, and policy influencers were held across the country. Finally, written submissions were encouraged, and dozens were received, from short emails sent by individuals to lengthy formal reports submitted by various organizations.[38]

Returning again to the example of the work of the federal Office of Nursing Policy on the health of nurses, the team undertook very purposeful stakeholder engagement. They were strategic in communicating extensively and positioning different key issues in the conversations and agendas of many outside groups. As a result, a range of salient issues that together represented the broad scope of the problem were able to accumulate in conversations across the country—with managers, unions, educators, scientists, hospital executives, the public, and more. Similar to the strategy undertaken at the political engagement level, stakeholder engagement was multi-pronged and included extensive private meetings with nursing and other system leaders across the domains of nursing practice across the country. Regular communication updates were provided in newsletters and journals of professional and union groups across Canada, 21 publications in peer-reviewed and professional publications (August 1999–August 2003), interviews with news organizations, and popular lay media such as *Chatelaine* magazine.

Step 7: Public Policy Deliberation

Kingdon suggested five conditions[39] that add up to a feasibility test, which may help predict whether all the work really will result in policy change:

1. Technical feasibility
2. Value acceptability (within the relevant system and policy community)
3. Tolerable cost
4. Anticipated public agreement (and/or agreement by those most affected)
5. Reasonable chance for elected officials (or the ultimate decision makers) to be receptive to it.

By the deliberation stage, Kingdon's conditions and issues should have already been fairly well considered. At this point, the knowledge is well developed, leaders are committed to doing something, and stakeholders have been consulted. This phase includes formal committee work and debate within governments around the wording of a new piece of legislation, or some other solution such as a health accord. This phase of work may be mirrored in a similar period of deliberation when organizations, boards, or regions are developing policy.

The deliberation stage is one of nailing down the final solutions that are feasible at costs the relevant system can bear—and is the time to prepare the wording and legalities before a bill or other policy proposal goes forward for final approval in any setting. It should be noted that this stage of work might take a very long time. In recent memory, however, Canadians watched the complicated issue of assisted dying move quite rapidly through the phase of deliberation, under a timing deadline imposed by the Supreme Court of Canada.

Step 8: Adoption, Legislation

At a formal political level, Step 8 is the time when bills in parliament undergo final debate, are revised after a careful reading, passed into legislation, and as necessary revised again in the future. For the Office of Nursing Policy example threaded through this chapter, the formal adoption phase took several forms within formal government structures and beyond.

When the Honourable Anne McLellan was appointed the new minister of health in January 2002, the conversation about nursing picked up some pace again, after waning in the collective anxiety and distraction across the country after the events of September 11, 2001. When the nursing renewal proposal was again put on the table, the office team was directed to propose a more formal position paper or brief laying out what the program would entail and what it might cost. Although a rough estimate was in the $1.4 billion range, there was, with a possible federal/provincial/territorial health accord looming ahead in September of the same year, reason to hope that an injection of funds might indeed be forthcoming (given all the attention on nursing at the time). Ultimately the policy victory was less lofty: the First Ministers' Accord on Health Care Renewal in 2003 included $90 million in funding for all health human resources over the next five years—not just nursing. However, language developed by the team appeared in the accord, and funds were allocated to support health human resources planning, recruitment, and retention, and to strengthen interprofessional education and practice across the country.

In another example, an initial private meeting of Office of Nursing Policy staff in 2001 with Elma Heidemann, then chief executive officer of what is now Accreditation Canada, led to an honest and uncomfortable question when discussing emerging evidence about nursing and its relationship to quality outcomes: "How can any hospital with the highest accreditation rating for quality of care be such an apparently unhappy place to work?" The links among patient, organizational, and provider outcomes were questioned. Heidemann and her successor, Wendy Nicklin, engaged their organization deeply in the work, helping partners like CFNU and CNA to establish what would become the Quality Workplace—Quality Healthcare Collaborative, and developing workplace quality indicators within the accreditation program. While accreditation is not the same as legislation, it is a similar end point for the policy work, which in this case pushed for the measurement of nursing workplace indicators that would force attention to the issue of nursing workplace health by employers.

With so much of the agenda moved forward, the next generation of the Office of Nursing Policy was able to focus on some new issues and agendas—knowing that very capable players in the field were coming together to help advance the work important to governments in the area of nursing.

Phase III: Implementation and Change

Miljan defined policy implementation as "the process of transforming the goals of a policy into results."[40] In this stage comes the hard work of actually implementing legislation, regulation, rules, and procedures that are the results of the policy that has been developed. A simplified summary of the steps in this complex stage of policy work is shown Figure 9.8. There are countless models of change that could be used; the high-level steps shown here underpin the process suggested by the Change Management Learning Center.[41]

Policy implementation can be a drawn out and bumpy process to say the least. It is best driven by a well-developed project management team; this recommendation is especially important with anything as complex as the sorts of system-level changes being raised in this text. However, even within a small work team, it must be said that short of becoming trapped by *paralysis through analysis*, one really cannot overplan something as complicated as a policy change.

Public policy change may require behavioural changes by professional groups, and might even have the expectation that millions of citizens will change their behaviours. Change is all about people; the Change Management Learning Center defines change management as "the application of a structured process and set of tools for leading the people side of change to achieve a desired outcome."[42]

Since there are entire books and graduate programs focused on change management theory, models, and strategy, they are not explored in detail here. However, regardless of the model ultimately followed, there are some basic steps that should be part of any policy implementation project. The Change Management Learning

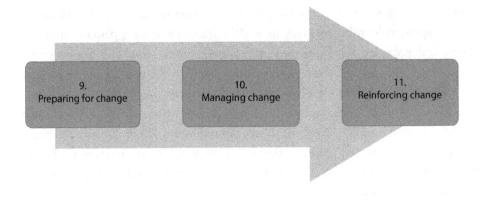

Figure 9.8: Phase III Steps in Policy Development: Policy Implementation and Change

Center lays out a number of actions within each of its theoretical steps for policy implementation; these anchor the steps shown in Table 9.2 (see page 284).[43]

Sometimes decision makers and change leaders generalize or downplay the potential impacts of resistance to change. Negotiating the policy implementation process may become clearer if the reasons people resist policy change are understood and addressed up front. As part of its Influencing Public Policy workshop developed for novice policy students,[44] CNA offered tips that may be of help to nurses and others engaging in policy development and implementation. The Change Management Learning Center notes that, while resistance is normal, "persistent resistance" can sink a project. People may resist change if they:

- do not see it as being in their interest to change, or they think the change is the wrong thing to do;
- are skeptical about the possibility of success or the people leading the change;
- do not understand why change is happening or what change is required;
- feel the change is not relevant to them;
- do not have the time or resources to engage in the change;
- want to change but don't think that they will be able to change; and
- feel change was imposed, that they were not involved in the process, and/ or feel disenfranchised.

Leveraging support from allies may temper the impact of resistors or even help to engage them in the change. Before projects begin, it would be valuable for change leaders to:

- analyze how and where allies might like to be involved, and invite or empower them to participate;
- build allies within and beyond health and social services;
- identify influential local champions;
- develop common goals and objectives and work together around high-priority issues;
- provide opportunities for allies to be publicly supportive;
- practice regular and open communication, and provide allies with ongoing updates on the status of the project so they feel informed and keep the work top of mind;
- ask for input and feedback on the work to clarify vision and provide input into the approach, plan, and strategy;
- seek advice on how to better market or sell the policy change; and
- stay positive and focused.

Table 9.2: Steps and Actions in the Change Management Process

PREPARING FOR CHANGE	MANAGING CHANGE	REINFORCING CHANGE
1. Define the change management strategy. 2. Prepare the change management team. 3. Identify and develop champions and a strong project sponsor. 4. Identify likely points of resistance.	1. Develop a comprehensive change management plan with clear objectives, timelines, milestones, and budget. 2. Execute the change management plan.	1.Seek and analyze feedback at each step. 2. Diagnose gaps, manage resistance, and implement corrective actions. 3. Identify and celebrate successes.

Source: Change Management Learning Center. (2014). *Change management: The systems and tools for managing change.* Retrieved from http://www.change-management.com/tutorial-change-process-detailed.htm.

Phase IV: Policy Evaluation and Revision

Finally, the phase of evaluation and revision arrives. Like the other three stages of policy development that have been introduced, there are many models and frameworks that can be used to explain and predict the steps involved. The Centers for Disease Control and Prevention defines policy evaluation as "the systematic collection and analysis of information to make judgments about contexts, activities, characteristics, or outcomes of one or more domain(s) of the Policy Process," with the aim to inform and improve policy development, adoption, implementation, and effectiveness.[45]

Of course, evaluation should be an ongoing and iterative process during each step of policy development, but this particular evaluation is the formal phase to determine the outcomes of the entire process. Evaluation methods may include collection of both quantitative and qualitative data, may involve some or all of the actors who have been part of the larger process, and may capture outcomes for the sorts of population health and system performance measures discussed in Chapter 8. The design and methodology of the different phases of evaluation will vary widely, and should be appropriate for each element assessed.

The National Center for Injury Prevention and Control in the United States undertakes complex policy evaluation on an ongoing basis and suggests a three-step framework that could be helpful to nurses at this stage of work. As shown in Figure 9.9, the centre's framework forces users to think about evaluation of policy in three areas: (1) the actual content of the policy; (2) the effectiveness of its implementation; and (3) the effect of the policy on its intended audiences.[46]

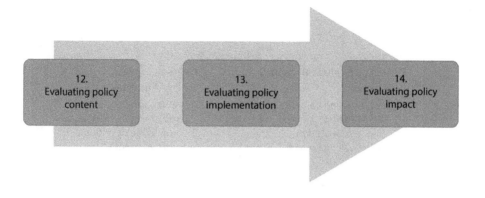

Figure 9.9: Phase IV Steps in Policy Development: Policy Evaluation
            and Revision

The National Center for Injury Prevention and Control speaks about the three phases this way:

1. The evaluation of policy content refers to assessing the actual goals of the policy and its intended outcome(s). Elements of the policy, internal logic, and context all should be taken into consideration.

2. The evaluation of policy implementation focuses on the way the policy was executed and applied (or not). This aspect of evaluation should examine the enablers and barriers encountered, and should undertake comparative outcomes of the various sub-steps of implementation.

3. The evaluation of policy impact attempts to measure whether the original policy actually resulted in the intended outcomes, and to what degree. Were there positive or negative side effects, or unintended consequences? This phase of evaluation may entail assessment of short-, medium-, and long-term measures, and may involve comparative policy analysis (pre- and post-implementation and/or cross-jurisdictional comparisons).

SUMMARY AND IMPLICATIONS

Chapter 9 has described a theoretical policy model that has been subjected to some practical testing over a period of time, and has proven useful in thinking about, understanding, explaining, and teaching principles underlying policy development (see Figure 9.10). Policy is a messy process, and as stated earlier is not precise or linear. Although laid out here as a cycle of events, in the real world the work may be more akin to juggling—because in some ways, and in many cases, pieces of all these

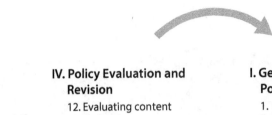

IV. Policy Evaluation and Revision
12. Evaluating content
13. Evaluating implementation
14. Evaluating impact

I. Getting to the Policy Agenda
1. Values and beliefs
2. Problem/issue emerges
3. Knowledge development
4. Public awareness

III. Implementation and Change
9. Preparing for change
10. Managing change
11. Reinforcing change

II. Moving into Action
5. Political engagement
6. Stakeholder activiation
7. Policy deliberation
8. Policy adoption

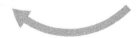

Figure 9.10: Stages and Steps in the Policy Cycle: An Evolving Model

phases and steps are likely to be happening concurrently. Understanding these stages and steps may help nurses understand where any given issue sits in the evolution of policy, and provide guidance around when and how to intervene—key steps in developing policy competency.

DISCUSSION QUESTIONS

1. What are the key elements and stages in public policy development that should inform the policy work of nurses?
2. What steps can nurses take to facilitate the evolution of public concerns from vague problems to focused issues on political agendas?
3. How should nurses collaborate with others to resolve policy challenges? What interest groups are natural allies of nurses, and who might oppose nursing policy work?
4. Discuss an example illustrating the effectiveness of nurses in influencing public policy. Why was the initiative effective? Are there areas of the work that could have been strengthened, and if so, how could they be informed by policy theory and/or policy models?

ADDITIONAL POLICY RESOURCES

THINK TANKS AND ADVOCACY ORGANIZATIONS

Broadbent Institute	http://www.broadbentinstitute.ca
Caledon Institute of Social Policy	http://www.caledoninst.org
Canadian Centre for Policy Alternatives	http://www.policyalternatives.ca
Canadian Doctors for Medicare	http://www.canadiandoctorsformedicare.ca
Canadian Institute for Advanced Research	http://www.cifar.ca
Canadian Labour Congress	http://canadianlabour.ca
C.D. Howe Institute	https://www.cdhowe.org
Centre for Health Economics and Policy Analysis	http://www.chepa.org
Centre for Health Services and Policy Research	http://www.chspr.ubc.ca
Conference Board of Canada	http://www.conferenceboard.ca
Couchiching Institute on Public Affairs	http://www.couchichinginstitute.ca
Council of Canadians	http://canadians.org
Fraser Institute	http://www.fraserinstitute.org
Frontier Centre for Public Policy	https://fcpp.org
HEAL (Organizations for Health Action)	http://www.healthactionlobby.ca
Institute for Research on Public Policy	http://irpp.org
Mowat Centre	http://mowatcentre.ca
Patients Canada	http://www.patientscanada.ca
Public Policy Forum	http://www.ppforum.com
Wait Time Alliance	http://www.waittimealliance.ca
Wellesley Institute	http://www.wellesleyinstitute.com

CHAPTER 10

Tools and Strategies to Support the Work of Policy

CHAPTER HIGHLIGHTS

- Tools of Policy Analysis and Synthesis
- Tools of Policy Development
- Tools of Policy Engagement and Consultation
- Tools of Policy Communication
- Summary and Implications
- Discussion Questions
- Additional Policy Resources

LEARNING OUTCOMES

1. Describe key examples of tools of policy analysis and synthesis, development, engagement and consultation, and communication.
2. Demonstrate skills in health policy interpretation and analysis techniques that can be used by nurses.
3. Describe the key elements of an effective briefing note.
4. Discuss tips for working effectively with interest groups, stakeholders, and members of the media.

Policy Influencer: Sheila Dinotshe Tlou

Sheila Tlou, RN, MAEd, MSc, PhD, is a distinguished nurse from Botswana who has enjoyed a soaring global career in education, politics, and health and social policy for the past 40 years. Presently the director of the Regional Support Team for Eastern and Southern Africa for UNAIDS, Tlou provides leadership and oversees support in the area of HIV/AIDS across 21 nations in the region. After serving as a nursing professor, she went on to be elected as a member of Parliament in Botswana and was the country's minister of health for five years. In that role she led a program in HIV prevention, treatment, care, and support still used as a model today.[1] She served as chair of the Southern African Development Community and the African Union Ministers of Health, and was on the board of the Global Fund to Fight AIDS, Tuberculosis and Malaria, where her nursing leadership was brought to bear in many areas of health, including sexual and reproductive rights. In her current role as the United Nations Eminent Person for Women, Girls, and HIV/AIDS in Southern Africa, she is focused on working at the grassroots level to eliminate child marriages across Africa. She is a fiercely intelligent, tireless, and humorous advocate for human rights, and in her spare time has acted on stage in the role of Precious Ramotswe from the Alexander McCall Smith Ladies' Detective book series.

"Very often you have bad alternatives and you are trying to choose between them.... Intelligence is never perfect and it might, in fact, be wrong. The fact is, in decision–making, you don't always have all the information that you want or need.... Never forget how hard it is to make complex decisions when you don't have all the information that you'd like, but you don't have the luxury of not making a decision."

—*Condoleeza Rice, Director, Global Center for Business and Economy, Stanford University Graduate School of Business and former US Secretary of State*[2]

It is valuable for nurses to become familiar with the many tools and techniques that support policy analysis, synthesis, development, and communication. Some have very precise meanings and follow rigid rules—briefing notes within governments, for example—while others vary more widely in their definition and content. All of them may be encountered routinely in the course of policy work; examples that will be covered in this chapter are shown in Figure 10.1.

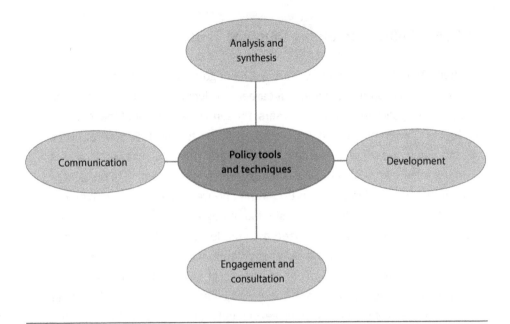

Figure 10.1: Policy Tools and Techniques

TOOLS OF POLICY ANALYSIS AND SYNTHESIS

Scans

Constant scanning is the first duty of any savvy policy analyst. Scanning may take the form of looking through a select group of resources every day—perhaps key news or targeted health sciences sites online, all depending on the nature of the policy work. Whether undertaking daily scanning to simply increase awareness of issues, or preparing a formal scan—such as an environmental scan for a board or leader—there is value to having some structure to guide the work. Scans should be carried out with an intention to ask honest questions (especially of oneself and one's organization), analyze evidence and opinion around a range of issues and needs, consider options for organizational response and/or policy solutions, and understand the costs of action or inaction.

A scanning tool often used by organizations and boards is the PEST tool, representing factors in the *political, economic, socio-cultural,* and *technological* spheres. There are variants of the tool that include other factors, such as PESTEM, which includes *environmental* and *management* sectors. Whatever factors are considered, the tool is valuable in providing a framework that forces a more careful examination of several sectors of information.

Policy analysts typically search for key scanning findings and messages, and think about urgency, degree of likely impact on the organization, and so on. Tools such as the SWOT analysis—*strengths, weaknesses, opportunities,* and *threats*—can help to understand the possible impact of any one issue and strategies to respond to or manage it. The Start-Stop-Continue-Change exercise essentially asks the question, "To manage this issue, what should the organization *start* doing, *stop* doing, *continue* to do, and/or *change*?" and is another way to think about scanning, analysis, and presentation of results. Many such tools exist to help policy analysts pour through information and estimate its importance and impact. An integrated scan, amalgamating all such findings, is normally presented to the leader(s) for a consideration of implications on mandate, budgets, future activities, and so on.

Briefing Notes

In its Public Policy certificate program, the Government of Newfoundland and Labrador[3] describes the purpose of briefing notes as being to provide the premier, ministers, and senior executive with:

- Communication about a new, or ongoing, issue
- Advice on a project or client file
- Preparation for sensitive or public issues
- Preparation for media interviews or news conferences
- Meeting preparation
- Information when seeking direction on some topic

Briefing notes are used similarly in many other sectors to share information with and/or seek direction from a leader or some other party. As the Newfoundland and Labrador team points out, these notes generally fall into common categories, including information, decision/direction, question and answer, and meeting preparation notes.

Just as the name implies, briefing notes are usually brief. The ability to synthesize complex documents into a concise briefing note is a highly valued skill for executives and other decision makers who must read extensive correspondence every day. Some governments and other organizations will not accept a note longer than two pages.

A well-written briefing note will reflect many of the elements of the policy cycle described in Chapter 9, and normally would include a statement of the original problem, research and information developed, the current state of affairs, who is involved (including political and public responses), special considerations, any legislation in place on this issue, and most importantly, clarity on what decision or outcome is being sought from the person receiving the note. It may be helpful to think through the "who, what, where, when, why, and how" questions when synthesizing issues and reports to translate them to briefing notes.

Evidence Briefs and Issue Briefs

Evidence and issue briefs are a newer tool of analysis and synthesis, different from briefing notes. The WHO describes evidence briefs for policy as "research syntheses in a user-friendly format, offering evidence informed policy options ... to convince the target audience of the urgency of the current problem and the need to adopt the preferred alternatives or strategies of intervention."[4] Understanding the time pressures of their audiences, the Canadian Foundation for Health Improvement

Effective Briefing Notes

- Be objective, factual, and concise—a briefing note is not a creative writing assignment.
- Assume the reader knows little about the issue, but don't waste words teaching a leader his or her role or business.
- Be very clear about any options you suggest and/or about what you are asking for.
- Write in an active voice, be professional, check spelling and grammar, and do it all within two pages.

Typical elements of a briefing note would include:

- *Statement of the issue*: one to two sentences maximum
- *Background*: The essential details, history of topic, and evolution of options that a stranger would need to know to understand this issue.
- *Current status or context*: Who is involved? What has happened to this issue—for example, since a report was released?
- *Key considerations*: What needs to be considered right now? What are the threats, opportunities, risks, and benefits for this organization?
- *Options or next steps*: Provide one to three options that should be considered. Be concise and set down clear actions and targets. Recommend one option and support with rationale.

and Health Council of Canada were both early adopters of the technique—sometimes even requiring that writers of their reports use a 1–5–25 paging model, meaning a 25-page (maximum) main report, a 5-page summary/brief, and a single page of key messages.

In its description of evidence and issue briefs, the McMaster Health Forum described an issue brief as being "similar to the evidence brief in terms of mobilizing research evidence about a problem, possible options for addressing it, and key implementation considerations."[5] The forum differentiates the two as shown in Table 10.1.

TOOLS OF POLICY DEVELOPMENT

Resolutions

A resolution is a motion that is submitted to an organization and voted on by its members according to procedures established by the organization. Examples have been shared throughout this text. Bringing resolutions forward to organizations—often in the setting of an annual general meeting—provides a chance for members, employees, and/or the public to influence the policy direction of an organization. Resolutions normally are received as advice and are non-binding for the organization. Examples of resolutions brought to the assembly of the Canadian Nursing Students' Association, for example, include topics such as interprofessional nursing education, complementary therapy, harm reduction, and creating a partnership for Aboriginal health promotion. Like many associations, the CNSA provides guidelines for writing resolutions and position statements on its website.[6]

Table 10.1: Typical Content of Evidence Briefs and Issues Briefs

EVIDENCE BRIEF	ISSUE BRIEF
Start with a policy issue, and then identify the available research evidence. Elements of each brief should include:	Undertaken on policy issues where either:
• what is known about the underlying problems;	• an evidence synthesis has already been prepared, so a comprehensive search for research evidence is not needed; or
• possible policy and program options to address the problem, including an outline of the known benefits, harms, and costs of these options; and	• a "one-stop shop" for systematic reviews doesn't exist, so a comprehensive search for research evidence could not be conducted in a timely way.
• a review of the barriers to implementation and strategies to address them.	

Position Statements

A position statement presents a viewpoint on a particular issue and provides documented background data on that issue. It is often used to explain, justify, or recommend a particular policy to an organization. The Canadian Association of Occupational Therapists (CAOT), for example, describes their position statements as quick reference sheets to "help you to understand CAOT's position on issues that affect occupational therapists and their clients."[7]

The International Council of Nurses publishes position statements in five categories:

1. Nursing roles in health care services
2. Nursing professions
3. Socio-economic welfare of nurses
4. Health care systems
5. Social issues

Examples of the organization's position statements include: *Reducing Travel-Related Communicable Disease Transmission* (2011), *Tobacco Use and Health* (2012), and *Distribution and Use of Breast Milk Substitutes* (2013). Position statements in nursing typically have a one- or two-page statement of the organization's position on an issue, often followed with an appendix that equates to an evidence or issue brief, as described earlier.

Position Papers

A position paper presents one or several positions on a focused issue or policy problem. Simon Fraser University likens a position paper to a debate, saying it "presents one side of an arguable opinion about an issue" with a goal "to convince the audience that your opinion is valid and defensible."[8] A position paper may expand on a position statement, but is a very different document. It may also expand upon and explore options presented in a briefing note. Position papers may be developed by an organization to serve as "trial balloons," in a sense to float policy ideas and observe reactions.

In the work of policy analysis and position papers, nurses may run into the technique of *comparative policy analysis*. These studies or papers are intended to compare and contrast "public policy making across sectoral, regional and national boundaries in order to overcome challenges in the formulation, implementation and evaluation of public policy."[9] This area of analysis and research requires use of more advanced methodological techniques.

Nurses also may hear the terms *green paper* and *white paper* during the course of policy work. These are types of position papers escalating in the seriousness of the position being presented. A green paper is a firmer laying-down of potential policy directions than the basic position paper. It usually has a somewhat consultative tone (in that the writer usually expects to hear reactions) and may start to clarify an intended policy direction of a government or organization. The first such paper is thought to have been tabled in the United Kingdom in 1967.[10]

A white paper is the most advanced of the three types of position papers, in that it describes a fairly entrenched policy direction while still allowing some wiggle room before being moved into a legislative or regulatory development process. These sorts of papers are often floated by country governments, political unions such as the European Union, and larger private organizations. A recent example of a Canadian white paper is the Canadian Medical Association's *Assisted Reproduction in Canada: An Overview of Ethical and Legal Issues and Recommendations for the Development of National Standards*.[11] As the title implies, the paper offers a review of issues in assisted reproduction and recommends national standards; it would be expected that with the paper's release there would be reactions to and input on the suggested standards.

Commissions—Royal and Otherwise

Commissions of Inquiry are struck to advise on or investigate major issues. At the federal level, a Commission of Inquiry—often called a Royal Commission—is "established by the Governor in Council (Cabinet) to fully and impartially investigate issues of national importance" and "has the power to subpoena witnesses, take evidence under oath and request documents."[12] The head of a Royal Commission may wield significant power but recommendations are non-binding.

Profession-led inquires, like the National Expert Commission of the CNA cited earlier, are struck with a mandate developed by the funding organization, and may be operated at arm's length from the host association. In the United Kingdom, *The Lancet* launched the Lancet Commission on Nursing in 2014 to address the image of nursing and influence the future of nursing practice and education.[13] Not unlike a Royal Commission, these sorts of broad national inquiries are usually charged with providing advice to or conducting an investigation for the funding organization.

TOOLS OF POLICY ENGAGEMENT AND CONSULTATION

Public Engagement

Engaging the public can be an important step in public policy development and eventual uptake. Public involvement may be invited for consultation on any given issues, deliberation of policy options, and/or to engage the public in rolling out new laws or procedures, for example. Public engagement may take the form of in-person meetings, surveys, and/or formal polls on specific issues.

The term *the public* refers to community members and leaders, people in

Cross-Country Consultations

For the National Expert Commission, the task of public consultation was initially daunting; Canada's geography alone leads to immediate cost implications when undertaking public consultations in person. The commission's fiscal investment in the services of MASS LBP, a small and creative Toronto firm specializing in public consultation, led to a creative and very helpful partnership. YMCA Canada was delighted to partner with nurses and offered up free space in its facilities across the country, trained its employees to participate in and even lead some of the consultations, and recruited members of the public to attend. It was an effective and energizing partnership that connected the commissioners with people right across Canada. Where there was no YMCA facility, commissioners undertook a number of direct consultations using facilities offered by communities, such as with the health team and town council in Fort Smith, Northwest Territories.

The enthusiasm of the public, including during three consultations with youth, were lessons too. When the issue of an honorarium for public participants was raised, the MASS LBP team was insistent in its response: "No. They should pay you for the chance to talk with nurses and the Commission." And with nothing more offered than Tim Hortons coffee and snacks, Canadians turned out across the country. Even in late-day sessions with youth, participants were engaged and shared insightful, smart, and innovative ideas about nursing and health care.

To read more about the cross-country consultations of the National Expert Commission, go to http://www.cna-aiic.ca/~/media/cna/files/en/mass_lbp_summary_e.pdf.

businesses and institutions, celebrities, and experts on the issue. Public engage-ment may be aimed at including any of the people who know about an issue, will have to approve policy, oversee its implementation, and/or be affected by it.

Engaging celebrities, who may include anyone from a local television news anchor to a music or film star, can, of course, bring significant attention to an is-sue. Their participation—whether paid or as volunteers—can attract attention that can accelerate any policy agenda dramatically. Experts like the head of a nursing or medical association, for example, are an important ingredient in public en-gagement, especially paired with a celebrity, because they bring credibility that enhances the reliability of messages in the minds of the public.

Polls and Surveys

Polls and surveys may take the form of informal surveys using one of many simple online tools, such as SurveyMonkey, or may entail large-scale national surveys such as the Health Care in Canada Survey conducted by Pollara Strategic Insights. That survey is marketed as "helping stakeholders understand what Canadians think about their own health and the quality of their health care system since 1998" and reports opinions of providers, administrators, and the public.[14] The CNA has represented nurses, along with other major providers and groups, throughout the survey's history and at the decision-making table regarding the questions and sub-sequent analysis.

Small surveys are inexpensive and can return data on selected issues quickly; they make very handy tools for surveying a group of nurses on a given topic, for example. These informal opinion polls can also be tremendously valuable when infrastructure or resources do not permit carrying out a formal poll.

Larger surveys come with a fiscal and time cost, but have the benefit of more generalizability and reliability. Large polling firms use random (or more random) samples and unbiased questions. They can be expensive for a small organization, but the costs may be shared by two or more organizations, and

Canadians' Opinion on Health

To learn more about the polling of Canadians by Nanos Research for the National Expert Commission, check out the summary report, *Canadians' Opinion on Health*, at: https://www.cna-aiic.ca/~/media/cna/files/en/2012-171_cna-june_omni_report.pdf.

they may provide much-needed exposure for an issue and return highly valuable data difficult to obtain another way. If several groups were to enter into a contract with a polling firm, the costs and results could be shared and co-marketed. Nurses using this tool would normally work with the polling firm to develop the specific questions of interest.

Engaging with Media

Members of the media are part of the public, and their business is to shape messages for the public in many formats—popular media such as television, radio, newspapers, and social media, and more targeted and issue-specific media. All of these can influence decision makers and the public.

Reporters are always looking for stories that contain new information. It is useful to think through what different types of media might help to advance any given policy initiative, which people could be helpful, and what the messages could be. The messages must be compelling to attract attention of journalists, and the journalists must believe the messages will attract, or at least inform, the public—and generate revenue.

For nurses who may not be used to working with members of the formal media it can be useful to simply invite a reporter or journalist to an organization to meet and talk. Ask them professionally about their work, how to attract their attention, and how they decide on what news stories are covered. In Ottawa, for example, local health reporter Pauline Tam, from the *Ottawa Citizen*, was very open to spending an hour simply giving some advice and tips as efforts were made to draw media into nursing work on an ongoing basis; these sorts of opportunities need not be prohibitively expensive or complicated to arrange.

Maintaining relationships with members of the media and acknowledging their efforts related to one's agenda is important. The CNA, for example, first presented its annual Media Awards to journalists in 1988. The association normally invites prominent members of the media to its major meetings, not just in a reporting role but also to participate on panels or moderate policy debates. Celebrity journalists and commentators such as Evan Solomon, Chantal Hébert, and Andrew Coyne—the latter two being regular members of CBC's iconic At Issue panel—have participated in numerous CNA conferences and conventions and are always a popular draw for participants. Ongoing relationships with these well-connected people provide the additional opportunity to pick up the phone or send an email and simply ask for advice on a policy issue and the media. These relationships are invaluable and worthy of time and fiscal investment over a period of years. They mean that the activities of an association and the names and faces of its leaders are kept regularly in the minds of journalists who have access to and influence on many disparate audiences.

Formal Lobbying

Lobbying in its broadest sense is the process of making views known to elected representatives and other decision makers, with the intention of influencing their decisions. The federal government has a narrower view of the term, describing it as "communicating, with public office holders, for payment" around issues such as bills, resolutions, regulations, legislation, policies or programs, or activities involving awarding of money.[15] Governments at all levels typically insist now that lobbyists are registered and activities are tracked; certainly this rule applies to nurses doing policy work with governments during the course of their jobs with health care associations across Canada.

Lobbying may take place in private meetings with officials or in organizational events, such as the Association of Registered Nurses of British Columbia's Nursing Day at the Legislature or the CFNU's topic-focused Breakfast on the Hill series with members of Parliament and senators in Ottawa. There are several issues and strategies it is valuable to keep in mind before diving successfully into formal lobbying:

- Read about the politicians, political staff, and bureaucrats with whom you plan to work. Learn to properly pronounce names. Look up their photographs online so you clearly know who they are when they enter a room.
- Learn about the personal and professional interests and priorities of the people you hope to engage and/or influence.
- Always arrive early and watch the time during the meeting so you do not linger (unless invited to do so).
- Maintain eye contact and listen well.
- Provide credible information using clear, discreet messages. Show that you understand the problems, issues, evidence, and solutions.

Ten Things You Should Know about Lobbying

To learn more about lobbying governments, read the federal government's document, *Ten Things You Should Know about Lobbying: A Practical Guide for Federal Public Office Holders*, at https://lobbycanada.gc.ca/eic/site/012.nsf/eng/00403.html.

- Identify and point out areas of common ground.
- Consider the impact of every element of policy on other (possibly competing) issues.
- Thank officials and their team members for their time, including the administrative staff that facilitated the meeting. Always follow up with written, formal thanks.

Public Rallies and Marches

Public rallies and marches are a popular strategy among some activist groups, although their impact on policy is not always clear. They may help groups and public observers feel that something active is being done, and in turn may attract more followers to a cause. For some groups, the act of carrying signs, chanting, marching, and sometimes swarming a decision maker is a *de facto* part of their culture. Knowing that most governments pay attention to public opinion, certainly these kinds of activities may draw media attention, depending on the competing stories of the day. However, overall their effectiveness in actually influencing policy is tricky to gauge. Teaching public policy to graduate students at the University of Toronto, Raisa Deber always offered a strong word of caution about this form of policy activity, saying, "If you're marching down Main Street to the legislature, you've already lost." What Deber meant was that people who march are on the wrong side of the policy door, and that one should be involved, if at all possible, in the shaping of any given initiative from the get-go. Nevertheless, this strategy can attract massive attention, and is now a given in many international settings—G20 meetings, for example, are typically accompanied by mass rallies and marches in protest that draw in significant, but not always positive, media attention.

Election Campaign Tools

Election participation tools are a popular product of many professional associations, designed to help members to vote, be involved in campaigns, and be equipped with key messages. Typically these sorts of tools provide:

- the key messages and positions of the sponsoring organizations;
- the key messages from the platforms of major parties;
- suggestions for questions to ask when candidates come to the door or in settings such as public, all-candidates meetings;
- backgrounders and suggestions for key health messages tied to the

sponsoring organization that individuals may use if an opportunity arises to lead a public meeting or speak with media; and

- logistical information, such as the names of ridings and candidates, and instructions on how to vote.

TOOLS OF POLICY COMMUNICATION

Developing Effective Messages

Nothing is more important to effective messages than simplicity and clarity. Creativity matters, but only after the simplest, clearest possible message has been developed. The phrase mentioned earlier—"Nurses are the sickest workers in the country"—provides us with a valuable example of very complicated information translated into a fairly simple sentence. Consider the example shown in Table 10.2 about ways one could target a public health policy message about head injury to different audiences:

Table 10.2: Public Policy Messages Adapted for Different Audiences

CHILDREN	ADULTS	ELECTED OFFICIALS
• Look both ways before you cross the street. • Wear a helmet when you ride your bike.	• Trauma is the leading cause of death in all age groups from 1 to 25.	• Childhood brain injury happens to x children every day and costs $x million for each case in lost lifetime productivity and social costs.

Images, anecdotes, and stories are important ways to communicate messages, but, as the saying goes, the plural of anecdote is not data. It is important in messaging to be factual and clear, and to communicate messages that are rooted in evidence. They should translate scientific information using plain language that will be relevant and meaningful for the intended receivers of the information. While not all messaging should include stories, the experiences of patients and families can be particularly compelling to the media, and in turn the public, simply because most of us can relate to them on a personal level. They can also instantaneously capture political attention (and sometimes drive a rapid response) in ways no amount of evidence ever could.

The CFNU has been very effective in developing and communicating its messages. Its 2015 report on the shrinking federal role in health care, for example, included some complicated statistical calculations. But the CFNU didn't speak about the math: they pointed to "what the cuts to federal funding mean for our health care system in terms of real tangible losses: fewer home care visits, fewer primary care centres, fewer long-term care beds, and fewer nurses in our communities providing care."[16] Its interactive online tool, based on a map graphic, asked the question, "How will this affect your province?" and allowed users to click on simple, compelling, and meaningful statistics for each jurisdiction.[17] Even in complex messages developed for the federal, provincial, and territorial health ministers in January 2016, CFNU translated factual information in an issue brief[18] to much more user-friendly documents that included a summary of the brief[19] and separate documents that summarized each major issue in graphic format—for example, a national prescription drug plan.[20]

Finally, in policy work it is valuable to always have in mind a small number of easy-to-understand messages about one's work and agendas that can be shared whenever an opportunity arises to do so. In policy circles these often are called *elevator messages* because they could be shared in a two-minute elevator ride or hallway encounter with a policy influencer. For nurses new to the work, practice helps: always be ready to be able to state a problem or issue needing resolution, a policy solution, and a piece of evidence to inform the conversation.

Press Releases

Press releases are often developed and released by organizations; some have been cited in this text. To bolster the exposure of an organization and its messaging, services such as the Canadian Press Wire Network (using Marketwired) will deliver press releases for a fee "directly into the editorial systems of hundreds of newspapers, radio and TV stations and websites across Canada."[21] While there is no guarantee that a media agency will follow up with a request for more information and/or an interview, widely circulated press releases have the potential to reach much broader audiences than those published by stand-alone organizations.

Social Media

Social media offers a relatively inexpensive mechanism to share messages widely and quickly. The position of the International Council of Nurses is that social media "can be a powerful tool for rapidly communicating, educating and influencing and has a significant potential to strengthen the nursing profession," particularly noting its usefulness "to enrich practice and to dialogue with the professional community and the public."[22] Most major nursing organizations—CNA and the American Nurses Association, for example[23]—have offered up positions, policies, and toolkits to help nurses consider issues related to social media use, such as confidentiality and some of the downsides of rapid mass communication.

The OECD notes that while political personalities, including heads of state, have been quick to see the power of social media, governments and some other actors have been slower to react.[24] Significantly, OECD noted that the purposes and returns of social media use by institutions are not so clear as in the case of political personalities, but argued that they have the potential to "make policy processes more inclusive." Canadian nurse Robert Fraser has developed a text—*The Nurse's Social Media Advantage*—that may help to guide nurses as they engage in policy work using social media.[25]

Paid Advertorial Space

If funds allow, many organizations pay for what is known as an *advertorial*—essentially a paid advertisement that is structured to look like editorial content rather than advertising. The CNA has used this strategy for several years to attract attention during National Nurses Week, for example, with opinion and editorial pieces as well as other information about nurses and nursing published in a *Globe and Mail* insert that looks like the rest of the paper. While the intent is not always to advertise a product as one might do a car or drug store chain, an advertorial is paid for by the sponsor and uses their narrative, images, and messaging, which is quite different from the usual news vetting and editorial processes.

SUMMARY AND IMPLICATIONS

The policy model presented in Chapter 9 suggested a series of variables and dynamics that should be in the "to do" list of groups or individuals undertaking policy work. The tools of policy work in this chapter should help nurses think about ways to go about tackling the various domains of policy work, including practical tools of analysis and synthesis, development, engagement and consultation, and communication.

DISCUSSION QUESTIONS

1. How might nurses engage effectively with stakeholder groups to think through how nursing reform could support better care for the growing number of seniors in Canada?
2. What is the difference between data and information? How could nurses most effectively use data and evidence to prepare policy briefs and position papers to influence public policy?

3. How could nurses more effectively engage policy decision makers in responding to the evidence on the impact of nursing staffing on outcomes?

4. In the lead-up to the 2015 federal election, the CFNU produced an interactive online map pointing to the impact of budgets on health care services (see https://nursesunions.ca/political-action/financing-map). Look at the map for your province (data for territories is not available). Why are tools like this effective in engaging Canadians in the policy work of nurses? What lessons can be applied to other areas of nursing policy work?

ADDITIONAL POLICY RESOURCES

TOOLS TO SUPPORT POLICY ANALYSIS

A Framework for Analyzing Public Policies: Practical Guide	http://www.ncchpp.ca/docs/Guide_framework_analyzing_policies_En.pdf
Advocacy & Policy Development: An HPC Resource List	http://phabc.org/wp-content/uploads/2015/07/Advocacy-and-Policy-Development.pdf
HC Link policy development resources	http://www.hclinkontario.ca/resources/14-hclink/resources/46-resources-policy-development.html
McMaster Health Forum evidence/issue briefs	https://www.mcmasterhealthforum.org/stakeholders/evidence-briefs-and-stakeholder-dialogues
National Collaborating Centre for Healthy Public Policy	http://www.ncchpp.ca
Social Media	Fraser, R. (2011). *The nurse's social media advantage.* Indianapolis, IN: Sigma Theta Tau International.

CHAPTER 11

Forces Influencing Policy Development, Priority Setting, and Allocation of Resources

CHAPTER HIGHLIGHTS

- How Do We Decide Where to Spend Public Dollars?
- Forces Influencing Policy Development and Allocation Decisions
- The Impact of Nurses and Nursing on Public Policy Development
- Summary and Implications
- Discussion Questions
- Additional Policy Resources

LEARNING OUTCOMES

1. Describe examples of the dynamics, actors, and forces that influence policy cycles and that, in turn, shape health policy development and implementation.
2. Demonstrate an understanding of ways resource allocation decisions are made and the different levels of allocation decisions.
3. Explain differing priorities in allocating limited health care resources using examples from nursing and/or current government policy.
4. Link the policy cycle and the forces having an impact on it to the ways resource allocation decisions are finally made.

Policy Influencers: Maureen A. McTeer and André Picard

Maureen A. McTeer, BA, MA, LLB, LLM, LLD (hons), is a renowned Canadian lawyer, teacher, scholar, author, philanthropist, and social activist. Over her lengthy career in and around politics and policy she has developed a remarkable policy savvy and rich network of influential friends and policy leaders. For several decades she has used her knowledge and influence to support many health and social initiatives, published four bestselling books, and has been a beacon of advocacy around gender rights, equity, and equality. Among many esteemed institutions, McTeer has taught at the American University in Washington, DC, University of California, Berkley, and at universities across Canada. A vocal champion of Canadian nurses, McTeer served as co-chair for CNA's National Expert Commission from 2011 to 2012, creating meaningful points of access to political, health, and social leaders across the country that nurses would not otherwise have had, all in the interest of seeing nursing more effectively deployed to achieve the health care triple aim.

Montreal-based *Globe and Mail* reporter André Picard is perhaps Canada's best-known investigative journalist, writer, and commentator in the area of health policy. A gifted and fair analyst of health systems performance and outcomes, he is the author of numerous books and publications, including *Critical Care: Canadian Nurses Speak for Change*; he also speaks out frequently about—and sometimes in support of—nurses. Among a long list of honours, Picard was awarded the Centennial Prize of the Pan-American Health Organization in 2002, naming him the top public health reporter in the Americas. A decade later, in his role as the 2012 CIBC Scholar-in-Residence, he wrote the landmark 2012 report *The Path to Health Care Reform: Policy and Politics*. Acknowledging his remarkable contribution to public policy debate through his media role and the esteem in which he is held, Picard has received numerous awards from nursing and health organizations, including the CNA Award of Excellence for Health Care Reporting.

"If you don't like change, you are going to like irrelevance even less."

—*General Eric Shinseki, Chief of Staff, United States Army, retired*

HOW DO WE DECIDE WHERE TO SPEND PUBLIC DOLLARS?

Singer and Mapa described resource allocation as "the distribution of resources among competing programs or people."[1] Three levels of decision-making often are involved—typically macro, meso, and micro, referring generally to governments, regions, and organizations. But these definitions vary widely in the ways they are used, and are not rigidly defined. Some models, for example, speak to macro, meso, and micro levels of allocation and decision-making within individual organizations or even programs; context is everything.

For the purposes of this discussion of the distribution of resources and forces influencing policy development, it might be helpful to expand the list slightly and consider five distinct levels of allocation decision-making, as shown in Table 11.1. These levels and activities cover the gambit from the highest level of government decision-making to the allocation of resources within programs or service delivery units. Making meta-, macro-, and meso-level choices to shift the focus of Canada's public health care system away from acute treatment care creates a major hurdle: assuming there is a limit to the size of the purse, how is it decided which activities to fund, how much funding they will receive, for how long, and for what expected return on investment?

Canadians bear significant private costs and are experiencing rising costs for health care through their taxes, and therefore we are all making allocation decisions

Table 11.1: Levels of Allocation of Health Care Resources

LEVEL OF ALLOCATION	ACTIVITY	RESPONSIBILITY
Meta	Allocation of resources to health care and other health determinants from among all government expenditures	Executive branches (cabinets) of federal, provincial, and territorial governments
Macro	Allocation of resources to major programs within health care (e.g., acute care, public health)	Ministries of health in federal, provincial, and territorial governments
Meso	Allocation of resources within regions and programs	Regional health authorities, First Nations bands
Micro	Allocation of resources within organizations	Organizational executives, directors, and managers
Nano	Allocation of resources within service units and among individual recipients of health care services	Care delivery teams and individual providers

all the time. People living in poverty may have to choose food over getting a prescription filled—a troubling allocation decision. Commissioner Romanow in 2002, and then the first ministers in 2003 and 2004, agreed on the need to put programs in place to transform the types, places, and funding of care to improve it and rein in costs. Evidence suggests that Canadians could rein in costs by putting in place national pharmacare, long-term care, and home care plans within medicare, for example. The first ministers agreed to these allocation decisions within the system and the federal government injected more than $41 billion additional tax dollars into the system between 2004 and 2014 to make them happen. Many would argue that, ethically, these are also the correct things to do, which would close the loop on these allocation decisions being based in evidence, economics, and ethics. However, decision makers have not seemed willing or able to make those decisions. The hold of acute care on the public imagination and on political allocations is seemingly as strong as ever. A short examination of the kinds of forces that may be influencing those policy and financing choices is in order.

FORCES INFLUENCING POLICY DEVELOPMENT AND ALLOCATION DECISIONS

"Scientific evidence is not the only recognized foundation for decision making, nor is it the only one with value."

—*Lamarche, Pineault, Rochon, and Sullivan*[2]

In Chapter 9, a policy cycle model was presented, explaining the theoretical steps in the development of public policy from idea to legislation. However, few things in life are that linear; the forces influencing the phases and steps of the policy cycle are myriad and can be turbulent. They may rapidly accelerate policy development through any given cycle or stall it permanently; recall the examples from Chapter 2 where it was 50 years after the Statute of Westminster (1931) before Canada's Constitution was repatriated from Britain, and 40 years after the Weir Report that nursing education finally moved fully from hospitals into colleges and universities.

As discussed previously, many factors affect the policy cycle and there are also many approaches to examining public policy. We've looked in some detail at economics and costs, both major influences on policy. This chapter identifies and introduces some of the other major influences on policy development at the federal, provincial, territorial, and Aboriginal governance levels. Nurses who want to be involved in policy development need not become experts in each of these forces, but should think of them as a checklist of important variables that should be considered during planning for policy development and implementation.

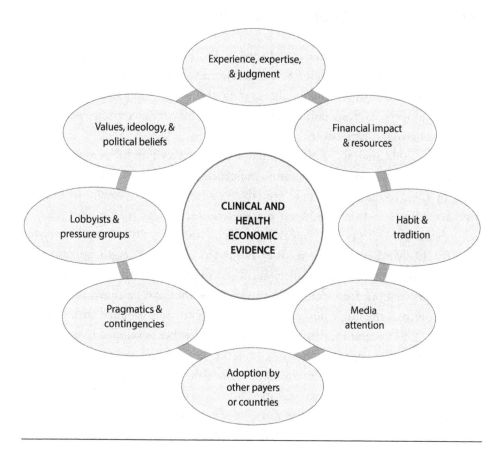

Figure 11.1: Adaptation of Davies's Evidence-Based Policy Framework

In their 2013 discussion of evidence-based health care policy in reimburse-ment decisions, Van Herck, Annemans, Sermeus, and Ramaekers adapted a model originally proposed by Davies, who has been cited earlier in this text.[3] Davies's model suggests that good clinical and economic evidence, which one might assume is the main driver of policy decision-making, is influenced by a whole range of factors, which may include (but are not limited to) lobbyists, ideology, habits (institutions), and the media (see Figure 11.1). Some of the forc-es Davies identified as influencing the use of evidence have been introduced throughout the book; others are described in the following section of this chap-ter. Just as policy is rarely linear, these forces and dynamics are rarely completely discreet; they tend to blur and overlap, as indicated in the Davies model adapted by Van Herck and colleagues. Nevertheless, for the sake of simplicity, they are treated individually in this discussion.

Economic Drivers: Budgets and Costs

This book has included a frequent focus on economics and dollars, looked at high-level government revenues and expenditures, and examined the notion of value and return on investment. Thus, with the assumption that the impacts of costs, budgets, and economics on policy choices are becoming clearer, the topic is not covered extensively again here.

In their 2007 analysis for the International Monetary Fund, Hsiao and Heller opened their paper saying, "Economic policymakers often measure their success solely by their country's economic growth. As a result, they devote most of their time and efforts to thinking about macroeconomic policy" to the detriment of sectors such as health policy.[4] Speaking to those links in a 2004 commentary for the OECD, Mexico's health minister reminded readers, "Health performance and economic performance are interlinked," noting that "wealthier countries have healthier populations for a start."[5] He cited evidence at the time showing that economic growth in the range of 0.35 points in one year was correlated with a 10 per cent rise in life expectancy; that evidence has been further developed in the decade since he wrote that paper. In addition, targeting certain high-cost areas of health care and attending to other determinants of health reduces overall costs and can free up funds to make more prudent investments in other areas.

However, the Mexican minister also spoke to the challenge of balancing investments in health care with national spending and competitiveness, and noted

Economics Lessons for Policy Students

Evans believes that economic and fiscal drivers are fundamental to allocation decisions; in a somewhat mischievous 2010 commentary in *Healthcare Policy*, he offered up seven serious economics lessons for students of policy[6]:

1.   Every dollar of expenditure on health services (or anything else) is a dollar of someone's income.
2.   Winners and losers are always unevenly distributed.
3.   It's the prices, stupid!
4.   Rising health costs are not a law of nature, like the tides. They are responsive to well-crafted policy.
5.   Cost containment is primarily a political, not an economic, problem.
6.   In the health services sector, regulation works. Markets don't.
7.   All six of these lessons apply across the whole health system.

that spending on health means not spending on programs that are priorities for someone else. Gibson, Martin, and Singer said in 2005 that "cost-effectiveness analysis is the most prevalent economic approach used by decision-makers," noting that "when resources are scarce, an economic approach to priority setting seeks to optimize health (and non-health) benefits to the general population within available resources."[7]

Although economics may seem to be the purview only of economists, the voice of nurses can be transformational in shaping economic analyses and resulting policy. In their analysis of nursing shortages[8] as part of a larger OECD study on health systems performance, health and social economists initially pointed to salary as the first and leading variable driving the labour market imbalances among member nations. Pulling the team back to the fundamental question in research (what is going on here?) it was the nurses that said, "No, this can't be salary, or just salary, because nurses aren't talking about that. Something else is going on here." The nurses proved to be correct; as discussed in Canadian examples throughout this book, there were all sorts of dynamics at play in nursing practice settings, many of which continue today. Nurses must engage with health and social economists and others who are part of shaping or informing fiscal policy.

Finally, as decisions are made about allocation of resources to nursing and other providers, outcomes must always be considered—think *inputs* and *outputs*. In a presentation to Canadian safety and quality leaders in November 2015, Needleman cautioned, "Looking only at the increased cost of nursing and ignoring the offsetting cost savings provides a misleading picture of the net cost of safe staffing levels." He went on to conclude, based on his 2006 analysis of the business case for nursing (discussed further in Chapter 12), that "direct regression of per admission cost on staffing levels finds no statistically significant increase in cost per admission in hospitals with higher staffing per patient," and that "given the offsetting cost savings, safe staffing levels can be achieved with little or no net cost to the hospital."[9] Nurses must be equipped to bring these sorts of data and perspectives to bear at policy decision-making tables.

Ethical Considerations

Differing markedly in spirit from economic drivers, Gibson, Martin, and Singer said in 2005 that an ethical approach to setting priorities "focuses on fairness in allocating resources to meet health needs," and "seeks a fair distribution of available resources among competing health needs."[10] Nurses have ethical training as part of most education programs and certainly have ethical behaviour obligations as a condition of registration. Ethical dilemmas arise in every setting, from the triage desk in a walk-in clinic to the withdrawal of life support in a critical care unit to meta-level decisions about whether to allocate funds to a pharmacare program.

Singer and colleagues suggest a five-element framework that may inform ethical organizational allocation decisions; see Table 11.2, which uses these same variables to shed light on ethical considerations in policy development.

Table 11.2: Variables to Inform Allocation Decisions and Policy Development

	ORGANIZATIONAL ALLOCATION DECISIONS	POLICY DEVELOPMENT
1. Mission	What difference does an organization hope to make?	What is the difference a new or revised policy hopes to make?
2. Quality	How is quality defined? How are disputes regarding measurements resolved? How does the definition of quality change in a stronger versus weaker fiscal environment?	What will be the impact of the policy on quality outcomes? How are they defined and by whom? How important will quality be as a variable based on the fiscal environment?
3. Efficiency	What is the value for dollars invested, and what is the additional investment one needs to make for what additional health gain? Note that "efficiency approaches do not provide guidance regarding the distribution of resources across different individuals (or different programs serving different individuals). The same resources can achieve identical net health gains by producing a small gain for many people, or a large gain for a few people." "Second, efficiency approaches do not provide guidance with respect to overall program costs, and the resulting access issues. A program can be very cost effective, but at the same time so expensive that it cannot be offered to all who might benefit."	What is the intended improvement in value for dollars invested? How is efficiency defined and distributed, and how will it be balanced with affordability? Will the policy drive change that is affordable for all the people who might benefit from it?

4. Need	The influence of life and death on resource allocation: "Responding to the needs of dying patients can be inefficient, but is also an important part of how an organization represents itself to its community."	How will the policy consider need at the individual and population levels, and how does the policy balance efficiency and need?
	Second, with respect to equality of access, needs-based approaches emphasize the total needs of the population served and associated program costs.	
5. Process	Who is involved in decision-making? What is the input of the community and patients served? Process is particularly important because substantive principles (based on efficiency and need) may conflict.	How does the policy propose fair solutions to influence resolution of conflicts in processes?

Source: Adapted from Gibson, J., Martin, D., & Singer, P. (2005). Evidence, economics and ethics: Resource allocation in health services organizations. *Healthcare Quarterly, 8*(2), 50–59.

In undertaking and trying to understand policy development and decision-making, nurses may find direction in the works of nurse ethicists like Rosalie Starzomski and Janet Storch at the University of Victoria, and their colleague, Patricia Rodney, at the University of British Columbia. The three talked about the importance of a *moral horizon*, meaning a compass to help guide and direct ethical decision-making. They also argued that nurses bring needs and knowledge that build on, but are not all the same as, those of other ethical traditions.[11] Ethical decision-making is especially at play for nurse leaders when their allocation decisions create a conflict between personal (and/or professional) values and the concerns that fiscal choices may jeopardize patient safety or the basic quality of the care experience. As Storch and Rodney observed, "Healthcare providers can find it difficult to practice according to their professional ethical standards and many experience moral or ethical distress."[12]

The *Code of Ethics for Registered Nurses* may be helpful to nurses in policy work. Noting that "there may be situations in which nurses need to collaborate with others to change a law or policy that is incompatible with ethical practice," the code "can guide and support nurses in advocating for changes to law, policy or practice."[13] The code was developed in the context of real ethical challenges, including debate over the public/private mix of financing and services in health care delivery, difficult allocation decisions regarding resources for programs and services, and the possibility that personal or organizational fiscal or reputational gain could influence care delivery decisions. The 2008 version of the code provides a number of practical case examples that can help guide behaviour when ethical conundrums are encountered in policy decision-making.

Peter noted in 2011 that there were divergent views between ethicists and regulators when the code was revised in 2008. She observed that "ethicists believed strongly that the Code should emphasize nurses' roles in promoting social justice" but that regulators "argued that statements in the Code related to social justice should *not* be used to evaluate nurses' ethical conduct," believing that "the expectation was … too high and too difficult to inform regulatory decisions."[14] Nurses too have wrestled at times with their social justice and advocacy roles, especially when juggling them with immediate task expectations within the tight constraints of institutions like hospitals, where the majority of them work.

Evidence

"Evidence based policy implies that policy makers make well informed decisions about policies, programs and projects by putting the best available evidence from research at the heart of policy development and implementation."
—*Van Herck, Annemans, Sermeus, and Ramaekers, 2013*[15]

Much has been written about the place of evidence in policy making. Speaking about evidence-based medicine as a tool in resource allocation, Gibson, Martin, and Singer noted that "when resources are scarce, clinical evidence can help to make allocation decisions that minimize waste of resources on ineffective or inappropriate treatments and maximize use of resources on 'the right treatment for the right patient at the right time.'"[16] Evidence-informed policy has similar goals—to help choose the best policy, bolster the impact of allocation decisions, and reduce waste.

For better or worse, evidence is often given a very high value; in their analysis of public policy in England, for example, Katikireddi and colleagues opened their paper saying that the "use of robust evidence to inform public health policy is likely to ensure the greatest and most equitable population health gains."[17] Indeed, despite the criticisms put forward in their analysis of evidence, Greenhalgh, Howick, and Maskrey concluded, "Much progress has been made and lives have been saved through the systematic collation, synthesis, and application of high quality empirical evidence."[18] Others, however, have framed the issue differently, saying for example that "research findings hardly ever directly influence or predict policy" and that "interpretations of research relationships and policy prescriptions" reflect the other forces discussed in this chapter—economics, politics, and interest groups, for example.[19]

A wide variety of data sources have been cited throughout this book. In a 2009 discussion of evidence-based policy, Brownson, Chriqui, and Stamatakis suggested that policy development typically should take into account evidence in the three domains shown in Table 11.3. However, how much evidence is really used or even sought in policy decision-making is not clear—and the forces in this chapter suggest that many other influences may rapidly overpower data. In fact, while evidence typically features in all policy models, "it is not a certainty that scientific evidence will carry as much weight in 'real world' policymaking settings as other types of evidence."[20] As Brownson and colleagues concluded, "Policymakers operate on a different hierarchy of evidence than scientists, leaving the 2 groups to live in so-called parallel universes."

Some observers felt that the issue of using—or more specifically selectively using—evidence became so extreme under the Stephen Harper government that the *Globe and Mail*'s national health reporter André Picard flipped the issue on its head and called the strategy "decision-based evidence."[21] Keynes famously wrote that "there is nothing a government hates more than to be well-informed: for it makes the process of arriving at decisions much more complicated and difficult."[22] Whether that was the case with the Harper government, or whether the issue was simply ideology, the prime minister was accused of waging war on experts and evidence with accusations like the one from the *Toronto Star* that his government was willing to "ignore, manipulate, even eliminate problematic facts" to meet its own ends.[23] Provoking scientists to march in a "death of evidence" rally in Ottawa in

Table 11.3: Domains of Evidence-Based Public Health Policy

DOMAIN	OBJECTIVE	DATA SOURCES	EXAMPLE
Process	To understand approaches to enhance the likelihood of policy adoption	• Key informant interviews • Case studies • Surveys of setting-specific political contexts	• Understanding the lessons learned from different approaches and key players involved in state health reforms
Content	To identify specific policy elements that are likely to be effective	• Systematic reviews • Content analyses	• Developing model laws on tobacco that make use of decades of research on the impacts of policy on tobacco use
Outcome	To document the potential impact of policy	• Surveillance systems • Natural experiments tracking policy-related endpoints	• Tracking changes in rates of self-reported seat belt use in relation to the passage of seat belt laws • Describing the cost-effectiveness of child immunization requirements

2012,[24] the government's use of evidence in decision-making had the left-leaning Broadbent Institute—admittedly not a likely ally—saying "bend it like Harper."[25] Myles, a senior fellow at the School of Public Policy and Governance, University of Toronto, opened his commentary for the Broadbent Institute saying, "Ideologues don't like evidence. They know what the problem is and what to do about it." He asserted that both sides of the political spectrum manipulate data, but that the Harper government's decisions were in particular "silencing the disadvantaged"— and called its message control "the most egregious form of evidence suppression we've witnessed under Mr. Harper's watch."[26] The strategy of simply using "alternative facts" under the Trump regime in the United States has exposed the extent to which evidence can be manipulated, ignored, or denied altogether when ideology is in the driver's seat.

The pressure to use evidence to inform policy has forced researchers to rethink some of their methodologies, study designs, and communication strategies. Policy decision makers may not have a good understanding of research, typically don't have a lot of time to wait to make decisions, and may be more apt than scientists to be satisfied with *good enough* data depth and quality. Walt and colleagues spoke about the problem as the "tension between the long-term nature of policy development and implementation and the short-term nature both of funding for policy research and of policy-makers' demands for quick answers and remedies."[27] The same holds true for research, which often is necessarily a multi-year undertaking resulting in exceedingly long and complex scientific reports. Certainly the emergence of techniques such as comparative policy analysis and rapid reviews show that the scientific community understands the need for change and is able to respond effectively without overly compromising principles of research rigour.

Responding to the pressures for shorter reports that translate research in more understandable ways, organizations such as the Canadian Foundation for Healthcare Improvement have established templates like the one cited in Chapter 10, requiring research to be reported in documents 25 pages long or less. The Canadian Institute for Health Information also provides a variety of separate reports (as did the now defunct Health Council of Canada) that, beyond the longer main report, include shorter executive summaries, key message briefs, data sets, and PowerPoint slide decks that can be used by those in policy development.

Finally, it is important to revisit comments made in the preface to this book. The use of evidence is often emphasized in the belief that it informs decisions in more objective ways than other variables. But Giacomini and colleagues remind us "evidence is not value-free."[28] They cautioned users of research that "value-laden choices guide the training of researchers, posing research questions, selecting methods for answering research questions, providing the resources to pursue the answers, distilling the answers into facts to be reported, and creating an audience for research reports."[29] Contrast the spin put on data when presented by the politically conservative Fraser Institute versus the politically liberal Canadian Centre for Policy Alternatives, for example; in the House of Commons, listen to Question Period and the interpretation of evidence presented by the Conservative Party versus the New Democratic Party.

The need to "read between the lines" extends to research,[30] especially given damning arguments of scientists like Greenhalgh, Howick, and Maskrey that the evidence-based *quality mark* has been "misappropriated" by the "hidden hand of vested interests."[31] Among these interests they name the drug and medical devices sectors, whom they accuse of having a growing influence in setting the research agenda. Alongside that concern, they argue that, with the low-hanging fruit long since picked, evidence-based medicine is increasingly about "marginal gains" where statistically significant research outcomes may in fact have only marginal, if any, clinical effect. Furthermore, their view is that medical science has drifted over the years toward "spurious certainty" in a search for non-diseases to treat. As a remedy, the authors champion the need for a campaign to redefine evidence-based medicine, with "ethical care of the patient" as its top priority.[32]

Globalization

Globalization speaks to the growing integration and interdependence of every sector of economies, not just with other business sectors within provinces and territories, but across them and internationally. Canadian governments have already signed or are exploring multi-national trade agreements within North America, the European Union, and Pacific region nations. The Canadian economy is tightly bound to the American one, to the value of the United States dollar, and to forces such as the price of oil in the Middle East and on the world market.

As important as economies are, the Global Policy Forum points to the rapidly increasing globalization—or interdependence—of cultures, laws, and politics. While acknowledging that there may be benefits, it warns that globalization also "sweeps away regulation and undermines local and national politics, just as the consolidation of the nation state swept away local economies, dialects, cultures and political forms."[33] These sorts of agreements may all impact health system variables such as drug prices, the migration of human resources, the use of technologies that enable care to cross borders, medical tourism, and the spread of private, for-profit providers[34]; they may also carry with them serious concerns about issues such as quality and safety.[35] In their discussion of global health and global economics, Benatar and colleagues tie these concerns and outcomes to "neoliberal economic policies and governance," which tend to "deepen the already extreme inequalities of income and wealth, and thus will likely further intensify current global health inequalities."[36]

Kickbusch further argued that "foreign policy can endanger health when diplomacy breaks down or when trade considerations trump health"[37] and asserts that "health is on the radar of foreign policy" as a result of three agendas:

1. Global security (e.g., pandemics, natural disasters, conflicts)
2. Economic (e.g., the effect of health on development)
3. Social justice (e.g., health as a human right, global health initiatives)

To counteract or avoid some of the negative effects of foreign policy and globalization, Kickbusch urged ministers of health to "insist on intersectoral mechanisms that create coherent policy between government departments." She argued that governments need to be prepared to "advocate strongly against positions which endanger health" and noted the value of a strong international health department.[38]

Ideas and Ideology

New and old ideas may inform policy development. In fact, policy making has been described as "essentially a search for the best ideas—even the 'right' idea—to solve a problem or achieve a public goal."[39] Ideology is made up of sets of ideas and beliefs about some aspect of life, society, or culture. Groups of people—citizens, professional groups, religious groups—come together around a common ideology or belief about the way they see the world. In addition, ideology brings people together in political groups that may go on to form governments. Of course, conflict is inherent in governing, because a government of one ideology is still expected to govern and meet at least some of the needs of all citizens. Public servants are expected to maintain a neutral political stance in their roles, informing and supporting the work of the elected government. Some of these ideas were introduced in the Chapter 1 discussion of policy theory.

Federal government responsibility, at its core, is really about protecting borders, defending the nation from attack, protecting citizens from assault, and generally maintaining public order. But looking at different federal political parties, often one sees different and broader mandates reflected in their language. On the far right, for example, libertarians align along the ideology of less government intervention and highly value individual rights. The Libertarian Party of Canada opens its website with the words, "The Libertarian Party of Canada stands for free market economic policies, property rights and entrepreneurship."[40] On the far left, the Communist Party of Canada "strives to unite in its ranks the most politically advanced and active members of the working class and of other sections of the people exploited by monopoly who are prepared to work for the achievement of working class state power and the building of a socialist Canada."[41] Of course, Canada has many political party ideologies between the two, most notably the Conservative Party of Canada on the political right, the New Democratic Party on the political left, and the Liberal Party of Canada generally falling more or less in the political centre.

As discussed in Chapter 1, nursing groups themselves have ideologies, tending through socialization to land on the political left in favour of social justice and care of the poor and vulnerable. In policy development, nurses must take into consideration the political ideologies of governments from the municipal to federal level, each of which might be different. Finding points of common ground is essential to successful input in the policy process.

Innovation and Technology

Innovation—new ideas or ways of doing things—and constantly evolving technology both may exert an impact on and be influenced by policy decisions. This is especially true in health care, where innovations and new technologies drive so much change in education, clinical practice, health human resources management, and in the vast sector of data collection, management, and analysis. Governments invest heavily in technology and innovation in all these areas, and in the past have dedicated funding programs solely to health care innovation. Today innovation is a main pillar of the work of the Council of the Federation.

The ubiquitous presence of very pricy clinical technologies is an important driver of the extensive conversations about how to control these expenditures. Wallner and Konski argued that vendors of new technologies "understandably desire early market penetration of any new device or technology, but often this may be accomplished before significant evidence of benefit is available."[42] Here in Canada, some decision makers have observed that the adoption and spread of innovative technologies have not really resulted in their promised cost reductions and that more government intervention might help. Such a line of thinking leads back to a primary driver: economics and costs.

Institutions

In this context, *institutions* refers not to brick-and-mortar buildings but to traditions—to the "significant customs, practices, laws or relationships accepted in society" as Merriam-Webster defines the term.[43] Here *tradition* refers to the "givens" at play in any policy setting. The institutionalism theory, which considers institutions as a force and speaks to the influence of the structure of the state and its political institutions, was introduced in Chapter 1. In a Canadian study of allocation decision-making by regional health authority senior decision makers, it was found that about a quarter of them reported that these sorts of "political or historical factors were predominant" in their allocation decisions.[44] Others no doubt would believe that those numbers are conservative. The federated structure of Canada and its Parliament, the Royal Canadian Mounted Police, and medicare are examples of institutions that may impact public policy. These forces can create tremendous inertia because there is a view that they have always been there, should always be there, and/or cannot be changed.

Interests and Interest Groups

Nurses and all other Canadians may have interests in any number of policy issues, and sometimes may come together to form interest groups or special interest groups. Parents of special-needs children, for example, may have an interest in public policy related to home and education supports without belonging to any formal group. Older Canadians may have interests in pensions and government plans for expanding long-term care. Interests tend to lie on the personal side; when they are lumped together, the people sharing those interests may be called an interest group. Thus, the parents of children with special needs may be called a special interest group. Seniors are certainly considered a special interest group by governments. In this context, the term may refer simply to a group of people who share a collection of interests.

Seniors may also belong to the Canadian Association for Retired Persons, for example, which is an interest group with paid membership and in most circles is considered a more formal lobby group. While a group of patients suffering from a certain disease may be called an interest group, the tobacco industry, on the other hand, also is an interest group, albeit a very different and much better funded one that casts it as a powerful lobby group.

All of these groups and interests may drive policy forward or grind it to a halt. The plan to implement a new sexual health curriculum in Ontario was brought to a screeching halt in 2010 when there was an outcry from religious groups. The same fight unfolded again in 2015. Governments, quite legitimately, have a policy interest in helping shape an informed public, and providing information that evidence suggests helps to reduce unwanted pregnancy and sexually transmitted disease, and in turn the utilization of health and social services. The Campaign Life Coalition, on the other hand, which defines itself as "the national pro-life organization working at all levels of government to secure full legal protection for all human beings, from the time of conception to natural death," has pitched the sexual health education as Ontario's Radical Sex Ed Curriculum[45] and is calling again for its withdrawal. In this case, the interest group is a formal lobby group with paid members, and its reference to "working at all levels of government" refers to lobbying all levels of government.

Whether their interests are personal, moral, religious, or commercial, these sorts of forces may exert powerful influence on policy decision makers. President Obama commented in 2016 that, in his government's efforts to implement the Affordable Care Act in the United States, certain "special interests pose a continued obstacle to change."[46] He said that the government had "worked successfully with some health care organizations and groups, such as major hospital associations" but "others, like the pharmaceutical industry, oppose any change to drug pricing, no matter how justifiable and modest, because they believe it threatens their profits."

That dynamic is similar to the lobbying by Canada's pharmaceutical industry against efforts to harmonize drug formularies and bring down costs across the country. On this side of the border, Busby and Blomqvist called the Canadian situation "policy gridlock," which they described as "a general reluctance to try new things to get more efficient services."[47] Akin to Obama's assertion about the American situation, they placed the blame on vested interests for entrenching the situation and "effectively preventing change."

Groups of interest groups sometimes come together at a global level in what have been called *global health networks*. In their analysis of these networks, Shiffman and his team described them as "cross-national webs of individuals and organizations linked by a shared concern to address a particular health problem global in scope."[48] While acknowledging that differences in some of the issues surely drive some of the differences in effective outcomes across problems as diverse as maternal health, tobacco use, and tuberculosis, they note the importance of the individual actors associated with them. As a result they presumed that "some of these networks are more capable than others in securing global agreements, attracting funding, producing policies, developing interventions and generating national commitment to scale up these interventions."[49] This analysis points to the importance of the policy actors involved, their leadership and governance, the way they frame issues and strategies, and the way they approach global policy conditions, including allies and opponents.

Intuition, Politics, and Timing

"Be ready when opportunity comes.... Luck is the time when preparation and opportunity meet."
> —*The Right Honourable Pierre Elliott Trudeau, former prime minister, Canada*

It is sometimes said that in politics and policy, timing is everything—and despite its ubiquitous presence in health care discussions, evidence definitely isn't everything. In fact, during his time in the Government Social Research Unit in the United Kingdom, Davies commented that "evidence-based decision-making is no substitute for thinking-based decision making."[50] The crushing effect of the terrorist attacks of September 11, 2001, on the then-burgeoning nursing policy agenda in Canada was noted earlier in this book, as was the accelerating effect of SARS on the creation of a Public Health Agency after years of discussion. In the latter case, within two years of her appointment as secretary of state for public health, the Honourable Carolyn Bennett "set up the Public Health Agency of Canada, appointed the first Chief Public Health Officer for Canada and established the Public Health Network" to enable federal, provincial, and territorial collaboration on population health.[51]

After campaigning on health care in 1992 with the goal that reform would be a legacy of his presidency, the United States was not ready for a health care reform discussion under President Clinton. He had won the presidency decisively, but the plan to overhaul health care started to unravel nearly from the get-go in early 1993. The appointment of Hillary Clinton as the task force chair was met with a tepid response that did not warm up. It took just 18 months to move Clinton's dream from hope to defeat, brought down in part by his own Democratic party. Health care reform would not come back to the most senior American policy tables for another 15 years, when President Obama took it on in 2009—and while the road was rocky, the Patient Protection and Affordable Care Act was finally signed into law in March 2010: an example of the relationship between politics and timing. Even before the inauguration of Donald Trump as president in January 2017, the Republican-dominated Congress had set the wheels in motion to dismantle the act—and on his first day in office, Trump signed an executive order to repeal it; again, a different time, and different political timing.

In her analysis for the OECD, Cerna cited the work of Reich,[52] which suggests three models that may shed some light on the interplay between politics and timing (see Table 11.4).[53] Certainly we have seen elements of these dynamics at play across and even within governments in Canada.

Table 11.4: Examples of Political Models Influencing Policy

POLITICAL WILL MODEL	POLITICAL FACTIONS MODEL	POLITICAL SURVIVAL MODEL
"Decisions by political leaders are necessary and sufficient for a major policy change. This model emphasizes a technocratic approach with a rational actor model of decision-making, but it tends to ignore political constraints to policy reform. This model is more likely under political circumstances such as 'a strong mandate, strong state, narrow coalition, and strong leadership.'"	"Politicians seek to serve the desires of different groups (interest groups, political parties). Rational analysis is the main means to promote and serve organizational interests. Reform occurs when it corresponds to a preferred distribution of benefits to specific constituent groups of government leaders."	"Government officials seek to protect individual interests (as power holders) in order to maintain or expand their existing control over resources. It assumes that politicians operate opportunistically, in which decision makers manipulate policies to achieve desired means. Reform occurs when it serves personal political survival or the personal interests of political leaders."

Source: Cerna, L. (2013). *The nature of policy change and implementation: A review of different theoretical approaches*. Paris: OECD, p. 15

The public service also has a role in all this, because the most senior members work closely with elected politicians and their political staff (meaning staff who are employed and work outside the public service). Savoie talked about the notion of work that goes on *above the fault line*, where he describes politicians and public servants collaborating "to define the public interest, to shape new policies, and to manage the blame game." Public servants at this level are still supposed to be non-partisan and, as Savoie argues, to have "good political judgment" and be able to "defuse a crisis that could put the government in a bad light."[54] But now, as he points out, cabinet members may also turn to large political staffs, advisors, think tanks, lobby groups (such as nurses), and even the Internet. He argues that the public service has lost some prominence as a "powerful policy resource," and here lies an opportunity for nurses wanting to help shape policy in the public interest. It was interesting to note Justin Trudeau's comment that "government by cabinet is back" and his action early in his mandate to free public service scientists to speak more freely; the pendulum may be swinging away from centralized control of policy.

Regardless of these dynamics, nurses need to be well connected with political and public service staffs if they hope to take advantage of the key variables of luck and timing. To be practical, policy influencers need to think about the potential spread and impact of any given issue, whether is it one that is emerging, growing, affecting a lot of Canadians, or bringing a sense of urgency. Before the outbreak of SARS in 2003, it had been a long time since politicians had worried about influenza; therefore the response in 2009 to H1N1 was very different than the response to SARS. It would be prudent to think about likely media interest, awareness of the problem among the public, and whether there is political interest or uptake.

At the national level, CFNU has been particularly adept at monitoring political developments and pouncing rapidly and effectively on timing opportunities; a policy intervention led by CFNU in 2016 may serve as a helpful exemplar for nurses. On October 20, 2015—the morning after the election of the Justin Trudeau government—the CFNU president proposed that the organization host a roundtable of health and social system stakeholders to agree on key elements and principles of a new health accord; this work would include striving to have all the stakeholders sign on to the same accord in a show of solidarity, and then presenting that work to the federal, provincial, and territorial health ministers at their first meeting with the new federal minister present. Within hours the work was underway. Outside consulting help was engaged to support the small CFNU operational team, stakeholders were invited into the process, and robust background materials were generated and distributed. The roundtable was held on December 12, 2015, and the outcomes were presented to the ministers on January 20, 2016, in a one-hour closed session scheduled as the opening of a two-day meeting in Vancouver. Ministers were fully attentive in the presentations by CFNU and CNA, and engaged thoughtfully in the follow-up conversation. Nursing organizations—informed, sophisticated, and ahead of all other professions—effectively positioned themselves with a small set of key messages at the ministerial policy table early in the process and before the skeleton of any future deal was crafted (or at least fully crafted) by bureaucrats and ministers.

Six months later, the impact of nursing was still visible in policy conversations. For example, in the lead-up to the July 2016 Council of the Federation meeting in Whitehorse, the Honourable Leo Glavine, Nova Scotia's minister of health and wellness and minister for seniors, said in a July 2016 column that "nurses across our province and indeed the country have presented key positions for consideration for the next accord. They want the new health accord to be driven by an integrated health and social approach to improving population health."[55] He went on to say, "Nurses see the need for improved population health, access to better care where and when it is needed. They are asking for a bold new vision, incorporating their four priorities in a new health accord." Clearly the nursing message was heard.

THE IMPACT OF NURSES AND NURSING ON PUBLIC POLICY DEVELOPMENT

"Power is what calls the shots, and power is a white male game."
—*Ann Richards, former governor, Texas, United States*

"Power only tires those who don't exercise it."
—*The Right Honourable Pierre Elliott Trudeau, former prime minister, Canada*

As discussed throughout this text, nurses may exert a significant influence on the development, adoption, implementation, and evaluation of policy. The regulated nursing professions as a block—more than 400,000 strong—would be a potentially powerful force if they came together around common messages during elections, for example. Individual nurse leaders are also in key positions to influence policy, and can be key players in the policy agenda. The influence of nursing and nurse leaders closes out this chapter's exploration of forces affecting policy.

Whatever may be theorized about the influences of nursing on policy, it cannot be denied that "despite the many profound changes in the delivery of health care over the last hundred years, the transformation in education systems around the world, and the revolution in the workplace in terms of gender politics (at least in Western countries), nursing remains resolutely gendered."[56] Most other occupations—especially professional ones—have made efforts to become more gender balanced, sometimes having been strong-armed into doing so. But nursing in most Western nations has remained stubbornly gender-segregated. Of course, gender is strongly related to power, pay, and influence. The fact that Justin Trudeau's appointment of a cabinet made up equally of men and women in November 2015 made news around the world speaks volumes about some of the realities that confront Canadian nurses, who remain about 94 per cent female in the registered nurse category. No concerted or sustained effort has been made by nursing to include more men in the profession, and as long as seats in schools of nursing continue to be oversubscribed there is little incentive to engage in the hard work of attracting non-traditional recruits, including men, Aboriginal people, or visible minorities. At the same time, it must be said that unlike the case of women wanting to enter medicine, for example, there is no line of men demanding entry into nursing or an indication that their applications are being treated unfairly when they do apply.

Shortly after September 11, 2001, the Global Nursing Partnerships: Strategies for a Sustainable Nursing Workforce meeting was held at the Carter Center in Atlanta, hosted by Marla Salmon, then dean of the Nell Hodgson Woodruff School of Nursing at Emory University. It would become the "first ever global invitational forum involving representatives from both governments and nursing associations, including government chief nursing officers, national and international nursing association leaders, and human resource directors/health planners."[57] When opportunities arose for nurses to speak, the stark reality of the gender/power issue was revealed when pairs of advisors, who had travelled together to the meeting from various nations, stood to speak—and from some countries it would always be the male. Some of the pairings even involved a male physician with a female nurse; even then, in a forum for nursing, the male voice was the only one heard. It was an important reminder of the need to continue pushing for those roles—and for events like the Atlanta meeting that provide role model opportunities, not just for women in so many countries, but for the men who watched it unfold.

The relative invisibility of nurses in the public policy of so many nations—and sometimes our own—is puzzling given the sheer numbers and levels of education of nurses. In most nations nurses are the largest group of educated, professional women and provide the bulk of care. It is only in a tiny minority of countries where physicians, usually men and much better paid, outnumber nurses. But while numbers and education are on the side of nurses, the high public perception and trust of nurses enjoyed in Canada and the United States is hardly universal; in some nations nurses may be teenagers equipped with essentially a high school education and some basic skills training. So on a global scale, the notion that "a nurse is a nurse is a nurse" is, of course, not true.

Here in North America, the high trust of nurses is an interesting phenomenon, because some nurses say the public "trusts us but doesn't respect us," as shown in behaviours, working conditions, and so on. When the head of a major polling firm was pushed for his thinking on why nurses came out ahead of physicians, his response was immediate: "Because nurses aren't that well paid, and they are salaried public employees, so they are not seen as having anything to gain by not telling the truth." What an interesting comment on the perception of nurse remuneration among the public—and a powerful piece of information.

While nurses certainly are not without formal power positions—think back to the Alberta governance example shared in Chapter 2—there is still a long way to go to beat down nursing images perpetuated in media and popular culture, and sometimes by nurses themselves. Centuries of competing and polarizing images of nurses as either angels or devils, virgins or prostitutes, nerds or clowns, unfit for other work, and certainly suspect if male, continue to play out in films and television programs; these images are damaging to nurses in ways they are not to physicians when they are portrayed in the media. Of course, it's easier to ignore such issues when one is in the dominant group and not under threat—there is little risk. What is more, physicians, dentists, pharmacists, and other health care providers have never been sexualized in popular media, popular myths, and pornography as pervasively as nurses.

It is the deep concern about nursing's image and its impact on political seats of power and policy influence that has caused such an uproar about a generation of nurses wearing what some have labelled as *pyjamas* to work, often capped off with dirty running shoes. Hearts, cuddles, and teddy bears still dominate images of nurses and nursing more than brains, skills, and professional caring. Nurses themselves sometimes have perpetuated these impressions, down to wearing uniforms and pieces of equipment draped in the same images. Why this all matters, of course, is because these images can become entrenched in cultures and in the minds of leaders—and it may take generations of courage to move nurses and nursing into a different societal mindset. A complicating factor is that other caregivers wear the same uniforms. Thus, if nurses do not wear readable name badges and/or do not introduce themselves professionally to patients and families, patients say it can be hard to distinguish "my nurse" from the rest of the team providing a range of care services.

Liaschenko and Peter cautioned, "Aspects of associating themselves with a caring identity may misrepresent the [nursing] profession because caring is often believed to be overly feminine and sentimental—women's work of often trivial significance and work that anyone can do."[58] In the early 1990s, Tronto talked about caring as a complex social practice requiring knowledge and competence[59] and, more recently, Needleman described nurses' work as being "cognitively, intellectually and managerially demanding."[60] We know that nursing is based in a rich body of science. Nurses need to keep searching for ways to translate and market all these parts of their profession, weaving care and cure messages strategically "to provide counterstories that represent the caring of nurses as skilled and intelligent and that convey an image of [themselves] as powerful and ethical."[61]

Nurse Leadership in Formal Policy Roles

Nurses hold clinical operational management and executive roles in which they make allocation decisions from the meso down to nano levels of health care organizations across the country every day. However, the role of nurses in making and/ or informing policy and allocation decisions in governments and quasi-government settings (such as regional health authorities) from the meso level up to the meta level is much less studied and not as well understood. In fact, only one major study of country-level chief nurses has been published and that report was tabled in 1994.[62] From municipal to global levels, nurses are found in advisory and decision-making positions in many governments—and the role has a lengthy history in Canada.

The CNA began lobbying for the appointment of a chief nurse for Canada in 1948 with the establishment of the WHO, which had appointed a chief nurse. Some movement forward happened in 1953 with the appointment of a senior nurse advisor, Dorothy Percy, who served until her retirement in 1967. During the latter five years of Percy's tenure, Verna Huffman served as a public health nursing consultant (1962–1967); she always gave great credit to Dorothy Percy for paving the way for stronger roles for nurses and especially for the chief nurse role. Percy was known to have served the role of an interpreter of nursing conditions and issues to the department, helping to increase the employment of nurse consultants in various divisions, advising the National Health Grants Program (which was a predecessor to medicare), organizing the first federal-provincial nursing conferences (three were held 1960–1965), and representing Canada in various international forums.

Verna Huffman moved into Dorothy Percy's role just after Canada's 100th birthday, on July 15, 1967. She was moved to the deputy minister's office and had a direct line to senior staff. She travelled the country to establish new relationships and groom old ones, bringing useful information into the department. Those efforts enabled her, for example, to inform the work of the Office of International Health, where she helped establish programs of study for nurses coming to study in Canadian nursing schools under what was then the Colombo Plan (under the auspices of the WHO). Well ahead of her time, Huffman was fighting for change in nursing roles, saying that "one of our educational goals should be to prepare nurses who can function both inside and outside the hospital"[63] because she believed that home care programs showed that nursing could not be separated by environment.

After observing the policy effectiveness of Lyle Creelman, who had served as the WHO's chief nurse from 1954 to 1968 and had a spectacular influence on global health and nursing (see Chapter 1), successive federal governments in Canada came to understand the value of the role. So on the heels of Percy's retirement in 1967, and in combination with the rapid growth of social and health programs during Pearson's governments, finally the political timing for a chief nurse was right. Canada's first formally titled Principal Nursing Officer, Verna Huffman (later Huffman Splane), was appointed in 1968 and served in the role until 1972.

Since she came into the role in the year leading up to medicare legislation, Huffman acted as a focal point for 11 nurse consultants in various departments across Health Canada (e.g., health services, health insurance and resources, medical services). She was positioned at the assistant deputy minister level, reporting to the deputy minister. While she described the structure at the time as "a foot in the door,"[64] it was in fact a coup for nursing. The role was never again positioned so highly at Health Canada, and over the ensuing 25 years was gradually moved down in the hierarchy. Huffman Splane set a pioneering and enduring example for the chief nurse role in Canada and globally. Her influence continues to be felt amongst the people holding the role at the federal, provincial, and territorial levels today as well as in countries around the world. Her political acumen was renowned and she persisted in her involvement with leaders across the country up until her death at the age of 100 in January 2015.

Versions of the chief nurse role existed until the position was eliminated in 1994, by which time the role had been pushed further down in the hierarchy. The new Office of Nursing Policy was created in 1999 with its leader titled as an executive director who reported to an assistant deputy minister. But history has repeated itself, and over the past few years the office has again been moved down in the hierarchy, now effectively dismantled and leaving a couple of nurses sitting several organizational layers away from any senior decision-making authority. Nurses who have held the senior nurse role at Health Canada are named in Table 11.5.

In the era of reform following the mid-1990s, principal nursing advisor roles were established within governments in most jurisdictions by 2002. Mirroring some other federal structures, the Office of Nursing Policy served as a focal point and secretariat for the group, which met regularly during the early years of the decade and indeed still does. Titles and positioning of the roles within provinces and territories varied (and continue to vary) widely. In Ontario, for example, Kathleen MacMillan was a policy advisor to the minister (1997–1999) and then appointed provincial chief nursing officer (1999–2001) where she reported directly to the minister of health and long-term care. In British Columbia and Saskatchewan,

Table 11.5: Canada's Federal Senior Policy Nurses, 1953–2016

DATES	FEDERAL SENIOR NURSE	TITLE
1953–1967	Dorothy Percy	Senior Nursing Consultant
1968–1972	Verna Huffman Splane	Principal Nursing Officer
1972–1973	Rose Imai	Principal Nursing Officer (acting)
1973–1977	Hugette Labelle	Principal Nursing Officer
1977–1994	M. Josephine Flaherty	Principal Nursing Officer
1994–1999	Position eliminated	
1999–2004	Judith Shamian	Executive Director, Office of Nursing Policy
2004–2013	Sandra MacDonald-Rencz	Executive Director, Office of Nursing Policy
2013–present	Barbara Foster	Manager, Nursing Policy Unit

respectively, Anne Sutherland Boal and Marlene Smadu were both positioned at the assistant deputy minister level, with Sutherland Boal holding the additional title of chief nurse executive (2001–2005) and Smadu the additional title of principal nursing advisor (2000–2002). In other jurisdictions different titles and hierarchical positions were used, but it must be remembered that governments in many Canadian jurisdictions are quite small when compared to Ontario, for example. Titles may matter less when access to decision makers and advisors is rapid and less formal. Other titles emerged at that time, but importantly, the role tended to focus on policy advice and development to strengthen nursing and health systems in the interest of public health and better health care. There was a sense of real movement forward for nursing within the country and globally.

Today, the most senior government nurses in Canada make up the federal, provincial, and territorial Principal Nurse Advisors Task Force, an advisory group to the Conference of Deputy Ministers' Committee on Health Workforce (see Figure 11.2). It typically includes the most senior nurse in each government, led by a secretariat based at Health Canada. The most senior nurse at Health Canada normally shares the role of co-chair along with one of the provincial or territorial principal nurse advisors. Members of the task force in 2015 are shown in Table 11.6.

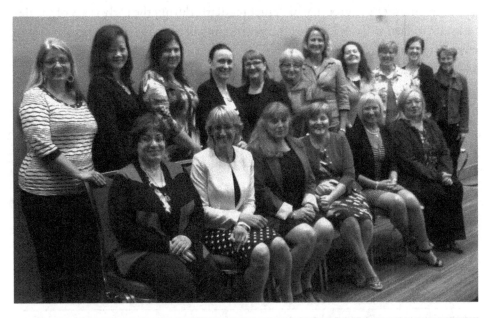

Figure 11.2: Members of the Federal/Provincial/Territorial Principal Nurse Advisors Task Force, Ottawa, June 2015

Source: Photo by Michael Villeneuve

Table 11.6: Members of the Principal Nurse Advisors Task Force, 2015

PROVINCIAL/TERRITORIAL PARTNERS	FEDERAL PARTNERS
Barbara Foster, co-chair	Joel Filion
Nurse Manager, Nursing Policy Unit	Head of Nursing Services, Canadian Forces
Health Canada	Department of National Defense
Mary Martin-Smith, co-chair	Donna Davis
Chief Nursing Officer	National Nursing Officer
Saskatchewan	Veterans Affairs Canada
Linda Smyrski, immediate past co-chair	Lucie Poliquin
Senior Analyst and Principal Nursing Advisor, Health Workforce Secretariat	Manager, Primary Mental Health Care/ Community Mental Health
Manitoba Health	Correctional Service Canada
Beverly Griffiths	Gina Howell
Director, Acute Health Services, Emergency Response & Nursing Policy Division	Director, Office of the Border Health Services
Department of Health and Community Services	Public Health Agency of Canada
Newfoundland and Labrador	
Heather Rix	Robin Buckland
Nursing Policy Analyst/Advisor, Health Systems Planning & Development	Executive Director, Primary Healthcare
Department of Health & Wellness	Health Canada
Prince Edward Island	
Francine Bordage	
Chief Nursing Officer and Nursing Resources Advisor	
Department of Health	
New Brunswick	
Cindy Cruickshank	
Director of Health Workforce Policies & Programs	
Department of Health & Wellness	
Nova Scotia	
Danielle Fleury	
Directrice conseil en soins infirmiers	
Quebec	

| Valerie Grdisa |
| Senior Nursing Advisor |
| Alberta Health |

| Kaiyan Fu |
| Provincial Chief Nursing Officer |
| Ontario |

| Debbie McLachlin |
| Director |
| Workforce Planning and Management Branch |
| British Columbia |

| Karen Archbell |
| Director, Community Nursing |
| Department of Health & Social Services |
| Yukon |

| Yves Panneton |
| Chief Nursing Officer |
| Manager, Primary Community and Acute Care Services |
| Northwest Territories |

| Barbara Harvey |
| Registrar, Acting Director of Professional Practice Community Health Nursing Specialist |
| Nunavut Health and Social Services |

On the international stage, the role has come and gone over the years in various countries. The WHO notes that government chief nursing and midwifery officers operate "at the policy level of ministries of health where they can influence policy and support governments in strengthening the nursing and midwifery workforce."[65] The organization also noted that "accelerating progress towards the Millennium Development Goals and pursuing an ambitious post-2015 development agenda requires governments, civil society and professional associations to work with educational institutions, nongovernmental organizations and a range of international and bilateral organizations to ensure that the input of nurses and midwives is more actively sought and acknowledged."[66] They acknowledge that actual capacity to carry out these roles varies.

The tremendous nursing policy energy, and the strengths and gains of the late 1990s and early part of the past decade, are floundering or have been lost altogether in some quarters in Canada. Some of the highly visible nursing voices in government policy circles have been quieted, and in some cases, silenced into inaction. Some of these leaders are not visible to or engaged with nurses or others outside immediate policy work. However, in nations where nurses may have few or no formal vehicles to influence public policy—or indeed even their own professional lives and working conditions—seeing nurses in formal policy roles within governments can go a long way as a beacon for nurses, as Splane and Splane found in their 1994 global study of chief nursing officers. And importantly, it can be a signal that nurses have something to offer in the development of domestic health policies.

SUMMARY AND IMPLICATIONS

The forces influencing policy development and allocation decisions described in this chapter complete this text's introductory examination of the stages, steps, and forces at play in a theoretical policy cycle that has been developed and tested by Canadian nurses in real policy settings. Reflecting the topics introduced in Chapters 9, 10, and 11, a final model of all the stages, steps, and forces is shown in Figure 11.3. It is critical for students and users to not lose sight of the fact that the process is

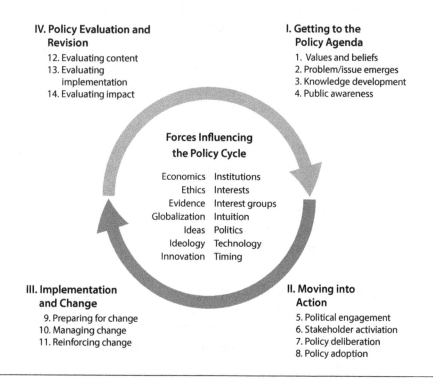

IV. Policy Evaluation and Revision
12. Evaluating content
13. Evaluating implementation
14. Evaluating impact

I. Getting to the Policy Agenda
1. Values and beliefs
2. Problem/issue emerges
3. Knowledge development
4. Public awareness

Forces Influencing the Policy Cycle

Economics   Institutions
Ethics   Interests
Evidence   Interest groups
Globalization   Intuition
Ideas   Politics
Ideology   Technology
Innovation   Timing

III. Implementation and Change
9. Preparing for change
10. Managing change
11. Reinforcing change

II. Moving into Action
5. Political engagement
6. Stakeholder activiation
7. Policy deliberation
8. Policy adoption

Figure 11.3: Stages, Steps, and Forces in the Policy Cycle: An Evolving Model

complex, complicated, and never as linear as the graphics might suggest them to be. Most policy work is a messy, convoluted beast where bits and pieces of every stage and step might be at play at the same time—and where different forces might be driving each of them in different directions. Witness the past 15 years of discussion, collaboration, outrage, political accords, political isolation, and the addition of tens of billions of taxpayer dollars into the funding pipeline, all in an effort to transform health care in areas most people seem to agree need to change. The inertia of policy development and implementation is excruciating, but is emblematic of just how challenging the game is—especially in a geographically huge federation. To wrap up this exploration, the closing chapter touches on trends and issues that still need resolution, and evolving health issues that could be amenable to policy leadership by courageous, informed nurses in the future.

DISCUSSION QUESTIONS

1. What is evidence-informed policy making? Discuss the role of evidence in policy decision-making today. Why has it become so prominent? How does evidence enable and/or hinder policy development?
2. If evidence were enough, we would already have very different health systems. So why don't we have those systems? What are the modifying and interacting roles of economics, ideology, and politics?
3. How should nurses approach policy decisions involving allocation and distribution of scarce resources? What factors should inform those decisions?
4. How might nurses utilize a policy cycle model to recast the dialogue about the nursing role in patient quality and safety going forward? What forces should be brought to bear to engage the public, governments, and employers in that discussion?
5. What innovations in health systems and nursing could most effectively impact the triple aim? What other forces could be manipulated to facilitate forward movement on those innovations?

ADDITIONAL POLICY RESOURCES

UNDERSTANDING THE FORCES AFFECTING POLICY DECISIONS

Canadian Medical Association list of readings on allocation of resources	http://www.cma.ca/ allocation-health-resources

Understanding Evidence-Based Public Health Policy	Brownson, R., Chriqui, J., & Stamatakis, K. (2009). Understanding evidence-based public health policy. *American Journal of Public Health, 99*(9), 1576–1583. Retrieved from http://www.ncbi.nlm.nih.gov/pmc/articles/PMC2724448.
"Real-World" Health Care Priority Setting Using Explicit Decision Criteria	Cromwell, I., Peacock, S., & Mitton, C. (2015). "Real-world" health care priority setting using explicit decision criteria: A systematic review of the literature. *BMC Health Services Research, 15,* 164. Retrieved from http://bmchealthservres.biomedcentral.com/articles/10.1186/s12913-015-0814-3.
From Efficacy to Equity: Literature Review of Decision Criteria for Resource Allocation and Healthcare Decision Making	Guindo, L., Wagner, M., Baltussen, R., Rindress, D., van Til, J., Kind, P., & Goetghebeur, M. (2012). From efficacy to equity: Literature review of decision criteria for resource allocation and healthcare decision making. *Cost Effectiveness and Resource Allocation, 9.* Retrieved from http://resource-allocation.biomedcentral.com/articles/10.1186/1478-7547-10-9.
Priority Setting: What Constitutes Success? A Conceptual Framework for Successful Priority Setting	Sibbald, S., Singer, P., Upshur, R., & Martin, D., (2009). Priority setting: What constitutes success? A conceptual framework for successful priority setting. *BMC Health Services Research, 9,* 43. Retrieved from http://bmchealthservres.biomedcentral.com/articles/10.1186/1472-6963-9-43.
Decision Maker Perceptions of Resource Allocation Processes in Canadian Health Care Organizations	Smith, N., Mitton, C., Bryan, S., Davidson, A., Urquhart, B., Gibson, J., et al. (2013). Decision maker perceptions of resource allocation processes in Canadian health care organizations: A national survey. *BMC Health Services Research 2013, 13,* 247. Retrieved from http://www.biomedcentral.com/content/pdf/1472-6963-13-247.pdf.
"Doing" Health Policy Analysis: Methodological and Conceptual Reflections and Challenges in Health Policy Analysis	Walt, G., Shiffman, J., Schneider, H., Murray S., Brugha, R., & Gilson, L. (2008). "Doing" health policy analysis: Methodological and conceptual reflections and challenges in *Health Policy Analysis, 23.* Retrieved from http://heapol.oxfordjournals.org/content/23/5/308.full.pdf+html.

CHAPTER 12

On the Horizon: Canada's Health Systems, Public Policy, and the Nursing Profession Going Forward

INTRODUCTION

- Better Health—Better Value
- Better Care—Better Value
- Better Nursing—Better Value
- Final Notes on Nursing and Policy
- Summary and Implications: Lessons and Thoughts from the Field
- Discussion Questions
- Additional Policy Resources

LEARNING OUTCOMES

1. Discuss examples of major health, system, and nursing challenges lying ahead and potential policy solutions to resolve them.
2. Summarize drivers, factors, and forces that are facilitating and impeding change in health care systems.
3. Describe ways the nursing profession could influence policy directions that would be beneficial to patients in future health systems, to population health, and to nurses themselves.
4. Imagine what the future health system might look like, and whether/how nursing must change to effectively meet and anticipate evolving population health needs.
5. Describe five basic lessons that may inform effective nursing policy work going forward.

Policy Influencer: Leigh Chapman

A doctoral candidate at the University of Toronto, Leigh Chapman, BScN, BA(Hons), MSc, is one of the young, new faces in an age-old nursing struggle: how to intervene to help vulnerable people living with the complex, interrelated challenges of addiction, homelessness, and mental illness. This trajectory of Chapman's career was not planned strategically; she was drawn into the policy fray in the wake of the death of her brother in August 2015. Brad Chapman, who had long-standing addiction and mental health problems, died several days after collapsing on a Toronto street and initially being resuscitated. Since then, Chapman has mounted tireless and effective advocacy efforts around homelessness and addiction, speaking out to media and municipal politicians in numerous appearances before Toronto City Council and its committees. Collaborating with others, her work has helped to consistently position the issues of shelters and safe injection sites on the policy agenda in Toronto and has moved those initiatives forward to action. In this work, Chapman joins a long line of iconic names in community nursing history, from Lillian Wald a century ago to nurses like Cathy Crowe today—the latter arguably being Canada's most well-known "street nurse" and herself a lifelong advocate for the most vulnerable people in Toronto.

For last year's words belong to last year's language
And next year's words await another voice.
... And to make an end is to make a beginning.

—T.S. Eliot[1]

INTRODUCTION

In the course of this text, a wide range of population health issues have been explored and key elements in the development, reform, and performance of health care in Canada were tracked. Throughout the journey, an attempt was made to link issues to nursing and the potential influence of nurses on policy development—or the ways they are affected by it.

Much has been accomplished in Canadian health care and there is much to celebrate. As Picard said in 2015, "The things we needed in the 1950s and 1960s are well covered."[2] But others are not, and as in most things, there is important work still to be done. Our monitoring of metrics has revealed interesting points in the journey of care where changes can and do make a huge difference. But data are a mixed blessing; partly as a result of our ability to capture so much, the amount of it is sometimes overwhelming. In some areas on the scientific front we've come to the point of conducting systematic reviews of groups of reviews in our struggle to sort through it all and make it accessible. As Andrea Baumann, associate vice president, global health, and past scientific director of the Nursing Health Services Research Unit, McMaster University, has said, "We are data rich and information poor" (A. Baumann, personal communication, April 19, 2006). There are consequences in real clinical settings: Greenhalgh, Howick, and Maskrey concluded that the "volume of evidence, especially clinical guidelines, has become unmanageable."[3] Carthey and her colleagues went further, saying that the information overload resulting from the proliferation of policies and guidelines "confuses staff, causes inefficiencies and delay and is becoming a threat to patient safety."[4]

As this book is being written, the federal, provincial, and territorial governments have entered into bilateral funding agreements but seem to have left the door open for negotiation of a future health accord with funding conditions. This third wave of health systems reform in Canada will, of course, include principles around smart spending of public dollars and should demand thoughtful conversations about how much money Canadians want to spend on health care. The proportion of financing that should be contributed by the federal government is always on the table and will be again; nurses have called for a scaling up to 25 per cent by 2025, using a "25 by 25" slogan in some materials. But many Canadians and health care providers seem to believe that more money is not the answer, and rather that emphasis should be placed on considering how and where money is spent.[5] As the CFNU noted in its briefing materials prepared for the federal/provincial/territorial health ministers meeting in January 2016, "the third wave of reform will be distinguished not by a singular focus on spending." Rather, they suggested,

> Impelled by the need to provide more and different services to a lot more people and a lot more diverse people, the largest number of seniors in history on the horizon, and the emergence of chronic disease as the seminal health challenge of this century, there is broad agreement that reform going forward must link health care services much more effectively to actual population health needs.[6]

The next wave of reform likely will include what Goodfellow called "watchwords" in health systems reform: integrated services, lean design, and patient-centred care. To achieve a sustainable and effective health system, he spoke about the potential impact of a "dramatic dehospitalization of health services"[7]—just the sort of major shift that has been batted around policy tables for more than 40 years, all the way back to Lalonde. Clearly if the ship is steered more forcefully in that direction then a major shift in the practices and work settings of nurses will have to fall in line accordingly. It will be helpful to have smart, informed nurses helping to turn the wheel—and not treading water in the wake.

As we close this probe of policy and nursing by looking at the challenges ahead, narrowing the exhaustive range of possible concerns for nurses to a meaningful list is no small feat. The modification of the triple aim framework used by the National Expert Commission (better health, better care, and better value) offers a helpful way to think about issues on the horizon to which nurses should pay attention. There is great overlap and blurred boundaries across the framework; for example, all improvements to health and care are intended to increase value. The fit of the framework with the overarching issues lying ahead is strong, because in truth those issues can be summarized in four simple points:

1. Canadians are living longer lives accompanied by some serious—and in some cases worsening—population health outcomes, including chronic diseases.
2. There are system performance problems in key areas that drive down quality and drive up costs. They can be fixed and nurses should be part of the solution.
3. There is a growing mismatch between our high-cost investments in health care and the actual health needs of the population.
4. Registered nurses are not deployed or employed effectively to achieve the maximum return on our shared investment in nursing.

BETTER HEALTH—BETTER VALUE

The population health issues confronting Canadians described in Chapter 8 include problems amenable to intervention by nurses. Moreover, most of the key elements needed to improve population health are fully within the domain of independent nursing practice *today* and do not depend at all on a future hope for expanded scopes. Among the nine actions recommended by the National Expert Commission[8] were to:

- Put individuals, families, and communities first
- Implement primary health care for all
- Pay closer attention to Canadians at risk of falling behind
- Invest strategically in the factors that improve health
- Think health in all policies

The fact that five of the nine commission recommendations fell strongly with-in the domain of "better health" reflects the importance accorded to it by the com-missioners (readers can refer to the commission's findings and recommendations rather than have them repeated here). It is worth reminding ourselves that there are areas where decisive action by nurses could make a transformational difference to health and its costs. Knowing where to start can be a challenge, but, as intro-duced in Chapter 6, the National Consensus Meeting in 2013 reached agreement on four population health goalposts that all are amendable to action by nurses:

1. Increase the percentage of primary care practices offering after-hours care.
2. Increase chronic disease case management and navigational capacity in primary care.
3. Reduce the prevalence of childhood obesity.
4. Reduce hospital admissions for uncontrolled diabetes-related conditions.

In addition to tackling these national priorities, nurses must act forcefully to help strengthen the particular health concerns of Aboriginal Peoples and aging Canadians. In a number of instances all of these variables interact with one anoth-er within the same populations.

Reconciliation

After years of work, the Truth and Reconciliation Commission tabled 94 actions and many more sub-actions in its June 2015 preliminary report. With the shock-ing truth and fallout of genocide now on the table, acknowledgement and recon-ciliation are in order. Among the commission's actions are seven recommendations about health, and others speaking to social issues including education and child welfare. Most notably for nursing is the need to work with Aboriginal Peoples to identify policy solutions that will help close the broad health status gaps between Aboriginal and non-Aboriginal communities. The gaps are so significant that they may indeed be a significant driver of our poorer overall national outcomes. If just those gaps could be closed, it may indeed be that Canada's overall population health rankings would change in a significantly upward direction.

As directed by the Truth and Reconciliation Commission, nursing education must include "Aboriginal health issues, including the history and legacy of residential schools, the United Nations *Declaration on the Rights of Indigenous Peoples*, Treaties and Aboriginal rights, and Indigenous teachings and practices."[9] Furthermore, nursing practice should embrace "skills-based training in intercultural competency, conflict resolution, human rights, and anti-racism," and should include Aboriginal healing practices in the routine care of Aboriginal people. The framework for cultural competence and cultural safety cited in Chapter 6 should be consulted in such work.

Although the Declaration on the Rights of Indigenous Peoples was passed by more than 140 countries after it was tabled in 2007, the Harper government refused to sign it. In public mandate letters to his cabinet ministers in November 2015, Justin Trudeau said, "No relationship is more important to me and to Canada than the one with Indigenous Peoples." In turn, during his government's first Speech from the Throne (February 2016) he said, "Because it is both the right thing to do and a certain path to economic growth, the Government will undertake to renew, nation-to-nation, the relationship between Canada and Indigenous peoples, one based on recognition of rights, respect, co-operation and partnership."[10] On May 9, 2016, Canada's justice minister, the Honourable Jody Wilson-Raybould, cited Nelson Mandela during a speech to the United Nations, saying, "Beyond the necessary truth telling and healing, reconciliation requires laws to change and policies to be rewritten."[11] It was then announced by the minister of northern affairs, the Honourable Carolyn Bennett, that Canada would signal an official change in policy direction on May 10, 2016, by removing its permanent objector status to the declaration and implementing it within the laws of Canada. Bennett went on to say that Canada would now offer unqualified support to the declaration, adding, "We intend nothing less than to adopt and implement the declaration in accordance with the Canadian Constitution."[12]

Nurses should respond immediately to the recommendations for nursing and offer help to Aboriginal Peoples, their leaders, and Canadian governments to develop policy that supports the other elements of reconciliation. These actions can begin immediately within nursing teams, health care organizations, professional and specialty associations, and unions across the country. To create synergies and reduce duplication of efforts nurses may wish to connect through a body such as the Canadian Indigenous Nurses Association, which is working in partnership with CNA; jurisdictional members of CNA may also, by extension, have policy work underway from which nurses could learn and/or to which they could connect.

Healthier Aging

In Canada, high levels of chronic disease, aging, and dying constantly bump up against a health care system set up for treatment, rescue, and cure. It is just not possible in emergency rooms, for instance, to mount more effective responses to the many different needs of the various populations coming through the door. Despite efforts to make improvements, users are still met with silos of sectors and specialization when we know that streamlining, simplification, and integration are important to the patient experience and to safety and costs. Naylor and his team concluded that as people in Canada age "there will be a greater premium on seamless delivery of multi-disciplinary care across diverse settings, not least the patient's place of residence."[13] We have a long way to go to reach that goal.

The needs of seniors, especially the oldest ones, fall nearly entirely within the domain of the nursing family. Chronic disease does not burden only seniors, of course, but the reality is that these conditions tend to appear and accumulate with age. Most of these Canadians are not lined up needing the care of surgeons; they have episodic acute health care needs that could be met by primary health care nurse practitioners and the other regulated nursing categories, deployed as appropriate to their competencies, in home and long-term care settings. These populations need help to manage the daily trials of chronic diseases, help that could be delivered very effectively by licensed practical nurses. Especially as people become frailer in their oldest years, they need many daily living supports that are safely within the domain of personal support workers.

The whole sector of supporting healthy aging could benefit from nursing models of care. However, there is no need to treat aging as a sickness, and nurses must be wary about trying to over-manage the lives of seniors. As an astute observer said at a conference of the Centre for Health Services Policy and Research, "it's only nurses who think they don't *medicalize* things for seniors; you nurses are as medical as everybody else"—a valuable perspective. If nurses do want to lay more claim to this large policy space, it should be with an intent to improve health and access to care in ways that support daily living but don't medicalize it.

BETTER CARE—BETTER VALUE

> "We're in a new place; we're not on the edge of the old place. We're not pushing the envelope; we're in a totally new envelope. So the rules have changed."
> —*Sister Elizabeth Davis, CM, Congregational Leader,*
> *Sisters of Mercy of Newfoundland and former Chief Executive Officer,*
> *Eastern Health Region, Newfoundland and Labrador*

Twenty years of reform have ostensibly all been about one important goal: ensuring that Canadians build a smart, safe, responsive, and effective public health care system at costs they can afford to sustain going forward. We have built a *not-for-profit* system that Canadians value, but as others have said, steadily rising costs have made clear that there is also value in running an efficient, *not-for-loss* system—and therefore we need to understand where and how we are spending public dollars and for what outcome.

The Not-For-Profit versus For-Profit Debate

The clinical and fiscal values in Canada's universal, not-for-profit system are sometimes not clear to the public, even when the public fights valiantly for their cultural significance. On the other hand, pro-private forces have argued vehemently in favour of more for-profit care despite meagre evidence that it is better in any way for patients or systems. In their 2007 analysis, Mark and Harless found that there is a "substantial but inconclusive body of research on quality differences between" for-profit and not-for-profit hospitals.[14] However, using data from the 1990s, they found lower case-mix adjusted registered nurse staffing levels in for-profit than not-for-profit hospitals—and as discussed in Chapter 8, more recent evidence shows that nurse staffing numbers and mix are directly correlated with outcomes.

While acknowledging that many individual factors may have an impact at the institution level, a 2004 systematic review and meta-analysis conducted by Devereaux and his team found, on average, higher risk-adjusted mortality rates and higher costs in for-profit hospitals in the United States.[15] Reflecting on the issue in an earlier commentary by Tanne, Devereaux said,

> Shareholders expect a 10% to 15% return and the hospitals have to pay taxes. Funding is fixed [from Medicare and other schemes in the United States and from national health insurance in Canada], so they cut corners on skills. It would be no different in Canada or Britain. If Canada opened its doors to private, for-profit hospitals, they would be the same US chains that generated the data included in our study.[16]

Hospitals are not the only settings that have been studied, of course. Another meta-analysis and systematic review found lower mortality rates in not-for-profit than for-profit dialysis centres in the United States.[17] Looking at long-term care, a 2009 Canadian systematic review and meta-analysis of evidence from 82 studies spanning four decades found that "on average, not-for-profit nursing homes deliver higher quality care than do for-profit nursing homes."[18] The quality link was based on more staff (or a richer staff mix) and lower rates of pressure ulcers in the not-for-profit nursing homes. There was no significant difference found on the other two most common measures, use of physical restraints and deficiencies in regulatory assessments (government surveys). A previous 2005 study had found similarly that quality of care was better in not-for-profit nursing homes.[19]

Fear about the potentially catastrophic health care costs that could be driven by the large cohort of seniors on the horizon began to ramp up as the first of the baby boomers, born in 1945, were about to turn 60 in 2005. The last of them will reach that age in 2025—now less than a decade away. As the new century began, little of substance had been done in health and social systems to prepare for this wave of new seniors. During consultations in 2005 for the Toward 2020 work mentioned in Chapter 6, Deb Grey—founder of the Reform Party—was asked about what governments had done to prepare; her answer was simple and memorable: "Nothing." Canada is now well into that seniors wave and starting to see some of the effects of a failure to plan—including an ongoing reliance on a range of acute care and curative services to treat the issues of aging, chronic disease, and dying.

One of the places seniors are affecting system performance is in hospitals. Sutherland and Crump called hospital beds "choke points" in the health care system because they are limited in number.[20] One of the canaries in the hospital bed coal mine is the number of alternate-level-of-care beds, beds occupied by patients who no longer require acute care but are awaiting transfer to some other level of care. Taking out obstetric and pediatric patients beds, in 2007–2008 patients in alternate-level-of-care beds made up 5 per cent of all hospitalizations and 14 per cent of acute hospital days—nearly 5,200 beds every day; a third of those beds were occupied by people with primary dementia or dementia with co-morbid conditions.[21] When those numbers are added to the 1,600-plus beds occupied by patients whose length of stay was extended after they were harmed during the course of their hospital care,[22] some 6,800 acute hospital beds across the system are occupied every day by patients who do not need them and/or should not have to be in them. What difference might it make to wait times and efficiency across the country if those 6,800 beds were opened up?

Many alternate-level-of-care patients are seniors, but change in the proportion of spending driven by seniors has not been significant (see Figure 12.1). As noted

Dementia

Dementia is a global-level problem affecting more than 46 million people in 2015 and set to affect more than 131 million by mid-century. Alzheimer's Disease International estimated in 2015 that dementia would become a trillion-dollar disease (annually) by 2018. A fulsome analysis of dementia prevalence, trends, and costs is provided in the *World Alzheimer Report 2015: The Global Impact of Dementia.*[23]

by the Canadian Institute for Health Information, "54% of seniors in acute care awaiting discharge to a more appropriate setting were discharged to a residential care facility"[24] and people with complex care needs and dementia, including challenging behaviours, were more likely to fall into that category. Climbing dementia rates are a particular challenge. While some leaders have called for funding more home care in favour of long-term care beds, that recommendation perhaps betrays a lack of understanding the realities of keeping people with dementia safe. Short of providing prohibitively expensive, 24-hour home care, for most families the answer does not lie there. There may be hope in some of the communal living models seen in Northern Europe and Scandinavia, but they still demand brick-and-mortar buildings, beds, and round-the-clock caregivers. The backup of seniors in acute care beds continues relatively unchecked, although initiatives such as the Home First program in Ontario have helped to drop the number of alternate-level-of-care beds in some hospitals.

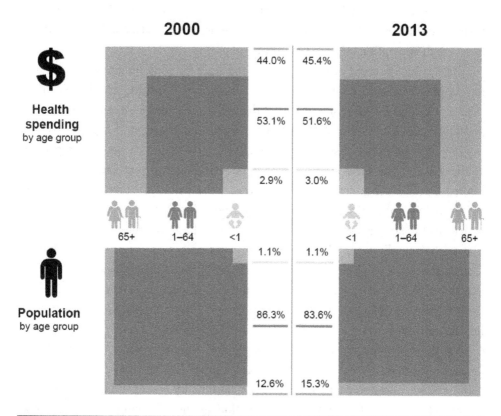

Figure 12.1: How Has Spending on Seniors Changed?

Source: Canadian Institute for Health Information. (2015). *National health expenditure trends, 1975 to 2015.* Ottawa: CIHI, p. 21.

The Right Care in the Right Place

The goal of having the right provider at the right place and time providing the right care across health systems has been a mantra across Canadian health care systems for 15 years; the failure to make this goal a reality beyond isolated boutique examples has grown tiring. Canada is not alone: OECD concluded in 2016 that "the main health workforce priorities in many OECD countries have shifted from concerns of widespread shortages towards more specific issues related to ensuring the right mix of health workers and a proper geographic distribution to provide adequate access to health services to the whole population."[25] The need to reorient publicly insured services away from their near singular focus on acute care and curing services to meet the needs of Canadians in this century is not in dispute; governments and providers seem to have reached agreement on that, which is an important start. But incrementalist strategies—the slow, safe, low-risk approaches to policy change discussed in Chapter 1—have not delivered the disruptive transformation needed to essentially turn the system on its head so that acute care, emergency visits, and hospital admissions are the exception and not the norm.

Reflecting on these realities, and in the light of some of the troubling system performance outcomes discussed in Chapter 8, a leading conclusion of the National Expert Commission was that the ability of acute treatment care to affect population health had been pretty much tapped out. However, making change is tough and is politically risky. President Obama also observed that it is especially challenging in the face of the sort of hyper-partisanship that characterized the United States during his tenure[26]—and that some would say casts a shadow over the Canadian political scene. An added, complicating factor impinging on change is that health care, as we understand the model today, remains tremendously popular with Canadians. In their study conducted to support the National Expert Commission, for example, Soroka and his team at McGill University noted that rising health care spending does exert a positive impact on public perceptions of health care—with spending on hospitals, drugs, and public health especially correlated with improved perceptions of health care quality.[27]

With those issues on the table, there is still a giant service gap in the broad areas of chronic/non-communicable disease, aging, long-term care, mental health, communities, and home care that could be claimed by nurses, should they choose to act before others fully take it over. Action in the following five policy areas could go a long way to advancing the better care agenda.

1. Help Frequent Users Find the Right Care

A small number of people tend to use a lot of services; they often have multiple co-morbid health problems or mental health issues, and very often live with other social and access conditions that drive their high use of emergency rooms and acute care. Browne, Birch, and Thebane remind us that these people are not hard to find—nurses and doctors know who they are because providers see them all the time. Their plea is that nurses find ways to pull those people aside and work with them in nurse-led clinics, away from doctors' offices and emergency rooms, to provide them with services that would actually make a difference to their high system utilization and related costs. Those costs are significant: projected nationally, Browne and her team estimated in 2012 that even a 10 per cent drop in the hospital care expenditures spent on these high users would realize some $2.4 billion in savings that could be re-allocated to other community care settings and could address broader determinants of health.[28]

2. Manage the Twin Challenges of Aging and Chronic Disease

Chronic/non-communicable diseases and injuries may not be entirely preventable, but prevention, health maintenance, wellness promotion, and managing the effects of disease or injury are logically within the scope of properly educated nurses. The evidence is clear that nurse-led models of chronic disease management and care are as effective as or more effective than the usual (physician-led) models of care for the same or lower cost.[29] Since chronic disease is the seminal global health problem of this century, nurses need to take the reins of this policy agenda for the betterment of health, care, and value. With the largest group of nurses still working in hospitals, and with so many resources allocated to the acute care sector, again we return to the imperative for a seismic shift in the orientation of the system, including where Canadians may access insured services and who provides them. More and more services have been moved out of the places where they can be accessed in the publicly insured model, increasing the burden for the populations needing and using a lot of these services (e.g., seniors, who often have fixed incomes).

3. Divert Avoidable Emergency Room Visits

A fifth of all patients discharged from Canadian emergency rooms without hospital admission present with problems that could be safely treated in a family practice setting.[30] Absent more accessible primary care available in communities around the clock, nurse-led clinics within or attached to emergency room settings could divert some 2.7 million avoidable visits every year, take some pressure off the lengthy wait times in many Canadian emergency rooms, and possibly reduce the estimated $400 million cost (assuming other settings would cost less than the hospital visit). Canadians have said repeatedly that they would seek care from nurses or other providers in non-emergency room settings, but first those settings have to exist. The next generation of policy work must include a focus on non-hospital after-hours care options and expand the scope of practice so nurses can meet the needs of patients in those settings.

Furthermore, while seniors living in long-term care settings represent only about 1 per cent of emergency room visits, their related costs (e.g., ambulance transfer) can be high and the visits uncomfortable and harmful to health. Many of the reasons for those visits are potentially avoidable—urinary tract and chest infections, dehydration, constipation, and falls, for example—and they are all under the care of nurses. Efforts to manage these conditions before they happen, and to drop the number of avoidable transfers when they do, usually fall to nurses. Mobile teams have proven successful in some urban settings, where nurses leave the hospital and go to the long-term care setting. At the Western Division of University Health Network in Toronto, 79 per cent of visits by mobile team nurses were with residents who otherwise would have been sent to emergency rooms, at a cost some 21 per cent lower than the emergency room visit. This model should be immediately scaled up and spread across the country, at least in areas having larger hospitals and a high density of long-term care beds. Expanding the scope of practice to allow nurses to deliver the primary care long-term care residents require (e.g., prescribe medications, suture minor wounds, order blood and other tests on site) also would go a long way to improve care.

4. Expand Discharge Options for Patients in Alternate-Level-of-Care Beds

Hospitalized patients in alternate-level-of-care beds, and in the places to which they are discharged, all have one thing in common: they need nursing care. Therefore their situation demands engagement by nurses to build solutions. Insured home care services and flexible institutional beds outside hospitals could go a long way to free up hospitals while providing safe, insured services for patients. As it stands there is limited surge capacity across the system, and a growing number of frail seniors, including those with dementia, are languishing in pricy hospital beds in the absence of a massive expansion in affordable home care services.

5. Expand Insured Care Options for Canadians at the End of Life

In their review of end-of-life care in Canada, Fowler and Hammer concluded that policy solutions to delay or reduce institutional care could diminish the high costs of health care at the end of life.[31] Given the lack of other options, most deaths happen in hospitals—precisely the place most Canadians say they do not want to die. There is no standardized approach to palliation and the myth persists that it is a "final days" approach instead of a potentially long trajectory that provides different options. As a result, hospitals are the only safe, reliable default when health status changes or when patients or families are frightened. Browne and her team estimated that moving just a quarter of Ontario's hospitalized palliative care patients to home care would save more than $15,000 per patient, or $90 million across the province. As a nation Canada needs an action plan that leads to the sorts of palliative care services that will help Canadians manage the ends of their lives in the way they say they want, including home care, hospice care, and acute care when it is needed. As in the case of seniors care and alternate-level-of-care in hospitals, all of this could relate to nursing practice should nurses wish to claim the territory and organize solutions.

The February 2015 Supreme Court decision decriminalizing medically assisted death and the subsequent federal legislation passed in June 2016 bring another dynamic to the story of dying and end-of-life care in Canada. But, complex as it is, the story does not end there. Within days of its Royal Assent, the British Columbia Civil Liberties Association declared the new law unconstitutional and filed a challenge in the British Columbia Supreme Court.[32] To further complicate matters, the emotional juggernaut that is *futile care*—treatment "seen to be non-beneficial because it is believed to offer no reasonable hope of recovery or improvement of the patient's condition"[33]—also has resulted in Supreme Court cases and should be part of our national dialogue on end-of-life care.

As often happens, technology has outpaced our ethical solutions to some of its effects—and many patients can be kept alive long after there is little indication that anything but vital signs are being sustained. The personal values and costs for families, the professional burden for providers, and the impact on scarce resources all are important factors that must be taken into account in a largely public health system.

Quality and Safety

Health care is a very high-risk industry. Other industries—commercial airlines, for example—have tackled safety pretty aggressively and in very public ways. The dramatic visual consequences of errors drive some of the public attention, and as a result, a culture of safety deeply permeates every aspect and process in the delivery of airline services. The outcomes, in terms of the number of people injured or killed by air carriers, are envious. Conversely, we know from the Canadian Adverse Events Study, cited earlier, that hundreds of thousands of Canadians experience adverse events in the course of their medical care every year, and thousands die.[34] In the United States, estimates suggest that medical error is the third leading cause of death.[35] And in the new Canadian study released in 2016, 1 in every 8 hospitalizations resulted in a harmful event—and those patients are four times more likely to die in the hospital.[36] By contrast, in the more than 30 million commercial flights globally in 2014, fewer than 500 passengers died. A key factor that has to be of concern to nurses, and prominent in policy development, is the impact of the constant drive in health care to do more, do it faster, and do it cheaper. In the United States, Mary Shiavo, then the inspector general of the Department of Transportation, warned about that mindset in the airline industry, saying, "With carriers, who are doing anything to save a dime, maintenance [and] safety take a back seat."[37] The results—plane crashes and loss of lives—speak for themselves.

A safe, high-quality, world-leading, and high-performing health system is completely dependent upon an equally high-performing nursing profession. While the positive impacts of nurses bring significant value to Canadians, there are quality and safety concerns that must be resolved going forward. Most urgently, if nurses are indeed everywhere in the system, then what is the message to or about nursing in the mediocre outcomes on so many measures? Nurses cannot claim to deliver more care than any other provider and at the same time divorce themselves from the poor communication, lack of patient-centred care, and embarrassing quality and safety outcomes that in some cases are sliding downward. These troubling outcomes cannot be blamed on *them* or *the system* because nurses are an integral part of that system.

Reflecting some of the findings laid out in this text, the National Expert Commission was particularly concerned about system safety and quality, the strangely inconsistent use of best evidence and care guidelines, and the best information and communication technologies. There is enormous duplication and wasted time and testing; these issues are especially problematic for frail seniors and anyone who cannot communicate and advocate well. Electronic health records may be one helpful solution. At the National Consensus Meeting in 2013, participants chose increased access to electronic health information and services as one of the top five goals, since, after billions of dollars already invested, there are still no inter-operable, portable records. And at the same time, nurses, through CNA, have joined the *Choosing Wisely Canada* initiative, which has opened a broad conversation among providers and patients about unnecessary treatments and tests.

It is a concern for the profession to have a high-visibility, nurse-friendly journalist like André Picard publicly call out communication with patients as "abysmal" and customer care as "virtually non-existent"[38] when nurses are responsible for so much of it. Importantly, care left undone often includes the kinds of tasks that patients value most, such as communicating, teaching, double checking, and answering requests. But beyond patient satisfaction, a call bell not answered is not just an annoyance to a patient or family; it may cause a fall when a patient climbs bedrails to reach a toilet, or is left sitting too long in a chair and stumbles while trying to get back to bed. These sorts of injuries during care can drive up length of stay, which in turn is a lead driver of institutional costs. All of this is the responsibility of nursing teams. Nurses must marshal the courage to step around the relentless jargon and self-praise to confront the harsh reality that actual experiences with nurses are troubling and dehumanizing for many patients across Canadian health systems.

BETTER NURSING—BETTER VALUE

In a 2014 presentation to the Wicked Leadership for Wicked Times forum at Dalhousie University, Shamian acknowledged the "rigorous bodies of return-on-investment evidence showing that nurses have economic impact and value, clinical/ care impact and value, cost/benefit impact and value, and social impact and value." But, as she commented, "the public cannot afford to have nurses sit back passively and wait to be acknowledged and recognized for the value we bring to solving some of the world's significant health challenges."[39]

Nurses are an expensive but effective link in the better value chain, but the evidence is clear that Canadians could realize much greater value from the more than $27 billion they invest in their nursing workforce. American nurse educator Tim Porter-O'Grady has commented that nursing historically has operated in what he calls a *volume equation*—essentially asking nurses, "What did you do, and how much of it did you do?"[40] and then measuring that ad nauseum. Although we are moving into a technological era, this model of work and management is clearly linked to the industrial era roots of modern nursing. We see the results of some of this mentality in the scurrying behaviour of hospital nurses, checking off lists of tasks while patients often rate their care experiences poorly in areas they value most like communication, coordination, and patient-centredness. As Needleman pointed out in an example in November 2015, nurses studied in one setting had 22 physical position changes in 50 minutes of one shift—and he wondered how they could possibly focus on delivering safe, individualized, high-quality, and professional care experiences.[41] In what other high-risk endeavour would that be considered appropriate? Most of the movement, as nurses will guess, was to two places: a medication room and a utility/ supplies room—begging the question why the tools and supplies nurses need most cannot be provided in the places they need them.

Porter-O'Grady posits that health care should move and is moving into a very different model—one that he calls a *values-driven social equation* where, quite differently from the volume equation, the test of nursing is, "What difference did you make and what impact did you have?"[42] This way of looking at value represents a major shift not just in nursing practice, but also in management practices and how to measure those very different outcomes. Similarly, in a 2012 study Snowdon and her team concluded that Canada's health systems are "focused on performance management in terms of costs, operational inputs, such as services delivered, or quality measures such as medication errors, readmissions to hospital, and mortality rates. Health system effectiveness is not evaluated in terms of delivering value to Canadians."[43] Of course, for the most part, nurses—like most workers—behave as they are asked to behave; they generally deliver what they are told to and what is measured.

With a baccalaureate degree required for registered nurse practice in all jurisdictions except Quebec being a fairly new reality for Canada, it's still early days to measure outcomes. However, despite evidence about the safety impact of more education on hospital patient outcomes, people receiving care still face ongoing safety and quality concerns. In a 2012 synthesis, Harris and McGillis Hall noted that as decision makers evaluate and redesign staff and skill mix, they may make use of task shifting, where certain tasks are "moved, where appropriate, to health workers with shorter training and fewer qualifications."[44] The zeal to save taxpayer dollars has led some decision makers to shift tasks within regulated categories, and others to move them from regulated nurses to unregulated workers. Both have caused alarm, with accusations levelled by nurses in all categories that these experiments are dangerous for patients.

Some of the changes in staffing, skill mix, and task shifting make sense; others seemingly fly in the face of the large and growing body of evidence about the impact of well-educated regulated nurses. The past 20 years have witnessed steady rises in patient acuity, pace and technical complexity of care, turnover of patients, and public expectations, all set against concerns that outcomes in quality, safety, compassion, communication, and overall patient experience have been eroded. No evidence has emerged to show that having less education, experience, or expertise, or fewer numbers on duty, improves outcomes in any of these areas. So it seems a paradox that now should be the time to deploy nurses or unregulated workers—whatever the category, who have less education, less experience, and/or less expertise—in skill mix models where they interact more with patients. At the same time, there are large elements of care and populations of patients for whom a properly educated personal support worker is an ideal care provider—think of the 14 per cent of acute care hospital beds occupied by people who do not require acute care, and long-term and home care where Canadians do not require the high intensity of care better delivered by a registered or advanced practice nurse.

When these allocation decisions are made, evidence and ethics should drive staffing decisions. Also frustrating is that most nurses with any experience know what needs to be done; it does not take advanced analysis to understand that more people with better training and experience tend to be able to provide more and better services in any industry. In some ways nurses have become caught in the same loop as people outside nursing, finding themselves needing to justify the obvious. As Maya Angelou—poet, not economist—advised, "You know what's right. Just do right. You don't really have to ask anybody. The truth is, right may not be expedient, it may not be profitable, but it will satisfy your soul."[45]

Some decision makers have questioned whether the baccalaureate entry policy and rhetoric matches performance outcome: What change did they buy with that investment? It is too early to reach conclusions, but there is no indication that the most educated generation of registered nurses in history has made a demonstrable impact on population health. More worrying is the fact that there is little evidence that nurses have demanded to do so—nor are they deployed or employed to achieve that. Most nurses are still taskmasters, whether in institutions or beyond their walls. And if Sister Elizabeth Davis is right in her assertion that our values are reflected in how we spend our time and money,[46] then the salary differential between hospital nurses and other settings makes plain that we still value hospital care above all.

Maybe this was the outcome some policy makers desired all along. But certainly some nurse leaders have expressed concern that, as Kathleen MacMillan puts it, "We are educating 21st century nurses in a 20th century education model to deliver an 18th century scope of practice." As she has commented wryly, "Florence Nightingale could drop into any hospital in this country and she'd know the routine" (K. MacMillan, personal communication, October 21, 2014). Going forward, to achieve better nursing, courageous and energized groups of nurses will need to take the knowledge they have, bolstered with evidence, to work with administrators, unions, and nurses in all categories across the domains of practice to create modern models of care delivery that meet the needs of patients, clients, and families in this century. It would be a huge boost to all of nursing if a modernized curriculum and pedagogy could similarly be developed to drive new models of practice across Canada; 50 years after the last comprehensive review, the world around nursing is rapidly transforming. Nursing deserves the opportunity to transform and Canadians need it.

Evolving Scopes of Practice and Models of Care

Nurses have yet to fully find their feet in a world of interprofessional teams and new providers coming into health care. What exactly is the place and value of nursing in interprofessional education and, sometimes, practice? Much of nursing practice has been cleaved off over the past 50 years to other health professionals, leaving some nurses struggling to define their appropriate roles on complex teams. At the same time, access to primary care is a strain for millions of Canadians, and nurses are uniquely poised to help close that gap. Providers outside of nursing certainly are eager to do so; witness, for example, the rapid spread of physician's assistants and paramedics in various home, community, clinic, and even emergency room roles—historically all parts of nursing.

Looking forward to resolving complicated access and delivery issues, registered nurses will need to mirror other health professionals and abandon long-standing habits by releasing their grip on the bottom of nursing's scope of practice. Nurses must confront nursing's own internal policy and regulatory challenges, and clamour *up* the scope ladder if they are going to be equipped to take on the valuable diagnostic and treatment services needed to meet evolving population heath needs. Responding to calls for change, including the Canadian Academy of Health Sciences work on optimizing scope,[47] these policy solutions could recast nurses with the authority needed to position them as much more effective players in primary, home, community, and institutional care for the 21st century.

Remembering that incrementalism has not worked, achieving better value will entail a major shift in the places nurses deliver care and the elements of care they deliver. More than four in five Canadians say they "don't care who provides their health care—doctor, nurse, or pharmacist—as long as they're qualified health care professionals" and 77 per cent are "comfortable allowing nurses to expand their scope of practice, for example by enabling them to write prescriptions for some types of medication."[48] In their initiative on optimal scope of practice, Nelson and colleagues concluded that health care in Canada "is underperforming relative to investment," leading to "widespread calls for change and the recognition that a new health care system must be built upon collaborative care models, where the right professional provides the highest quality of care in the right setting and at the right time based upon the needs of the individual patient." They concluded that "determining the optimal scopes of practice of these health care providers will be an essential element in leading health care transformation for the future."[49] Nursing needs to take part in the work to determine its optimal scope; while that work goes on, and to make good on the better care imperative and its link to better value, two fundamental changes in registered nursing practice (and in turn in the practice of other providers) must be put in place:

1. Even registered nurses with clinical master's degrees are not authorized in Canada to order the medications or treatments teenagers can purchase

over the counter in any drug store and administer themselves. As a starting point, properly educated registered nurses in all primary, community, and long-term settings should be licensed to prescribe independently from a formulary appropriate to treating the broad range of typical conditions encountered in those settings. A decade after the Toward 2020 work prompted an uproar over its scenario including registered nurse prescribing, change is appearing across Canada: in 2015, the *Framework for Registered Nurse Prescribing in Canada* was published to help frame and guide that evolution.[50] The work now needs to be vaulted forward and spread widely.

2. Canadians often need admission to hospitals and other settings, or transfers among them, to receive nursing care. In fact, it is often the only reason for admission, but physicians retain full control over who comes into the system, who leaves, and when. In the current model, even patients receiving nursing care in alternate-level-of-care hospital beds, waiting for transfer to another facility to receive more nursing care, require the approval and order of a physician to make the move. This antiquated model should be abandoned. Canadians are not owned by physicians nor are the institutional beds over which they retain so much control. Properly educated registered nurses should be licensed with full authority—and, of course, in communication with physicians and other providers—to admit, transfer, and discharge patients across and among care settings.

It goes without saying that prescribing authority and admission privileges require proper education. Indeed, modern, forward-focused nursing education is the base on which any possible transformation depends. With nurses graduating with generalist baccalaureate degrees, and no appetite to change to specialty streams in Canada, these added skills should be taught as part of professional development with rigorous certification after graduation and a period of clinical experience.

To make a difference in the value equation, nurses and the people managing systems will need to decide on the most effective deployment of nurses. As introduced earlier in this text, some leaders have advocated for all–registered nurse staffing in hospitals, for example, and indeed evidence has been presented to show that more registered nurses make a difference to morbidity and mortality. What is less clear is whether those nurses must provide every aspect of the care, or whether vigorous collaboration with other providers could achieve the same outcome.

Needleman and colleagues conducted a rigorous analysis of data in the United States in 2006, asking if there is a business case for nursing.[51] Their results showed that by raising the bottom 75 per cent of hospitals to the same staffing levels as the top 25 per cent, higher numbers of registered nurses and higher numbers of regulated nurses overall would both result in significantly fewer hospital days, adverse outcomes (including cardiac arrest and shock, pneumonia, upper GI bleeding, deep vein thrombosis, and urinary tract infection), and deaths. Importantly, while these two staffing changes came with some $8.5 billion (US) in new costs, offsets in avoided costs resulting from the improved staffing resulted ultimately in a total increased system cost of about 0.4 per cent, or $1.6 billion (US)—a relatively minor investment for the results it could realize.

What is certain is that there has been no political inclination to fund all–registered nurse staffing in hospitals, other institutions, or in ambulatory, community, and home care settings. Canadians won't pay for it all and nurses can't do it all. As a result, allocation decisions will have to be made, and nurses in various categories will need to decide, together, what their business is. If nurses want to make a difference to population health, many more need to move away from hospitals and work in different models of care much closer to the primary care end of the continuum.

The Health of Nurses and Their Nursing Organizations

To circle back to the question of the health of nurses introduced earlier in this text, despite more than 15 years of work, the problems of high absenteeism and high overtime continue to plague nursing. In its 2015 update of statistics,[52] CFNU revealed that in 2014 there were on average 21,000 public sector nurses absent due to illness or disability every week—a rise to 7.9 per cent from 7.5 per cent in 2012. At almost 8 per cent, the rate for full-time nurses is higher than any other occupation, just as it was back in 2000. Absenteeism comes to almost 25 million hours, or 14,000 full-time nurses, and is conservatively estimated to cost roughly $846 million per year.

Of course, absent nurses usually need to be replaced. Beyond using part-time staff and/or externally contracted staff (e.g., from nursing agencies), nurses worked roughly 19.4 million hours of paid and unpaid overtime in 2014—equivalent to 10,700 full-time nurse positions and costing nearly $872 million, of which $680 million was for paid overtime. Needless to say, these rates represent a terrible waste of human capital, to say nothing of the fiscal costs to taxpayers. They also constitute a glaring signal of a labour force in (ongoing) distress.

As noted, however, this is not a new problem; it's been discussed year after year, and has gone on unresolved for more than 15 years—in fact, some of the outcomes are worse than when they were first measured. The work must continue with a new generation, who must return to the policy cycle and carefully push the issue through again, under different leadership with different thinking and different strategies. The same groups of administrators and unions are not likely to solve the problem;

new thinking is required. There are models where workplaces are healthier and absenteeism and overtime rates are lower; why are they not duplicated across the country? As the Advisory Panel on Healthcare Innovation (and many others) observed, "Pockets of extraordinary creativity and innovation dot the Canadian healthcare landscape. Local, regional and even provincial programs worthy of emulation have simply not been scaled up across the nation."[53]

Persistent conflict within and across nursing organizations over the past decade mirrors in some ways the poor health of the workforce. A decade of increasingly disjointed and decaying professional representation has not served nurses or the public well—especially during a decade when the federal government largely recused itself from leadership in health care. The embarrassing public spectacle of a series of behind-closed-doors decisions, ignoring members, threats, and legal actions from nursing organizations whose mandates claim to be member-focused, "exemplify a blatant exclusion of important voices and views—those of the members of our profession."[54] The decision of the College of Registered Nurses of British Columbia to withdraw from CNA "sent shockwaves" through Canadian nursing[55] and the termination in 2016 of RNAO as the Ontario jurisdictional member did the same. Those and the other issues discussed through this book have left many nurses disappointed, discouraged, and angry.

The rancour between and within Canadian provincial and national nursing associations that has played out in public since the early 2000s is, in part, about challenging the power and influence of individuals and/or associations. In her discussion of policy theories, Osman explored power struggles "amongst interest groups within the structure of the health care system" and introduced Alford's (1975) theory of structural interests.[56] While Alford's focus was on the United States, his focus on "the relative power of interest groups and their interrelationships within the structure of a health care system" may help explain some of the recent events in our own federation. As Osman noted, Alford's theory speaks to dominant interests, and he positions medicine as having a monopolistic position as the most dominant interest. These dominant interests challenge those that are emerging to test them, along with repressed interests—those Alford posits have no institutions or mechanisms to ensure that their interests are served. His various tenets may help to explain changing and evolving balances of power and influence, including the dynamic of dominant influences being challenged across Canadian nursing organizations. Lenihan goes even further, observing that

> many of the most acrimonious public debates today are not so much the result of a real clash of ideas as an attempt to manipulate the process. An increasing amount of tension and disagreement stems from intransigence, grandstanding,

and wilful misrepresentation of facts, positions and views (spin). Irritants like these are often part of a "game" participants play to manipulate the public policy process and gain influence over the decision makers.[57]

Absent any other conspicuous explanation beyond personal power, the same issues may be at play in the conflicts within the nursing family in Canada. There are real consequences: in the concluding comments of their critical policy analysis of regulatory trends, Duncan, Thorne, and Rodney argued,

> The professional function is essential to the interests of professional nursing practice, patient care and public policy jurisdictionally, nationally and internationally. Further, nursing will thrive as a profession in the public interest only if it is well supported by effective regulatory, professional and union functions, and we are convinced that the demise of one will ultimately lead to the weakening of the others.[58]

Although professional nursing is rising in new organizations in British Columbia and now Manitoba, there is no resounding professional nursing voice across the provinces and territories. The fallout in Ontario could take years to correct as individual voices struggle to find a collective identity after more than 90 years represented by RNAO and CNA. Despite Shamian's plea in 2014 that the voices of nurses are more urgently needed than ever at high levels of policy formation and decision-making, nurses in Canada have been let down by distracting and divisive behaviours that have sidelined much more important policy and program work. Needless to say, it would be more constructive to have nursing associations work more closely than ever, and this whole issue requires urgent resolution and healing before nurses will be able to give other policy work the focus it needs.

A New CNA?

When RNAO decided to withdraw, CNA already was working to reinvent itself and secure its financial future in the wake of the decision of the Canadian Council of Registered Nurse Regulators to abandon the Canadian Registered Nurse Examination in favour of the NCLEX-RN examination. But despite facing serious threats to its future, the CNA board did not make the bold decisions required to redefine the organization's whole purpose and vault it forward into something new for the 21st century. Perhaps one of the most puzzling decisions was the failure to leap on the opportunity to open the door to licensed practical nurses and registered psychiatric nurses in a redefined and more inclusive Canadian nursing association. Those groups may not have wanted membership in CNA, but with both struggling for professional representation on a national level, they might at least have been invited. One might imagine that they could see a future as members of different divisions within the considerable collective resources of a redefined and redesigned CNA. The same may hold true for unregulated workers who provide aspects of nursing care and who seek affiliation and even credentialing.

Certainly the large number of small, poorly staffed (or volunteer) nursing associations nationwide is not a model we should choose to sustain. They struggle to stay afloat and some of their effectiveness is therefore harshly limited. For more than 20 years, a long line of nurse leaders have called for a revamped CNA that would be the home of all Canadian nursing, across the domains of practice, providing a hub of services that could strengthen the many Canadian nursing associations, at least those at the national level. Such an evolution would mean the family of nursing across the regulated categories and also across domains and functions, including union representation, all becoming a little more comfortable with and trusting of one another in a strong allied model.

The success of CNFU and the political attention it has attracted is no small feat. As noted earlier in this text, 20 years ago the situation was very different: unions at that time struggled to attract attention and in some ways were little more than an irritant (or accepted as a necessary evil) in workplaces and during contract negotiations. But by maintaining a small operational team, hiring content experts and credible researchers for specific topics, constantly positioning evidence in the conversation, and being fiercely nimble in acting quickly and consistently, CFNU has taken control of aspects of the nursing agenda that used to be wholly within the domain of a professional association. Even CFNU's taglines, "Canada's nurses" and "Where knowledge meets know-how," lay claim to a professional space that sounds very different from those of its provincial members—and that clearly at one time would only have come from a national professional association.

There are lessons in CFNU's success for other organizations, including CNA. The CNA has been forced to downsize considerably from its zenith in the past decade, but its transformation work is not done yet. For decades CNA was in many ways the only show in town—the unquestioned queen of the national nursing scene in Canada. But now, 25 years into the technological era, information moves globally in seconds and life is lived online. The old monarchical model that served many global nursing associations so well has suddenly crumbled. The information that may once have been part of their power is now in everyone's hands, and respect for the historic national leader is not the currency it once was in most circles. There is a long list of century-old companies that were dealt mortal blows by competitors, new technology, changing customer expectations, and risk aversion that stymies innovation. As Diamandis observed astutely in a 2012 *Huffington Post* blog, "The day before something is truly a breakthrough, it's a crazy idea. And experimenting with crazy ideas requires a high degree of tolerance for risk-taking."[59] Leaders at CNA know they face the same challenges: the world has changed and others are stepping up; the organization must find its footing in that new reality, and bring its considerable strengths, including tremendous popularity with nurses and its national and global reach, to define its purpose in this century and build its business into a new way forward. This will be especially important for supporting a professional nursing voice in the public policy process.

Global Health and Nursing Leadership

"In the broad church that makes up nursing we have not united on the central image we want to communicate to the public and our professional colleagues."

—*Alison Kitson, FRCN, Dean of Nursing, University of Adelaide, Australia*

The WHO has stated that "responding to global, regional and national needs requires a well-prepared health workforce at all levels of the health system,"[60] and Canada has a long history of leadership in global health through its links with that organization. Canada was the third member to ratify the Constitution of the World Health Organization (in 1946) and Brock Chisolm, who had been Canada's federal deputy minister of health, was the first director general of the organization (1948–1953).[61]

Structured in six regions and a series of offices all reporting to the director general (see Figure 12.2), there are more than 150 country members and 7,000 employees across the WHO. While the organization has a long history of staffing a busy Office of the Chief Nurse Scientist, it has not been staffed consistently since Jean Yan retired in the middle of the last decade.

There are a number of regular opportunities for nurses to connect with global colleagues through their government's chief nurses. For example, the WHO holds a global forum for government chief nursing and midwifery officers every other year. These forums are tied to themes being addressed in World Health Assembly (WHA) priorities and resolutions. And there is a Global Advisory Group on Nursing and Midwifery, established in 1992, with a mandate to serve "as a strategic, action-oriented body providing policy advice to the Director-General and the WHO Cabinet to strategically enhance the contributions of nursing and midwifery within the context of all WHO priorities and programmes."[62]

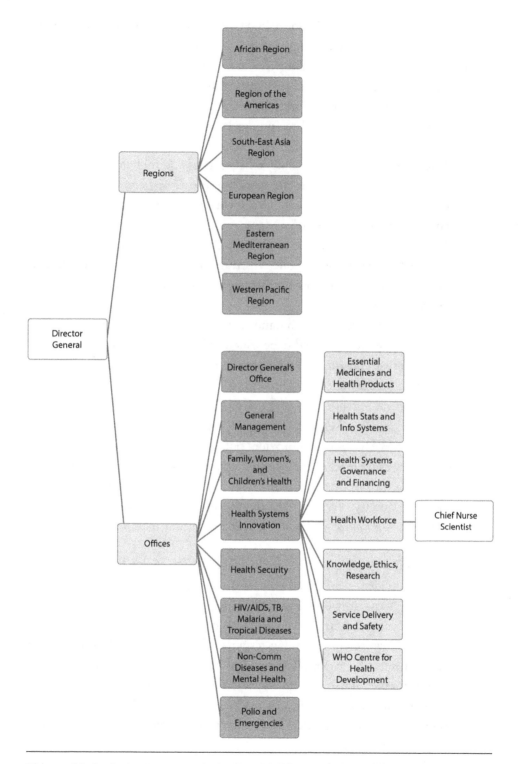

Figure 12.2: Organizational Structure, World Health Organization, 2014

Figure 12.3 shows the 2011 to 2015 WHO strategic directions for nursing and midwifery. Despite there being so many economic and cultural differences, the *WHO Nursing and Midwifery Progress Report 2008–2012* shows that Canadian nursing has many issues in common with other countries. They noted, for example, that "the nursing and midwifery workforce remains understaffed, undertrained and poorly deployed" and called for a three-pronged strategy:

1. "Member States must continue to help nurses and midwives to maximize their roles, not only as practitioners but also as leaders, in order to empower the profession to cope with the evolving health and demographic changes in society at large."

2. "Continuing to support the implementation and improvement of effective information systems and policy instruments … is vital to anticipate and improve strategic planning for nursing and midwifery services, education and workforce."

3. "Effective ways of enhancing and sustaining investments in nursing and midwifery services … need to be widely published and disseminated globally to ensure consistency and innovation in nurses' and midwives' contribution to health system strengthening."[63]

In its *Options Analysis Report on Strategic Directions for Nursing and Midwifery (2016–2020)*, the WHO hopes to provide "policy makers, practitioners and other stakeholders at every level of the health-care system with a flexible framework for broad-based, collaborative action to enhance the capacity of nurses and midwives to provide quality services."[64] In the meantime, going forward the *Global Strategy on Human Resources for Health* will focus on four main objectives:[65]

1. "To optimize performance, quality and impact of the health workforce through evidence-informed policies on human resources for health, contributing to healthy lives and well-being, effective universal health coverage, resilience and strengthened health systems at all levels.

2. To align investment in human resources for health with the current and future needs of the population and of health systems, taking account of labour market dynamics and education policies; to address shortages and improve distribution of health workers, so as to enable maximum improvements in health outcomes, social welfare, employment creation and economic growth.

3. To build the capacity of institutions at sub-national, national, regional and global levels for effective public policy stewardship, leadership and governance of actions on human resources for health.

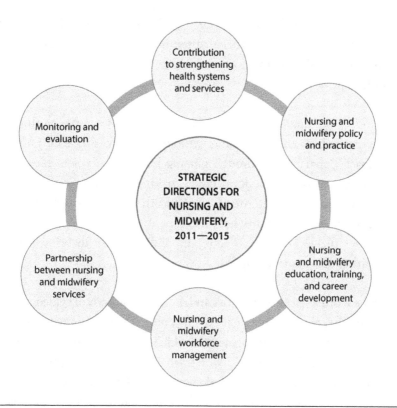

Figure 12.3: World Health Organization Strategic Directions for Nursing and Midwifery, 2011–2015

Source: Adapted from World Health Organization. (2013). *WHO nursing and midwifery progress report 2008–2012.* Geneva: WHO, p. 15. Retrieved from http://www.who.int/hrh/nursing_midwifery/NursingMidwiferyProgressReport.pdf.

4. To strengthen data on human resources for health, for monitoring and ensuring accountability for the implementation of national and regional strategies, and the Global Strategy."

FINAL NOTES ON NURSING AND POLICY

"Nursing cannot plan in isolation from government or other health disciplines. We [need] to consider major national nursing issues—how medical care will affect nursing, how to recruit nursing leaders in the face of population projections, and how we may work more closely with professional organizations, university schools of nursing, and nursing service agencies."

—*Verna Huffman Splane, former Principal Nursing Officer, Canada, 1968*[66]

As nursing moves forward and makes choices about whether and how to confront some of the challenges listed in this chapter, Judith Shamian, as president of the International Council of Nurses, offered her perspective that nurses should participate in four priorities:

1. "Impact the quality of nursing care and patient safety—without risking their own lives and safety, and without compromising their family life.
2. Impact global health through nursing knowledge, voice, experience, and participation both at policy decision-making tables and at the point of care.
3. Impact the social determinants of health by removing barriers and increasing access to quality health care.
4. Impact the level of knowledge and skills we use to bring about better health and better nursing."[67]

To augment other national inquiries and the immense body of evidence, Canadian nurses undertook a credible, national nursing commission that gave focus to health system transformation and nursing, and in which registered nurses have issued and been issued a strong call to political action by the public and other providers. Nurses, therefore, have a blueprint for policy action and are not starting from scratch.

To help think about how to approach policy and such daunting challenges, there are now some policy tools that were not as available to the pioneers that came before us. Shamian, after spending more than 25 years in executive and policy roles, serving as the president of the International Council of Nurses (2013–2017) and as a member of the United Nations Secretary-General's High-Level Commission on Health Employment and Economic Growth, is conceptualizing a new model of nursing policy influence (see Figure 12.4). While the model is still evolving, she observes that nurses often operate quite effectively within what she calls the "nursing bubble," while operating less vigorously and effectively in health care more broadly, at regional and domestic levels, and in the global health and policy sector. What is more, she believes nurses have not been as effective as they should be in forming the sorts of "strategic partnerships that could exert the desired impact on health policy, planning and delivery."[68]

Shamian argues that to be more effective, nurses need to think about engaging in policy in ways that bridge the four "bubbles" or spheres of health policy more strategically, more effectively, and with more collaboration. Her thinking is that nurses must be strong in the core business of nursing, and it should be the lens with which they carry out policy work. In a sense, nursing knowledge is nested at the base of the policy work, but from there she urges that nurses reach out and take on more purposeful and strategic relationships in spheres expanding outward, so

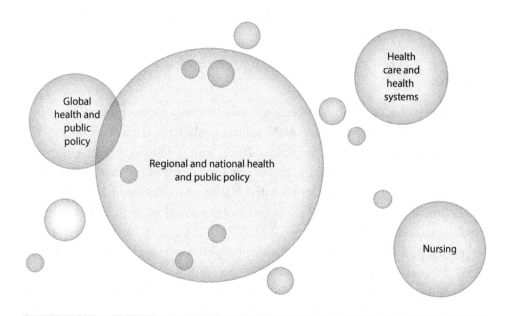

Figure 12.4: Traditional Spheres of Policy Influence—the Evolving Policy "Bubbles" Model, Judith Shamian

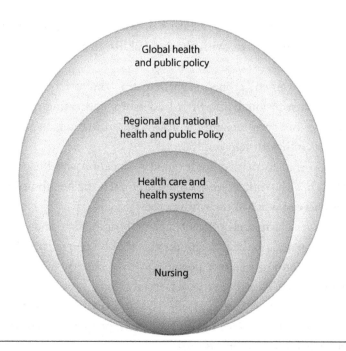

Figure 12.5: Conceptual Elements of an Evolving Model of Integrated Nursing Policy Influence, Judith Shamian

that the other spheres are much more tightly interconnected and build upon each other (as shown in Figure 12.5).

Closure

While they were not fully achieved, the Millennium Development Goals initiative has largely ended. Those eight global goals were developed during the United Nations' Millennium Summit in 2000, with specific outcomes targets for the year 2015.[69] Reaffirming an "unwavering commitment to ... transform our world for the better by 2030," the United Nations has identified 17 Sustainable Development Goals toward which it intends the world to work collectively between now and 2030 (see Figure 12.6).[70] With a focus on people, the planet, prosperity, peace, and partnership, heads of governments agreed in January 2016 on the 17 goals with 169 targets.

Intended in part to support that ambitious plan, the United Nations High-Level Commission on Health Employment and Economic Growth offered 10 recommendations to transform the global health workforce in its September 2016 report. Canadian governments and, in turn, nurses will be impacted by and have to take into consideration these directions going forward:[71]

1. "Stimulate investments in creating decent health sector jobs, particularly for women and youth, with the right skills, in the right numbers and in the right places.
2. Maximize women's economic participation and foster their empowerment through institutionalizing their leadership, addressing gender biases and inequities in education and the health labour market, and tackling gender concerns in health reform processes.
3. Scale up transformative, high-quality education and lifelong learning so that all health workers have skills that match the health needs of populations and can work to their full potential.
4. Reform service models concentrated on hospital care and focus instead on prevention and on the efficient provision of high-quality, affordable, integrated, community-based, people-centred primary and ambulatory care, paying special attention to underserved areas.
5. Harness the power of cost-effective information and communication technologies to enhance health education, people-centred health services and health information systems.
6. Ensure investment in the International Health Regulations core capacities, including skills development of national and international health

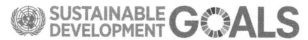

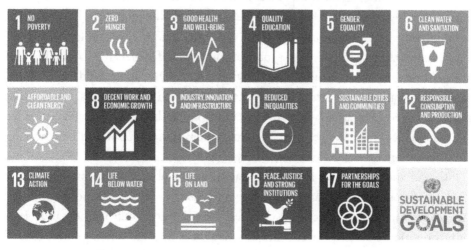

Figure 12.6: Sustainable Development Goals, United Nations, 2016

Source: Image used by permission of the United Nations. Retrieved from http://www.globalgoals.org.

workers in humanitarian settings and public health emergencies, both acute and protracted. Ensure the protection and security of all health workers and health facilities in all settings.

7. Raise adequate funding from domestic and international sources, public and private where appropriate, and consider broad-based health financing reform where needed, to invest in the right skills, decent working conditions and an appropriate number of health workers.

8. Promote intersectoral collaboration at national, regional and international levels; engage civil society, unions and other health workers' organizations and the private sector; and align international cooperation to support investments in the health workforce, as part of national health and education strategies and plans.

9. Advance international recognition of health workers' qualifications to optimize skills use, increase the benefits from and reduce the negative effects of health worker migration, and safeguard migrants' rights.

10. Undertake robust research and analysis of health labour markets, using harmonized metrics and methodologies, to strengthen evidence, accountability and action."

Nurses are now challenged, in a sense, by 17 new global "bubbles" of policy work to complicate the four mentioned earlier. To engage in these priorities, Canada needs an army of courageous nurses who are well educated in the policy game. Nursing education leaders have the opportunity to (and must) help to transform nursing from the ground up, from undergraduate to doctoral levels and beyond. Canadian nursing needs to groom a generation of leaders in all domains who are politics-, economics-, and policy-savvy, courageous, and confident. Nursing science must align with these challenges to inform and test solutions. In addition, nurses all need to imagine what new mechanisms can be put in place to galvanize the personal courage and confidence of individual nurses that would help nursing shine as a more effective, collective force.

Canadians trust nurses at levels that are the envy of every other profession; the field is wide open for brilliant, innovative nurse leaders to take the policy and system leadership reins. Collectively, Canada's nurses need to believe there must be a transformational systems-level change—they must marshal nursing's best brains, stamina, evidence, and numbers, and be deeply engaged in it. There are myriad points of entry through which to get involved: nurses may engage in policy work at the organization/employer level, become active in nursing associations, get involved in research and publishing, or as Michael Decter urged, through roles such as being a voter, a volunteer, a public servant, or serving on organizational boards.[72]

SUMMARY AND IMPLICATIONS: LESSONS AND THOUGHTS FROM THE FIELD

The content covered in this text offers up some key messages and lessons for nurses, as well as some practical advice from various leaders that may spur on those who want to wade into the world of policy development. To summarize just five of them:

1. Policy work is a human relationships game at every step of the process, and health care and health policy exist in a surprisingly small world. It is of value to approach the work with a sense of professional inquiry, joy, and collaboration. Be smart; nurture relationships; build professional friendships partnerships, and networks; leave a positive trail; and constantly reach out to build—never burn—bridges.

2. A lot of policy work entails a long, messy marathon, not a sprint. Things change slowly in most organizations, systems, and cultural institutions; stamina is required in the long term. Dorothy Wylie, one of Canada's iconic 20th century nurse executives, always advised graduate students

studying administration to aim for one to three cultural changes over five years in a complex organization like a hospital—and if a leader can make that sort of policy change happen, consider it an unqualified success (D. Wylie, personal communication, October 1989). A smart, steady leadership hand over a long period of time can be tremendously reassuring in organizations and systems, and can create the trust that is the wellspring of innovation and risk-taking. Policy work can benefit from the same thinking.

3. Florence Nightingale famously said that little can be accomplished "under the spirit of fear"—and the reality is that policy work can feel very intimidating. The data and information are massive in size, complicated, and constantly changing. Some of the players in the world of leadership, policy, and politics also can make the process daunting. Many of the settings—whether one is speaking out for the first time at a seminar in a workplace, making a presentation at a local town hall meeting, or testifying formally before a parliamentary committee and answering difficult questions—can leave the best of us feeling exposed and vulnerable to criticism. In her book *Lean In*, as well as in many of her lectures, Sheryl Sandberg counsels that we not give up before we start: "Don't leave before you leave," she advises—and she asks, "What would you do if you weren't afraid?"[73] Mustering courage for risk-taking and for the long game of policy is essential. Practice and repetition help, just as they do for mastery of clinical nursing skills. But developing content expertise—simply knowing one's area of content *cold*—is a remarkable form of confidence building and is a key to success.

4. As he neared the end of his eight-year presidency of the United States, Barack Obama concluded that pragmatism is necessary in both legislation and policy implementation, saying, "Simpler approaches to addressing our health care problems exist at both ends of the political spectrum."[74] In a country as vast as Canada with so many complicated variables, we should strive to not overcomplicate our policy solutions. Sometimes simple solutions really are the best.

5. Three-quarters of Canadians polled in 2015 said that health care is so complicated they don't know who to trust.[75] There is room for nurses to respond to that confusion, take advantage of the high trust of the public, and shape messages about the value of investments in nursing—including investments in the right providers from other professions to meet population health needs. Nurses need not and should not be self-serving in providing information about health systems to governments and the public,

but rather, simply and masterfully tell the story of practical steps leading to differently structured, less complicated, and more clinically effective and cost-efficient health care.

Citing years of chaos within Canadian health care—driven by forces such as constant restructuring, inadequate human resources set against high patient acuity, offloading of care to families, and the uncritical adoption of a rigid corporate business ethos—Rodney and colleagues used the bleak metaphor of a "moral winter" to describe the place nursing finds itself in today. By that term, they are referring to a "moral landscape of nursing practice that has become frozen, lying dormant and buried beneath layers of contextual constraints."[76] In contrast, nurse theorist Jean Watson has often positioned nursing as "the light in institutional darkness."[77] One might hope that nurses could be that light in the dreary image of a moral winter. To rekindle that kind of flame given current practice realities, nurses must galvanize their huge public support and find ways to be courageous, active, moral, and disruptive agents in an effort to improve outcomes in our current systems. They must also act aggressively to improve nursing itself.

In his 1902 book *Observations by Mr. Dooley*, American humourist Finley Dunne wrote that one role of newspapers was to comfort the afflicted and afflict the comfortable. Playing on those words today, Kathleen MacMillan is fond of saying that it's "the role of *nurses* to comfort the afflicted, and afflict the comfortable" (K. MacMillan, personal communication, October 21, 2014). Hopefully this text provides some of the tools needed to help nurses wade effectively into the tough and competitive playing field of "afflicting the comfortable."

DISCUSSION QUESTIONS

1. If you could change one thing about Canada's health systems today, what would it be and why?
2. What five changes to health systems would make the most significant difference to population health going forward?
3. If you could change one thing about nursing in Canada today, what would it be and why?
4. How could nursing be reformed to contribute to improvements in the performance of health care delivery in Canada?
5. Suggest basic elements of a nursing policy strategy to generate solutions to one key health systems performance challenge lying ahead.

6. How should Canadian nursing organizations engage with nurses, governments, and the public in the Sustainable Development Goals global initiative?
7. What implications for Canadian nursing arise from the recommendations of the United Nations High-Level Commission on Health Employment and Economic Growth? Who should respond to them?
8. What priority should be given to policy competency in undergraduate and graduate nursing education in Canada?

ADDITIONAL POLICY RESOURCES

INDIGENOUS PEOPLES' HEALTH

Canadian Indigenous Nurses Association	http://www.indigenousnurses.ca
Determinants of Indigenous Peoples' Health	Greenwood, M., de Leeuw, S., Lindsay, N.M., & Reading, C., (Eds.). (2015). *Determinants of Indigenous peoples' health in Canada: Beyond the social.* Toronto: Canadian Scholars' Press.
National Collaborating Centre for Aboriginal Health	http://www.nccah-ccnsa.ca
National Aboriginal Health Organization	http://www.naho.ca

LEADING CHANGE AND TRANSFORMATION

High-Impact Leadership: Improve Care, Improve the Health of Populations, and Reduce Costs	http://www.ihi.org/resources/pages/ihiwhitepapers/highimpactleadership.aspx
Top 10 Health Care Game Changers (Canada)	http://humanfactors.ca/wp-content/uploads/2011/08/Top-10-Canada-Health-Innovations_2011.pdf
Leading Change, Adding Value: Framework for Nursing, Midwifery and Care Staff	https://www.england.nhs.uk/wp-content/uploads/2016/05/nursing-framework.pdf

OTHER RESOURCES

Better Home Care: A National Action Plan	http://www.thehomecareplan.ca
Framework for Registered Nurse Prescribing in Canada	https://www.cna-aiic.ca/~/media/cna/page-content/pdf-en/cna-rn-prescribing-framework_e.pdf
Working for Health and Growth: Investing in the Health Workforce	http://apps.who.int/iris/bitstream/10665/250047/1/9789241511308-eng.pdf?ua=1

Transforming our world: The 2030 Agenda for Sustainable Development	https://sustainabledevelopment.un.org/post2015/transformingourworld
World Health Organization Human Resources for Health	http://www.who.int/hrh
World Health Organization Nursing and Midwifery	http://www.who.int/hrh/nursing_midwifery

NOTES

Preface

1. Hilson, M. (1999). *Presentation to Florence Nightingale International Foundation luncheon.* London, UK, June 30, 1999. Retrieved March 2014 from http://www.fnif.org/hilsonpresent.htm.

2. Canadian Nurses Association. (2000, May). Nursing is a political act—the bigger picture. *Nursing Now: Trends and Issues in Canadian Nursing, 8.* Retrieved from https://www.cna-aiic.ca/~/media/cna/page-content/pdf-en/nursing_political_act_may_2000_e.pdf?la=en.

3. Lewis, S. (2010). So many voices, so little voice. *Canadian Nurse, 106*(8), 40.

4. Picard, A. (2000). *Critical care: Canadian nurses speak for change.* Toronto: Harper Collins, p. 2.

5. Ipsos Reid. (2015, June). *Expectations of the health care system.* Presented at HealthCareCAN, Ottawa, Ontario.

6. Liaschenko, J., & Peter, E. (2016). Fostering nurses' moral agency and moral identity: The importance of moral community. *Hastings Center Report, 46*(S1), S18–S21, p. S20.

7. Presbyterian Historical Society. (2014). *Maggie Kuhn & women's history month.* Philadelphia: Presbyterian Historical Society. Retrieved from http://www.history.pcusa.org/blog/maggie-kuhn-womens-history-month.

8. Canadian Nurses Association. (1998). Nurses take over Ottawa. *CNA Today, 8*(4), 1.

9. Elliott, J., Rutty, C., & Villeneuve, M. (2013). *The Canadian Nurses Association 1908–2008: One hundred years of service.* Ottawa: Canadian Nurses Association.

10. National Expert Commission. (2012). *A nursing call to action: The health of our nation, the future of our health system.* Ottawa: Canadian Nurses Association, p. 1.

11. Picard, A. (2000). *Critical care: Canadian nurses speak for change.* Toronto: Harper Collins, p. 241.

12. Humphreys, K., & Piot, P. (2012). Scientific evidence alone is not sufficient basis for health policy. *British Medical Journal, 344*, e1316. Retrieved from http://dx.doi.org/10.1136/bmj.e1316.

13. Ibid.

14. Evans, R. (2004, May 26). Keynote address. Presented at the Canadian Association for Health Services and Policy Research Annual Meeting, Montreal, Quebec.

15. Spenceley, S., Reutter, L., & Allen, M. (2006). The road less travelled: Nursing advocacy at the policy level. *Policy, Politics, & Nursing Practice, 7*(3), 180–194.

Chapter 1

1. Guardian. (2014, 4 July). Good to meet you… Anne Marie Rafferty. *The Guardian.* Retrieved from http://www.theguardian.com/theguardian/2014/jul/04/good-to-meet-you-anne-marie-rafferty.

2. International Council of Nurses. (2012). *Spotlight interview with: Anne Marie Rafferty.* Geneva: International Council of Nurses. Retrieved from http://www.icn.ch/what-we-do/spotlight-interview-with-anne-marie-rafferty.

3. Davies, P. (2005, March 3). *Evidence-based government: How do we make it happen?* Keynote address, Seventh annual workshop of the Canadian Health Services Research Foundation, Montreal, Quebec.

4. Canadian Institute for Health Information. (2011). *CMDB hospital beds staffed and in operation, fiscal year 2009–2010: Quick stats.* Ottawa: CIHI; and Databank of Official Statistics on Quebec. (2011). *Beds, places, internal users and other indicators of service use in public and private facilities, by health region of the reporting institution.* Quebec: Government of Quebec.

5. Canadian Institute for Health Information. (2011). *Health care in Canada, 2011: A focus on seniors and aging.* Ottawa: CIHI.

6. Canadian Institute for Health Information. (2014). *Physicians in Canada, 2013: Summary report.* Ottawa: CIHI. Retrieved from https://secure.cihi.ca/free_products/Physicians_In_Canada_Summary_Report_2013_en.pdf.

7. Canadian Institute for Health Information. (2016). *Regulated nurses, 2015.* Ottawa: CIHI. Retrieved from https://secure.cihi.ca/free_products/Nursing_Report_2015_en.pdf.

8. Jacobson Consulting, Inc. (2015). *Trends in own illness- or disability-related absenteeism and overtime among publicly-employed registered nurses: Quick facts 2015.* Ottawa: Canadian Federation of Nurses Unions.

9. Organisation for Economic Co-operation and Development. (2016). *Health.* OECD. Stat. Paris: OECD. Retrieved from http://stats.oecd.org/index.aspx?DataSetCode=HEALTH_STAT.

10. Nightingale, F. (1892, November 25). Miss F. Nightingale on local sanitation: Letter to the editor. *The Times*; cited in McDonald, L. (Ed., 2004). *The collected works of Florence Nightingale.* (Vol. 6). Waterloo: Wilfred Laurier University Press.

11. Crowe, C. (2015, May 11). Where have all the nurses gone? *rabble.ca*. Retrieved from http://rabble.ca/blogs/bloggers/cathycrowe/2015/05/where-have-all-nurses-gone.

12. Cancer Care Ontario. (2010, January). *Changing rates in lung cancer reflect past levels of cigarette smoking.* Toronto: Cancer Care Ontario. Retrieved from https://www.cancercare.on.ca/common/pages/UserFile.aspx?fileId=60549.

13. Rydin, Y., Bleahu, A., Davies, M., Dávila, J., Friel, S., De Grandis, G., et al. (2012). Shaping cities for health: Complexity and the planning of urban environments in the 21st century. *The Lancet, 379*, 2079–2108.

14. United Nations. (2009). *United Nations convention on the elimination of all forms of discrimination against women.* New York: United Nations. Retrieved from http://www.un.org/womenwatch/daw/cedaw/text/econvention.htm.

15. Truth and Reconciliation Commission of Canada. (2015). *Truth and Reconciliation Commission of Canada: Calls to action.* Winnipeg: TRC.

16. Daveluy, M-C. (2003). Mance, Jeanne. *Dictionary of Canadian Biography* (Vol. 1). Toronto: University of Toronto/Université Laval. Retrieved from http://www.biographi.ca/en/bio/mance_jeanne_1E.html.

17. Library and Archives Canada. (2010). *Jeanne Mance.* Ottawa: LAC. Retrieved from https://www.collectionscanada.gc.ca/women/030001-1410-e.html.

18. Selanders, L. (2015). Florence Nightingale: English nurse. *Encyclopædia Britannica.* Chicago: Encyclopædia Britannica, Inc. Retrieved from http://www.britannica.com/biography/Florence-Nightingale.

19. Ibid.

20. Centre Screen Productions, Ltd. (2014). *Navigating Nightingale.* iTunes application. Cupertino, CA: Apple Inc. Retrieved from https://itunes.apple.com/us/app/navigating-nightingale/id420890908?mt=8.

21. Richards, L. (1902). The entrance of the nursing profession into reform and protective work. *The American Journal of Nursing, 2*(8), 591.

22. Mansell, D., & Dodd, D. (2005). Professionalism and Canadian nursing. In C. Bates, D. Dodd, & N. Rosseau (Eds.), *On all frontiers: Four centuries of Canadian nursing* (pp. 197–212). Ottawa: University of Ottawa Press.

23. Nelson, S., & Rafferty, A. (2010.) Introduction. In S. Nelson & A. Rafferty (Eds.), *Notes on Nightingale* (pp. 1–8). Ithica: Cornell University Press, p. 4.

24. Liaschenko, J., & Peter, E. (2016). Fostering nurses' moral agency and moral identity: The importance of moral community. *Hastings Center Report, 46*(S1), S18–S21, p. S18.

25. Ibid.

26. History of Nursing News. (2007). Lyle Morrison Creelman 1908-2007. *History of Nursing News, 18*(2), 1–4.

27. Attributed to the *Journal of the International Council of Nurses*, 1968.

28. Martin, S. (2012). *Working the dead beat: 50 lives that changed Canada.* Toronto: Anansi.

29. Government of Canada. (2006). *2003 first ministers' accord on health care renewal.* Ottawa: Government of Canada. Retrieved from http://healthycanadians.gc.ca/health-system-systeme-sante/cards-cartes/collaboration/2003-accord-eng.php.

30. Thumath, M. (2016, June 9). The role of street nurses in increasing access to health care for marginalized populations. *Association of Registered Nurses of British Columbia Blog.* Vancouver: Association of Registered Nurses of British Columbia. Retrieved from http://www.arnbc.ca/blog/the-role-of-street-nurses-in-increasing-access. The downtown eastside is a fascinating place to practice nursing with a rich history.

31. Merriam-Webster. (2015). *Politics.* Retrieved from http://www.merriam-webster.com/dictionary/politics.

32. Ibid.

33. Miljan, L. (2012). *Public policy in Canada: An introduction.* (6th ed.). Don Mills, ON: Oxford University Press, p. 6.

34. Skelton-Green, J., Shamian, J., & Villeneuve, M. (2013). Policy: The essential link in successful transformations. In M. McIntyre & C. McDonald (Eds.), *Realities of Canadian Nursing* (4th ed., pp. 87–113). Philadelphia: Lippincott, Williams & Wilkins.

35. National Collaborating Centre for Healthy Public Policy. (2010). *What we do.* Quebec City: Government of Quebec. Retrieved from http://www.ncchpp.ca/62/What_We_Do.ccnpps.

36. Brooks, S. (1989). *Public policy in Canada: An introduction.* Toronto: McClelland and Stewart, p. 16.

37. Canadian Association for Health Services and Policy Research. (2015). *What is health services and*

policy research? Ottawa: CAHSPR. Retrieved from https://www.cahspr.ca/en/community/whatishspr.

38. Oxford Dictionaries. (2015). *Procedure*. Retrieved from http://www.oxforddictionaries.com/definition/english/procedure.

39. Health Canada. (2011). *Eating well with Canada's food guide*. Ottawa: Health Canada. Retrieved from http://www.hc-sc.gc.ca/fn-an/food-guide-aliment/index-eng.php.

40. Alberta Health Services. (2015). *Cancer guidelines*. Edmonton: Alberta Health Services. Retrieved from http://www.albertahealthservices.ca/cancer-guidelines.asp.

41. Registered Nurses' Association of Ontario. (2015). *Nursing best practice guidelines*. Toronto: RNAO. Retrieved from http://rnao.ca/bpg.

42. Oxford Dictionaries. (2015). *Rule*. Retrieved from http://www.oxforddictionaries.com/definition/english/rule.

43. Miljan, L. (2012). *Public policy in Canada: An introduction*. (6th ed.). Don Mills, ON: Oxford University Press, p. 6.

44. Canadian Institute for Health Information. (2015). *Regulated nurses, 2014*. Ottawa: CIHI.

45. Department of Economics and Social Affairs, Population Division. (2005). *Population challenges and development goals*. New York: United Nations. Retrieved from http://www.un.org/esa/population/publications/pop_challenges/Population_Challenges.pdf.

46. World Health Organization. (1988, April 5–9). *Adelaide recommendations on healthy public policy*. Second International Conference on Health Promotion, Adelaide, South Australia.

47. National Collaborating Centre for Healthy Public Policy. (2010). *What we do*. Quebec City: Government of Quebec. Retrieved from http://www.ncchpp.ca/62/What_We_Do.ccnpps.

48. World Health Organization. (1988, April 5–9). *Adelaide recommendations on healthy public policy*. Second International Conference on Health Promotion, Adelaide, South Australia.

49. Melkas, T. (2013). Health in all policies as a priority in Finnish health policy: A case study on national health policy development. *Scandinavian Journal of Public Health, 41*(11 supp), 3–29.

50. Hoskins, E. (2015, November 4). *Remarks to the 2015 HealthAchieve conference*. Retrieved from http://www.videodelivery.gov.on.ca/player/download.php?file=http://www.media.gov.on.ca/fce819f6e34c7dad/en/transcripts/page.html.

51. National Center for Injury Prevention and Control. (n.d.). *Brief 1: Overview of policy evaluation*. Atlanta: Centers for Disease Control and Prevention. Retrieved from http://www.cdc.gov/injury/pdfs/policy/Brief%201-a.pdf.

52. Merriam-Webster. (2015). *Legislation*. Retrieved from http://www.merriam-webster.com/dictionary/legislation.

53. Malcolmson, P., & Myers, R. (2009). *The Canadian regime*. Toronto: University of Toronto Press, p. 13.

54. Centers for Disease Control and Prevention. (n.d.). *Brief 1: Overview of policy evaluation*. Atlanta, GA: National Center for Injury Prevention and Control. Retrieved from http://www.cdc.gov/injury/pdfs/policy/Brief%201-a.pdf.

55. Dictionary.com. (2015). *Regulation*. Retrieved from http://www.dictionary.com/browse/regulation?s=t.

56. Health Canada. (2010). *Canada's health care system: Medicare*. Ottawa: Health Canada. Retrieved from http://www.hc-sc.gc.ca/hcs-sss/medi-assur/index-eng.php.

57. Center for Medicare & Medicaid Services. (2015). *How is Medicare funded?* Baltimore: Center for Medicare & Medicaid Services. Retrieved from https://www.medicare.gov/about-us/how-medicare-is-funded/medicare-funding.html.

58. Center for Medicaid and CHIP Services. (2015). *About us*. Baltimore: Center for Medicaid and CHIP Services. Retrieved from http://medicaid.gov/about-us/about-us.html.

59. Tholl, W., Bujold, G., & Grimes, K. (2013.) *Reframing the federal role in health and health care: A report to the Health Action Lobby*. Ottawa: Health Action Lobby, p. iv.

60. Simpson, J. (2012). *Chronic condition: Why Canada's healthcare system needs to be dragged into the 21st century*. Toronto: Penguin, p. 1.

61. Organisation for Economic Co-operation and Development. (2004). *Towards high-performing health systems: Policy studies*. Paris: OECD, p. 17.

62. Oxford Dictionaries. (2016). *Theory*. Retrieved from http://www.oxforddictionaries.com/definition/english/theory.

63. Merriam-Webster. (2015). *Framework*. Retrieved from http://www.merriam-webster.com/dictionary/framework.

64. Dictionary.com. (2016). *Conceptual model*. Retrieved from http://www.dictionary.com/browse/conceptual-model.

65. Brownson, R., Chriqui, J., & Stamatakis, K. (2009). Understanding evidence-based public health policy. *American Journal of Public Health, 99*(9), 1576–1583, p. xx.

66. Social Development Department, World Bank. (2008). *The political economy of policy reform: Issues and implications for policy dialogue and development operation*. Washington, DC: International Bank for Reconstruction and Development/World Bank.

67. Walt, G., Shiffman, J., Schneider, H., Murray, S., Brughas, R., & Gilson, L. (2008). 'Doing' health policy analysis: Methodological and conceptual reflections and challenges. *Health Policy and Planning, 23*, 308–317.

68. Ibid., p. 310.

69. Cairney, P. (2013, June). *How can policy theory have an impact on policy making?* Presented at the International Conference on Public Policy, Grenoble, France.

70. Ibid.

71. Government of Scotland. (2009). *Review of policymaking*. Edinburgh: Government of Scotland.

72. Cerna, L. (2013). *The nature of policy change and implementation: A review of different theoretical approaches*. Paris: OECD.

73. Bryant, T. (2009). *An introduction to health policy*. Toronto: Canadian Scholars' Press, Inc.

74. Decter, M. (1994). *Healing medicare: Managing health system change the Canadian way*. Toronto: McGillan Books.

75. Bryant, T. (2009). *An introduction to health policy*. Toronto: Canadian Scholars' Press, Inc.

76. Social Development Department, World Bank. (2008). *The political economy of policy reform: Issues and implications for policy dialogue and development operation*. Washington, DC: International Bank for Reconstruction and Development/World Bank.

77. Miljan, L. (2012). *Public policy in Canada: An introduction* (6th ed.). Don Mills, ON: Oxford University Press, p. 6.

78. Johnson, P. (2005). *Systems theory models of decision-making*. Auburn, AL: Auburn University, Department of Political Science.

79. Ibid.

80. Browne, A. (2001). The influence of liberal political ideology on nursing science. *Nursing Inquiry, 8*(2), 118–129.

81. Peter, E., & Liaschenko, J. (2014). Care and society/public policy. In B. Jennings (Ed.), *Bioethics* (Vol. 2), 4th ed., pp. 504–512). Farmington Hills, MI: Macmillan Reference.

82. The Mack Alumni Association. (n.d.). *Mack alumni association*. Retrieved from http://www.mack-alumni.org.

83. Association of Registered Nurses of British Columbia. (2015). *Who we are*. Vancouver: ARNBC. Retrieved from http://arnbc.ca.

84. Registered Nurses' Association of Ontario. (2015). *About RNAO*. Toronto: RNAO. Retrieved from http://rnao.ca/about.

85. American Nurses Association. (2015). *About ANA*. Silver Springs, MD: ANA. Retrieved from http://www.nursingworld.org/FunctionalMenuCategories/AboutANA.

86. Merriam-Webster. (2015). *Neoliberal*. Retrieved from http://www.merriam-webster.com/dictionary/neoliberal.

87. Collins Dictionary. (2015). *Neoliberalism*. Retrieved from http://www.collinsdictionary.com/dictionary/english/neoliberalism.

88. Monbiot, G. (2016, April 15). Neoliberalism—the ideology at the root of all our problems. *The Guardian*. Retrieved from https://www.theguardian.com/books/2016/apr/15/neoliberalism-ideology-problem-george-monbiot.

89. Ibid.

90. Osman, F. (2013). Public policy making: Theories and their implications in developing countries. *Asian Affairs, 24*(3), 45. Retrieved from http://www.cdrb.org/journal/2002/3/3.pdf.

91. Harrison, T. (2015). Reform Party of Canada. *The Canadian Encyclopedia*. Toronto: Historica Canada. Retrieved from http://www.thecanadianencyclopedia.ca/en/article/reform-party-of-canada.

92. Martin, L. (2016, July 12). As the boomers fade, Canada's hopes rise. *Globe and Mail*. Retrieved from http://www.theglobeandmail.com//opinion/as-the-boomers-fade-canadas-hopes-rise/article30861271.

93. Miljan, L. (2012). *Public policy in Canada: An introduction* (6th ed.). Don Mills, ON: Oxford University Press, p. 27.

94. Fekete, J. (2013, July 24). Why Prime Minister Stephen Harper steers clear of premiers' meetings. *The Ottawa Citizen*. Retrieved from http://o.canada.com/news/premiers-meetings-rarely-include-prime-minister-stephen-harper.

95. Picard, A. (2015, September 27). Life support: Medicare's mid-life crisis [radio broadcast]. *The Sunday Edition with Michael Enright*. Toronto: CBC.

96. Boucher, C. (2013). Canada-US values distinct,

inevitably carbon copy, or narcissism of small differences? *Policy Horizons Canada*. Ottawa: Government of Canada. Retrieved from http://www.horizons.gc.ca/eng/content/feature-article-canada-us-values-distinct-inevitably-carbon-copy-or-narcissism-small.

97. Poisson, Y. (2013). Comments on Boucher, 2013. Retrieved from http://www.horizons.gc.ca/eng/content/feature-article-canada-us-values-distinct-inevitably-carbon-copy-or-narcissism-small.

98. Adams, M. (2014). *Fire and ice revisited: American and Canadian social values in the age of Obama and Harper*. Toronto: Environics Institute.

99. Pew Research Center. (2012). *The American-Western European values gap*. Washington, DC: Pew Research Center. Retrieved from http://www.pewglobal.org/2011/11/17/the-american-western-european-values-gap.

100. Ibid.

101. Wu, S., & Keysar, B. (2007). The effect of culture on perspective taking. *Psychological Science, 18*(7), 600–606.

102. Adams, M. (2014). *Fire and ice revisited: American and Canadian social values in the age of Obama and Harper*. Toronto: Environics Institute.

103. Koon, A., Hawkins, B., & Mayhew, S. (2016). Framing and the health policy process: A scoping review. *Health Policy and Planning, 31*, 801–808, p. 802.

104. Mackenbach, J., Karanikolos, M., & McKee, M. (2013). Health policy in Europe: factors critical for success. *British Medical Journal, 346*, f533. Retrieved from http://dx.doi.org/10.1136/bmj.f533.

105. Ibid.

106. Trudeau, J. (2015). *Mandate letter to Minister of Health*. Ottawa: Government of Canada.

107. Lenihan, D. (2009). *Rethinking the public policy process: A public engagement framework*. Ottawa: Public Policy Forum, p. 7.

Chapter 2

1. Liberal Party of Canada. (2004). *The Liberal team in Quebec: The Honourable Lucie Pépin*. Quebec City: Liberal Party of Canada.

2. Keon, W. J., & Pépin, L. (2009). *A healthy, productive Canada: A determinant of health approach*. Final report of the Subcommittee on Population Health. Ottawa: Senate of Canada, Standing Senate Committee on Social Affairs, Science and Technology.

3. Clark, J. (2013). *How we lead: Canada in a century of change*. Toronto: Random House Canada, p. 2.

4. Statistics Canada. (2012). *Highlights of Canada's geography*. Retrieved from http://www.statcan.gc.ca/pub/11-402-x/2012000/chap/geo/geo-eng.htm.

5. Ibid.

6. Statistics Canada. (2014). *Population by year, by province and territory*. Ottawa: Statistics Canada. Retrieved from http://www.statcan.gc.ca/tables-tableaux/sum-som/l01/cst01/demo02a-eng.htm.

7. Greater Toronto Marketing Alliance. (n.d.). *Population forecast and growth rate*. Toronto: Greater Toronto Marketing Alliance. Retrieved from http://www.greatertoronto.org/why-greater-toronto/economic-overview/population.

8. Statistics Canada. (2014). *Canada's population estimates: Age and sex, 2014*. Ottawa: Statistics Canada. Retrieved from http://www.statcan.gc.ca/daily-quotidien/140926/dq140926b-eng.htm.

9. Merriam-Webster. (2015). *Aboriginal*. Retrieved from http://www.merriam-webster.com/dictionary/aboriginal.

10. The G20. (2015). *About G20*. Istanbul: The G20. Retrieved from https://g20.org/about-g20.

11. Statistics Canada. (2014). *Aboriginal peoples in Canada: First Nations people, Métis and Inuit*. Ottawa: Statistics Canada. Retrieved from http://www12.statcan.gc.ca/nhs-enm/2011/as-sa/99-011-x/99-011-x2011001-eng.cfm.

12. Aboriginal Affairs and Northern Development Canada. (2015). *First Nations profiles*. Aboriginal Affairs and Northern Development Canada, Retrieved from http://fnp-ppn.aandc-aadnc.gc.ca/fnp/Main/index.aspx.

13. Statistics Canada. (2014). *Aboriginal languages in Canada*. Ottawa: Statistics Canada. Retrieved from http://www12.statcan.gc.ca/census-recensement/2011/as-sa/98-314-x/98-314-x2011003_3-eng.cfm.

14. Statistics Canada. (2014). *Aboriginal peoples in Canada: First Nations people, Métis and Inuit*. Ottawa: Statistics Canada. Retrieved from http://www12.statcan.gc.ca/nhs-enm/2011/as-sa/99-011-x/99-011-x2011001-eng.cfm.

15. Aboriginal and Northern Affairs Canada. (2015). *Urban Aboriginal peoples*. Ottawa: Aboriginal and Northern Affairs Canada. Retrieved from http://www.aadnc-aandc.gc.ca/eng/1100100014265/1369225120949.

16. Canadian Museum of History. (2015). *Historical overview of immigration to Canada*. Ottawa:

Canadian Museum of History. Retrieved from http://www.historymuseum.ca/cmc/exhibitions/tresors/immigration/imf0301e.shtml.

17. Plamondon, D. (2013, June 5). *The truth about Pierre Trudeau and immigration. Macleans.* Retrieved from http://www.macleans.ca/news/canada/nothing-to-write-home-about.

18. Statistics Canada. (2014). *Immigration and ethnocultural diversity in Canada.* Ottawa: Statistics Canada. Retrieved from http://www12.statcan.gc.ca/nhs-enm/2011/as-sa/99-010-x/99-010-x2011001-eng.cfm.

19. Statistics Canada. (2014). *Linguistic characteristics of Canadians.* Ottawa: Statistics Canada. Retrieved from http://www12.statcan.ca/census-recensement/2011/as-sa/98-314-x/98-314-x2011001-eng.cfm.

20. Statistics Canada. (2014). *Immigration and ethnocultural diversity in Canada.* Ottawa: Statistics Canada. Retrieved from http://www12.statcan.gc.ca/nhs-enm/2011/as-sa/99-010-x/99-010-x2011001-eng.cfm.

21. The World Bank. (2015). *GDP ranking.* Washington, DC: The World Bank. Retrieved from http://data.worldbank.org/data-catalog/GDP-ranking-table.

22. The World Bank. (2015). *GDP per capita (current US$).* Washington, DC: The World Bank. Retrieved from http://data.worldbank.org/indicator/NY.GDP.PCAP.CD?order=wbapi_data_value_2014+wbapi_data_value+wbapi_data_value-last&sort=asc.

23. Organisation for Economic Co-Operation and Development. (2015). *Domestic product.* Paris: OECD. Retrieved from https://data.oecd.org/gdp/gross-domestic-product-gdp.htm.

24. Citizenship and Immigration Canada. (2014). *Canada's economy.* Citizenship and Immigration Canada. Retrieved from http://www.cic.gc.ca/english/resources/publications/discover/section-12.asp.

25. Statistics Canada. (2012). *Public sector employment, wages and salaries, by province and territory.* Ottawa: Statistics Canada. Retrieved from http://www.statcan.gc.ca/tables-tableaux/sum-som/l01/cst01/govt62a-eng.htm.

26. The Heritage Foundation. (2015). *2015 index of economic freedom: Canada.* Washington, DC: The Heritage Foundation. Retrieved from http://www.heritage.org/index/country/canada.

27. Forsey, E. (2012). *How Canadians govern themselves* (8th ed.). Ottawa: Minister of Public Works and Government Services Canada, p. 1.

28. Collins Dictionary. (2015). *Liberal democracy.* Retrieved from http://www.collinsdictionary.com/dictionary/english/liberal-democracy.

29. Plattner, M. (1998). Liberalism and democracy: Can't have one without the other. *Foreign Affairs, 77*(2), 171-180. Retrieved from https://www.foreignaffairs.com/articles/1998-03-01/liberalism-and-democracy-cant-have-one-without-other.

30. Ibid.

31. Plattner, M. (1999). From liberalism to liberal democracy. *Journal of Democracy, 10*(3), 121–134.

32. Oxford Dictionaries. (2015). *Federation.* Retrieved from http://www.oxforddictionaries.com/definition/english/federation.

33. Malcolmson, P., & Myers, R. (2009). *The Canadian regime.* Toronto: University of Toronto Press, p. 60.

34. Directorate-General for Communication. (2014). *How the European Commission works.* Luxembourg: European Commission, p. 3. Retrieved from http://bookshop.europa.eu/en/how-the-european-union-works-pbNA0414810.

35. Council of the Federation. (2013). *Founding agreement—December 2003.* Ottawa: Council of the Federation. Retrieved from http://www.canadaspremiers.ca/en/about/31-root-en/about-features/52-founding-agreement.

36. Smith, D. (2010). *Federalism and the constitution of Canada.* Toronto: University of Toronto Press, p. 17.

37. United States Senate. (2015). *Constitution of the United States.* Washington, DC: United States Senate. Retrieved from http://www.senate.gov/civics/constitution_item/constitution.htm.

38. The White House. (2015). *Our government.* Washington, DC: The White House. Retrieved from https://www.whitehouse.gov/1600/legislative-branch.

39. O'Brien, A., & Bosc, M. (2009). Parliamentary institutions. In A. O'Brien & M. Bosc (Eds.), *House of Commons procedure and practice* (2nd ed.). Ottawa: House of Commons. Retrieved from http://www.parl.gc.ca/Procedure-Book-Livre/Document.aspx?sbdid=73CC891E-0676-4773-850B-CCDC-B472AD8C&sbpidx=1&Language=E&Mode=1.

40. Parliament of Canada. (n.d.). Canada: A constitutional monarchy. Ottawa: Parliament of Canada. Retrieved from http://www.parl.gc.ca/About/Senate/Monarchy/senmonarchy_00-e.htm.

41. Royal Household, Buckingham Palace. (2015). *The Queen in Canada.* London: Government of the United Kingdom. Retrieved from http://www.

royal.gov.uk/MonarchAndCommonwealth/Canada/
TheQueensroleinCanada.aspx.

42. Royal Household, Buckingham Palace. (2015). *Her Majesty the Queen*. London: Government of the United Kingdom. Retrieved from http://www.royal.gov.uk/hmthequeen/hmthequeen.aspx.

43. The Commonwealth. (2015). *Our work*. London: The Commonwealth. Retrieved from http://thecommonwealth.org/our-work.

44. The Governor General of Canada. (2015). *Role and responsibilities*. Ottawa: The Governor General of Canada. Retrieved from http://gg.ca/document.aspx?id=3.

45. The Governor General of Canada. (2016). *Constitutional duties*. Ottawa: The Governor General of Canada. Retrieved from https://www.gg.ca/events.aspx?sc=1&lan=eng.

46. Malcolmson, P., & Myers, R. (2009). *The Canadian regime*. Toronto: University of Toronto Press, p. 13.

47. Harris, I. (2006). *Canadian influences on the constitutional and procedural development of the Australian House of Representatives*. Presentation for the Canadian Clerks-at-the-Table (CATS) Annual Professional Development Seminar, Whitehorse, Yukon. Retrieved from http://www.parliamentarystudies.anu.edu.au/pdf/harris_cats.pdf.

48. Government of Canada. (1982). *Constitution acts, 1867 to 1982*. Ottawa: Government of Canada. Retrieved from http://laws-lois.justice.gc.ca/eng/Const/page-4.html#h-19.

49. Malcolmson, P., & Myers, R. (2009). *The Canadian regime*. Toronto: University of Toronto Press.

50. Forsey, E. (2016). *How Canadians govern themselves* (9th ed.). Ottawa: Library of Parliament. Retrieved from http://www.lop.parl.gc.ca/About/Parliament/senatoreugeneforsey/book/assets/pdf/How_Canadians_Govern_Themselves9.pdf.

51. Department of Justice. (2016). *Where our legal system comes from*. Ottawa: Department of Justice. Retrieved from http://www.justice.gc.ca/eng/csj-sjc/just/03.html.

52. Department of Justice. (2015.) *Rights and freedoms in Canada*. Ottawa: Department of Justice. Retrieved from http://www.justice.gc.ca/eng/csj-sjc/just/06.html.

53. Government of Canada. (2013). *Section 32-33: Application of charter*. Ottawa: Government of Canada. Retrieved from http://canada.pch.gc.ca/eng/1468851006026.

54. Department of Justice. (2015). *Rights and freedoms in Canada*. Ottawa: Department of Justice. Retrieved from http://www.justice.gc.ca/eng/csj-sjc/just/06.html.

55. Department of Justice. (2015). *How does Canada's court system work?* Ottawa: Government of Canada. Retrieved from http://www.justice.gc.ca/eng/csj-sjc/ccs-ajc/01.html.

56. Goldenberg, E. (2006). *The way it works: Inside Ottawa*. Toronto: McClelland & Stewart, p. 71.

57. Privy Council Office. (2010). *About cabinet*. Ottawa: Government of Canada. Retrieved from http://www.pco-bcp.gc.ca/index.asp?lang=eng&page=information&sub=Cabinet&doc=about-apropos-eng.htm.

58. Privy Council Office. (2010). *The Queen's Privy Council for Canada*. Ottawa: Government of Canada. Retrieved from http://www.pco-bcp.gc.ca/index.asp?lang=eng&page=information&sub=council-conseil&doc=description-eng.htm.

59. Privy Council Office. (2014). *Clerk of the Privy Council*. Ottawa: Government of Canada. Retrieved from http://www.pco-bcp.gc.ca/index.asp?lang=eng&page=clerk-greffier; and Privy Council Office. (2014). *The role of the Clerk*. Ottawa: Government of Canada. Retrieved from http://www.clerk.gc.ca/eng/feature.asp?pageId=88.

60. Elections Canada. (2015). *Canada's federal electoral districts*. Ottawa: Elections Canada. Retrieved from http://www.elections.ca/content.aspx?section=res&dir=cir/list&document=index338&lang=e.

61. Broadbent, E., Himelfarb, A., & Segal, H. (2016, May 10). Only proportionality will fix our democratic malaise. *Globe and Mail*. Retrieved from http://www.theglobeandmail.com/opinion/only-proportionality-will-fix-our-democratic-malaise/article29944241.

62. Clemens, J., Jackson, T., LaFleur, S., & Emes, J. (2016). *Electoral rules and fiscal policy outcomes*. Vancouver: The Fraser Institute, p. 17.

63. Ibid.

64. Collins Dictionary. (2015). *Political party*. Retrieved from http://www.collinsdictionary.com/dictionary/english/political-party.

65. Parliament of Canada. (n.d.). *Role of the Speaker*. Ottawa: Parliament of Canada. Retrieved from http://www.parl.gc.ca/About/House/Speaker/role-c.html.

66. Standing Senate Committee on Social Affairs, Science and Technology. (2006). *Out of the shadows at last: Transforming mental health, mental illness*

and addiction services in Canada. Ottawa: Senate of Canada.

67. Carstairs, S. (2010). *Raising the bar: A roadmap for the future of palliative care in Canada*. Ottawa: The Senate of Canada.

68. Standing Senate Committee on Social Affairs, Science and Technology. (2006). *Time for transformative change: A review of the 2004 health accord*. Ottawa: Senate of Canada.

69. Parliament of Canada. (n.d.). *About the Senate*. Ottawa: Parliament of Canada. Retrieved from http://sen.parl.gc.ca/portal/about-senate-e.htm.

70. Stone, L., & Fine, S. (2016, June 17). Senate backs down, passes assisted-dying legislation. *Globe and Mail*. Retrieved from http://www.theglobeandmail.com/news/politics/senate-passes-assisted-dying-legislation/article30507549.

71. Supreme Court of Canada. (2014). *In the matter of a reference by the Governor in Council concerning reform of the Senate, as set out in Order in Council P.C. 2013-70, dated February 1, 2013*. Ottawa: Supreme Court of Canada. Retrieved from https://scc-csc.lexum.com/scc-csc/scc-csc/en/item/13614/index.do.

72. Axworthy, T. (2016, March 24). Justin Trudeau is taking the Senate into uncharted territory. *Toronto Star*. Retrieved from https://www.thestar.com/opinion/commentary/2016/03/24/justin-trudeau-is-taking-the-senate-into-uncharted-territory.html.

73. Centre for Constitutional Studies. (2015). *The Constitution and Canada's branches of government*. Edmonton: University of Alberta. Retrieved from https://ualawccsprod.srv.ualberta.ca/index.php/constitutional-issues/democratic-governance/818-the-constitution-and-canada-s-branches-of-government.

74. Parliament of Canada. (2014). *Supreme Court of Canada: Judges*. Ottawa: Parliament of Canada. Retrieved from http://www.parl.gc.ca/Parlinfo/compilations/SupremeCourt.aspx?Menu=SupremeCourt&Current=True.

75. S.B. (2013, July 16). The Economist explains: What is the difference between common and civil law? *Economist*. Retrieved from http://www.economist.com/blogs/economist-explains/2013/07/economist-explains-10.

76. Department of Justice. (2016). *Where our legal system comes from*. Ottawa: Department of Justice. Retrieved from http://www.justice.gc.ca/eng/csj-sjc/just/03.html.

77. Ibid.

78. Department of Justice. (2015). *The Canadian Constitution*. Ottawa: Department of Justice. Retrieved from http://www.justice.gc.ca/eng/csj-sjc/just/05.html.

79. Parliament of Canada. (2014). *Supreme Court of Canada: Judges*. Ottawa: Parliament of Canada. Retrieved from http://www.parl.gc.ca/Parlinfo/compilations/SupremeCourt.aspx?Menu=SupremeCourt&Current=True.

80. Savoie, D. (2015). *What is government good at? A Canadian answer*. Montreal: McGill-Queen's Press.

81. Statistics Canada. (2012). Public sector employment, wages and salaries, by province and territory. Ottawa: Statistics Canada. Retrieved from http://www.statcan.gc.ca/tables-tableaux/sum-som/l01/cst01/govt62a-eng.htm.

82. Savoie, D. (2015). *What is government good at? A Canadian answer*. Montreal: McGill-Queen's Press, p. 209.

83. Torjman, S. (2016, January). Farewell, Wizard of Oz. *Caledon Commentary*. Ottawa: Caledon Institute of Social Policy.

84. Foreign Affairs, Trade and Development Canada. (2015). *Canadian government offices abroad*. Ottawa: Government of Canada. Retrieved from http://www.international.gc.ca/cip-pic/description_bureaux-offices.aspx.

85. Brown, G. (1864). *George Brown describes the Charlottetown Conference, 1864*. Ottawa: Library and Archives Canada. Retrieved from http://www.collectionscanada.gc.ca/confederation/023001-7103-e.html.

86. Slattery, B. (2005). Aboriginal rights and the honour of the Crown. *Supreme Court Law Review, 29*, 433–445.

87. Ibid.

88. O'Brien, A., & Bosc, M. (2009). Parliamentary institutions. In A. O'Brien & M. Bosc (Eds.), *House of Commons procedure and practice* (2nd ed.). Ottawa: House of Commons. Retrieved from http://www.parl.gc.ca/Procedure-Book-Livre/Document.aspx?Language=E&Mode=1&sbdid=73CC891E-0676-4773-850B-CCDCB472AD8C&sbpid=55CF9BA9-6592-457E-92AE-B90437D47609.

89. Statistics Canada. (2012). *Public sector employment, wages and salaries, by province and territory*. Ottawa: Statistics Canada. Retrieved from http://www.statcan.gc.ca/tables-tableaux/sum-som/l01/cst01/govt62a-eng.htm.

90. Library and Archives Canada. (2005). *Canadian confederation*. Ottawa: Library and Archives Canada.

Retrieved from http://www.collectionscanada.gc.ca/confederation/023001-5006-e.html.

91. Intergovernmental Affairs. (2010). *Difference between Canadian provinces and territories*. Ottawa: Government of Canada. Retrieved from http://www.pco-bcp.gc.ca/aia/index.asp?lang=eng&page=prov-terr&doc=difference-eng.htm.

92. Ibid.

93. Legislative Assembly of the Northwest Territories. (2014). *What is consensus government?* Yellowknife: Legislative Assembly of the Northwest Territories. Retrieved from http://www.assembly.gov.nt.ca/visitors/what-consensus.

94. Statistics Canada. (2012). *Public sector employment, wages and salaries, by province and territory*. Ottawa: Statistics Canada. Retrieved from http://www.statcan.gc.ca/tables-tableaux/sum-som/l01/cst01/govt62a-eng.htm.

95. Council of the Federation. (2013). *About Canada's premiers*. Council of the Federation. Retrieved from http://www.canadaspremiers.ca/en/about.

96. Parliament of Canada. (n.d.). *Three levels of government*. Ottawa: Parliament of Canada. Retrieved from http://www.parl.gc.ca/About/Parliament/Education/OurCountryOurParliament/html_booklet/three-levels-government-e.html.

97. Plunkett, T. (2013). Municipal government. *The Canadian Encyclopedia*. Toronto: Historica Canada. Retrieved from http://www.thecanadianencyclopedia.ca/en/article/municipal-government.

98. Statistics Canada. (2012). *Public sector employment, wages and salaries, by province and territory*. Ottawa: Statistics Canada. Retrieved from http://www.statcan.gc.ca/tables-tableaux/sum-som/l01/cst01/govt62a-eng.htm.

99. Aboriginal and Northern Affairs Canada. (2015). *Inuit*. Ottawa: Aboriginal and Northern Affairs Canada. Retrieved from http://www.aadnc-aandc.gc.ca/eng/1100100014187/1100100014191.

100. Inuit Tapiriit Kanatami. (2015). *About ITK*. Ottawa: Inuit Tapiriit Kanatami. Retrieved from https://www.itk.ca/contact.

101. Aboriginal and Northern Affairs Canada. (2015). *Inuit*. Ottawa: Aboriginal and Northern Affairs Canada. Retrieved from http://www.aadnc-aandc.gc.ca/eng/1100100014187/1100100014191.

102. Nunavut Tunngavik Incorporated. (n.d.). *About NTI*. Iqaluit: Nunavut Tunngavik Incorporated. Retrieved from http://www.tunngavik.com/about.

103. Métis National Council. (n.d.). *What is the Métis National Council?* Ottawa: Métis National Council. Retrieved from http://www.metisnation.ca/index.php/who-are-the-metis/mnc.

104. Aboriginal Affairs and Northern Development Canada. (2013). *Harper government and the Métis National Council renew commitment to work together and improve financial accountability, transparency and predictability*. Ottawa: Government of Canada. Retrieved from http://www.aadnc-aandc.gc.ca/eng/1367263803477/1367263872186.

105. Statistics Canada. (2014). *Aboriginal peoples in Canada: First Nations people, Métis and Inuit*. Ottawa: Statistics Canada. Retrieved from http://www12.statcan.gc.ca/nhs-enm/2011/as-sa/99-011-x/99-011-x2011001-eng.cfm.

106. Aboriginal and Northern Affairs Canada. (2015). *Governance*. Ottawa: Aboriginal and Northern Affairs Canada. Retrieved from http://www.aadnc-aandc.gc.ca/eng/1100100013803/1100100013807.

107. Aboriginal and Northern Affairs Canada. (2015). *First Nations election act*. Ottawa: Aboriginal and Northern Affairs Canada. Retrieved from http://www.aadnc-aandc.gc.ca/eng/1323195944486/1323196005595.

108. Assembly of First Nations. (n.d.). *Description of the AFN*. Ottawa: Assembly of First Nations. Retrieved from http://www.afn.ca/index.php/en/about-afn/description-of-the-afn.

109. First Nations Studies Program. (2009). *The Indian act*. Vancouver: University of British Columbia. Retrieved from http://indigenousfoundations.arts.ubc.ca/home/government-policy/the-indian-act.html.

110. Truth and Reconciliation Commission of Canada. (2015). *Honouring the truth, reconciling for the future: Summary of the final report of the Truth and Reconciliation Commission of Canada*. Winnipeg: TRC. Retrieved from http://www.trc.ca/websites/trcinstitution/File/2015/Honouring_the_Truth_Reconciling_for_the_Future_July_23_2015.pdf.

111. Macdonald, N. (2016, July 29). Saskatchewan: A special report on race and power. *Macleans*. Retrieved from http://www.macleans.ca/news/canada/saskatchewan-a-special-report-on-race-and-power.

112. Congress of Aboriginal Peoples. (n.d.). *Our mandate*. Ottawa: Congress of Aboriginal Peoples. Retrieved from http://abo-peoples.org/our-mission.

113. Native Women's Association of Canada. (2015). *About us*. Akwesasne, ON: Native Women's Association of Canada. Retrieved from http://www.nwac.ca/

about-nwac/about-us.

114. Sandberg, S. (2010). Why we have too few women leaders. Subtitles and transcript. *TED*. Retrieved from https://www.ted.com/talks/sheryl_sandberg_why_we_have_too_few_women_leaders/transcript.

Chapter 3

1. Khera, K. (2016). *Kamal Khera: Your member of parliament for Brampton West*. Retrieved from https://kamalkheramp.liberal.ca.

2. First Nations Health Authority. (2015). *Our history, our health*. Vancouver: Nations Health Authority. Retrieved from http://www.fnha.ca/wellness/our-history-our-health.

3. Heller, M. (2008). The National Insurance Acts 1911–1947, the Approved Societies and the Prudential Assurance Company. *20th Century British History, 19*(1), 1–28.

4. Canadian Museum of History. (2010). *Making medicare: The history of health care in Canada, 1914–2007*. Retrieved from http://www.historymuseum.ca/cmc/exhibitions/hist/medicare/medic-1h12e.shtml.

5. Decter, M. (1994). *Healing medicare: Managing health system change the Canadian way*. Toronto: McGillan Books.

6. Hansard. (1919, April 10). House of Commons debates. Ottawa: Hansard, p. 1375.

7. Elliott, J., Rutty, C., & Villeneuve, M. (2013). *The Canadian Nurses Association 1908–2008: One hundred years of service*. Ottawa: CNA, p. 30.

8. Canadian Museum of History. (2010). *Making medicare: The history of health care in Canada, 1914–2007*. Retrieved from http://www.historymuseum.ca/cmc/exhibitions/hist/medicare/medic-1h15e.shtml.

9. Canadian Medical Association and Canadian Nurses Association. (2011). *Principles to guide health care transformation in Canada*. Ottawa: CMA and CNA. Retrieved from http://policybase.cma.ca/dbtw-wpd/Policypdf/PD11-13.pdf.

10. Elliott, J., Rutty, C., & Villeneuve, M. (2013). *The Canadian Nurses Association 1908–2008: One hundred years of service*. Ottawa: CNA, p. 5.

11. The Royal Commission on Health Insurance. (1921). *Report of the Royal Commission on Health Insurance*. Victoria: The Royal Commission on Health Insurance. Retrieved from http://www.llbc.leg.bc.ca/public/pubdocs/bcdocs_rc/461648/461648_report_rc_health_insurance.pdf.

12. Elliott, J., Rutty, C., & Villeneuve, M. (2013). *The Canadian Nurses Association 1908–2008: One hundred years of service*. Ottawa: CNA, p. 59.

13. Elliott, J., Rutty, C., & Villeneuve, M. (2013). *The Canadian Nurses Association 1908–2008: One hundred years of service*. Ottawa: CNA.

14. Simpson, R., Wilson, J., & Gunn, J. (1938). A submission to the Royal Commission on Dominion-Provincial Relations. *The Canadian Nurse, 34*(July 1938), 371–374.

15. Boan, J. (2006). Medicare. *The Encyclopedia of Saskatchewan*. Regina: University of Regina. Retrieved from http://esask.uregina.ca/entry/medicare.html.

16. Ibid.

17. Lalonde, M. (1974). *A new perspective on the health of Canadians: A working document*. Ottawa: Minister of Supply and Services Canada.

18. Chenier, N. (2002). *Health policy in Canada*. Ottawa: Government of Canada. Retrieved from http://publications.gc.ca/Collection-R/LoPBdP/CIR/934-e.htm.

19. Health Canada. (2012). *Canada's health care system*. Ottawa: Health Canada. Retrieved from http://www.hc-sc.gc.ca/hcs-sss/pubs/system-regime/2011-hcs-sss/index-eng.php.

20. Health Canada. (2004). *Royal Commission on health services, 1961 to 1964*. Health Canada Retrieved from http://www.hc-sc.gc.ca/hcs-sss/com/fed/hall-eng.php.

21. Silversides, A. (2007). *Conversations with champions of medicare*. Ottawa: Canadian Federation of Nurses Unions, p. 42.

22. Chenier, N. (2002). *Health policy in Canada*. Ottawa: Government of Canada. Retrieved from http://publications.gc.ca/Collection-R/LoPBdP/CIR/934-e.htm.

23. Ibid.

24. Government of Canada. (1980). *Health Services Review: Canada's national-provincial health program for the 1980's: A commitment for renewal*. Ottawa: Health and Welfare Canada.

25. Elliott, J., Rutty, C., & Villeneuve, M. (2013). *The Canadian Nurses Association 1908–2008: One hundred years of service*. Ottawa: CNA, p. 102.

26. Chenier, N. (2002). *Health policy in Canada*. Ottawa: Government of Canada. Retrieved from http://publications.gc.ca/Collection-R/LoPBdP/CIR/934-e.htm.

27. Elliott, J., Rutty, C., & Villeneuve, M. (2013). *The*

Canadian Nurses Association 1908–2008: One hundred years of service. Ottawa: CNA, p. 106.

28. Health Canada. (2012). *Canada's health care system.* Ottawa: Health Canada. Retrieved from http://www.hc-sc.gc.ca/hcs-sss/pubs/system-regime/2011-hcs-sss/index-eng.php.

29. Parliament of Canada. (2005). *The Canada Health Act: Overview and options.* Ottawa: Parliament of Canada. Retrieved from http://www.parl.gc.ca/content/lop/researchpublications/944-e.htm#ajustificationtxt.

30. Ibid.

31. Canadian Intergovernmental Conference Secretariat. (2015). *Agreement—A framework to improve the social union for Canadians.* Retrieved from http://www.scics.gc.ca/english/conferences.asp?a=viewdocument&id=638.

32. Ibid.

33. Palmer, K. (2015). Backgrounder: A primer on the legal challenge between Dr. Brian Day and British Columbia—and how it may affect our healthcare system. *Making Evidence Matter.* Winnipeg: The Evidence Network. Retrieved from http://umanitoba.ca/outreach/evidencenetwork/archives/25738.

34. Ibid.

35. Health Canada. (2011). *Canada Health Act.* Ottawa: Health Canada. Retrieved from http://www.hc-sc.gc.ca/hcs-sss/medi-assur/faq-eng.php#a3.

36. Parliament of Canada. (2005). *The Canada Health Act: Overview and options.* Ottawa: Parliament of Canada. Retrieved from http://www.parl.gc.ca/content/lop/researchpublications/944-e.htm#ajustificationtxt.

37. Ibid.

38. Canadian Foundation for Healthcare Improvement. (2011). *Myth: Medicare covers all necessary health services.* Ottawa: CFHI. Retrieved from http://www.cfhi-fcass.ca/SearchResultsNews/11-05-12/dd2b140f-7405-461c-a077-06ad45256fb1.aspx.

39. The Standing Senate Committee on Social Affairs, Science and Technology. (2002). *The health of Canadians — The federal role,* vol. 6, *Recommendations for reform.* Ottawa: Senate of Canada. Retrieved from http://www.parl.gc.ca/Content/SEN/Committee/372/soci/rep/repoct02vol6-e.htm.

40. Parliament of Canada. (2005). *The Canada Health Act: Overview and options.* Ottawa: Parliament of Canada. Retrieved from http://www.parl.gc.ca/content/lop/researchpublications/944-e.htm#ajustificationtxt.

41. The Standing Senate Committee on Social Affairs, Science and Technology. (2002). *The health of Canadians—The federal role,* vol. 6, *Recommendations for reform.* Ottawa: Senate of Canada. Retrieved from http://www.parl.gc.ca/content/sen/committee/372/soci/rep/repoct02vol6part7-e.htm.

42. Health Canada. (2011). *Canada Health Act.* Ottawa: Health Canada. Retrieved from http://www.hc-sc.gc.ca/hcs-sss/medi-assur/faq-eng.php#a3.

43. Canadian Museum of History. (2010). *Making medicare: The history of health care in Canada, 1914–2007.* Retrieved from http://www.historymuseum.ca/cmc/exhibitions/hist/medicare/medic-1h12e.shtml.

44. Dunsmuir, M. (1991). *The spending power: Scope and limitations.* Ottawa: Library of Parliament (Law and Government Division). Retrieved from http://www.parl.gc.ca/Content/LOP/researchpublications/bp272-e.htm.

45. Dickin, C. (2014). Public health. *The Canadian Encyclopedia.* Toronto: Historica Canada. Retrieved from http://www.thecanadianencyclopedia.ca/en/article/public-health.

46. Parliament of Canada. (2010). *Government response to the Standing Committee on Health's report: Promoting innovative solutions to health human resources challenges.* Ottawa: Parliament of Canada. Retrieved from http://www.parl.gc.ca/HousePublications/Publication.aspx?DocId=4677841&Language=E&Mode=1&Parl=40&Ses=3.

47. Health Canada. (2008). *Activities and responsibilities.* Ottawa: Health Canada. Retrieved from http://www.hc-sc.gc.ca/ahc-asc/activit/index-eng.php.

48. Canadian Institute for Health Information (2011). *CMDB Hospital beds staffed and in operation, fiscal year 2009–2010: Quick stats.* Ottawa: CIHI; and Databank of Official Statistics. (2011). *Beds, places, internal users and other indicators of service use in public and private facilities, by health region of the reporting institution.* Quebec City: Government of Quebec.

49. Institute of Public Administration of Canada, MNP, & Fasken Martineau. (2013). *Healthcare governance models in Canada: A provincial perspective.* Toronto: IPAC, MNP, & Fasken Martineau. Retrieved from http://www.ipac.ca/documents/ALL-COMBINED.pdf.

50. Born, K., & Sullivan, T. (2011, June 29). LHINs and the governance of Ontario's health care system. *HealthyDebate.* Retrieved from http://healthydebate.ca/2011/06/topic/cost-of-care/lhins-2.

51. Closson, T. (2015). The Goldilocks principle and Canadian healthcare system governance. *Law and*

Governance, 17(2). Retrieved from http://www.long-woods.com/content/24188.

52. Public Health Agency of Canada. (2014). *Health portfolio*. Ottawa: PHAC. Retrieved from http://www.healthycanadians.gc.ca/minister-ministre/portfolio-eng.php.

53. Ontario Ministry of Health and Long-Term Care. (2014). *Public health units*. Toronto: Ontario Ministry of Health and Long-Term Care. Retrieved from http://www.health.gov.on.ca/en/common/system/services/phu.

54. Public Health Agency of Canada. 2015). *Who delivers public health services?* Ottawa: PHAC. Retrieved from http://www.phac-aspc.gc.ca/about_apropos/faq-eng.php.

55. Department of Health and Community Services. (2015). *Services in your region*. St. John's, NL: Government of Newfoundland and Labrador. Retrieved from http://www.health.gov.nl.ca/health/findhealth-services/in_your_community.html.

56. Deber, R., Millan, K., Shapiro, H., & McDougall, C. (2006). A cautionary tale of downloading public health in Ontario: What does it say about the need for national standards for more than doctors and hospitals? *Healthcare Policy, 2*(2), 60–75.

57. Health Canada. (2007). *History of providing health services to First Nations people and Inuit*. Retrieved from http://www.hc-sc.gc.ca/ahc-asc/branch-dirgen/fnihb-dgspni/services_e.html.

58. Health Canada. (2015). *First Nations and Inuit Health: Nursing*. Ottawa: Health Canada. Retrieved from http://www.hc-sc.gc.ca/fniah-spnia/services/nurs-infirm/index-eng.php.

59. Town of Fort Smith. (2015). *Health services*. Fort Smith, NT: Town of Fort Smith. Retrieved from http://www.fshssa.hss.gov.nt.ca/our-health-and-social-services-centre.

Chapter 4

1. Sermeus, W., Aiken, L., Van den Heede, K., Rafferty, A., Griffiths, P., Moreno-Casbas, M. ... RN4CAST Consortium. (2011). Nurse forecasting in Europe (RN4CAST): Rationale, design and methodology. *BMC Nursing, 10*(6). doi: 10.1186/1472-6955-10-6.

2. Statistics Canada. (2012). *Public sector employment, wages and salaries, by province and territory*. Ottawa: Statistics Canada. Retrieved from http://www.statcan.gc.ca/tables-tableaux/sum-som/l01/cst01/govt62a-eng.htm.

3. Statistics Canada. (2015). Distribution of employed people, by industry, by province (Canada, 2014). Ottawa: Statistics Canada. Retrieved from http://www.statcan.gc.ca/tables-tableaux/sum-som/l01/cst01/labor21a-eng.htm.

4. Canadian Nurses Association & Canadian Medical Association. *Toward a pan-Canadian planning framework for health human resources. A green paper.* Ottawa: CNA & CMA. Retrieved from https://www.cna-aiic.ca/~/media/cna/page-content/pdf-fr/cma_cna_green_paper_e.pdf?la=en.

5. Health Action Lobby. (2013). *Welcome to the Health Action Lobby*. Ottawa: Health Action Lobby. Retrieved from http://www.healthactionlobby.ca.

6. Health Canada. (2012). *Supply of health providers*. Ottawa: Health Canada.

7. Advisory Committee on Health Delivery and Human Resources. (2009). *How many are enough? Redefining self-sufficiency for the health workforce*. Ottawa: Health Canada.

8. Advisory Committee on Health Delivery and Human Resources. (2007). A *Framework for collaborative pan-Canadian health human resources planning*. Ottawa: Health Canada. Retrieved from http://www.hc-sc.gc.ca/hcs-sss/pubs/hhrhs/2007-frame-cadre/index-eng.php#a3.

9. Ibid.

10. Canadian Health Human Resources Network. (n.d.). *About us*. Ottawa: CHHRN. Retrieved from http://www.hhr-rhs.ca/index.php?option=com_content&view=section&id=5&Itemid=33&lang=en.

11. Health Canada. (2016). *Health human resources*. Ottawa: Health Canada. Retrieved from http://www.hc-sc.gc.ca/hcs-sss/hhr-rhs/index-eng.php.

12. Tomblin Murphy, G., MacKenzie, A., Alder, R., Langley, J., Hickey, M., & Cook, A. (2012). Pilot-testing an applied competency-based approach to health human resources planning. *Health Policy and Planning, 28*(7), 739–749.

13. Ibid.

14. Canadian Institute for Health Information. (2012). *Canada's health care providers: Provincial profiles—2012*. Ottawa: CIHI.

15. Berridge, V. (1990). Health and medicine. In F. Thompson (Ed.), *The Cambridge social history of Britain 1750–1950*, vol. 3, *Social agencies and institutions* (pp. 171–242). Cambridge: Cambridge University Press, p. 183.

16. Splane, R., & Splane, V. (1994). *Chief nursing officer positions in national ministries of health: Focal points*

for nursing leadership. San Francisco: University of California.

17. Elliott, J., Rutty, C., & Villeneuve, M. (2013). *The Canadian Nurses Association 1908–2008: One hundred years of service*. Ottawa: CNA.

18. College of Registered Nurses of British Columbia. (2016). *Three nursing colleges joining to co-create new regulator*. Vancouver: CRNBC. Retrieved from https://crnbc.ca/crnbc/Announcements/2016/Pages/new_college_all_nurses.aspx.

19. Canadian Council of Registered Nurse Regulators. (2014). *Adult/Paediatric NP exam frequently asked questions from Canadian universities*. Beaverton, ON: CCRNR. Retrieved from http://www.ccrnr.ca/assets/np-exam-university-faq.pdf.

20. Canadian Council of Registered Nurse Regulators. (2016). *NCLEX-RN 2015: Canadian results*. Beaverton ON: CCRNR, p. 5. Retrieved from http://www.ccrnr.ca/assets/np-exam-university-faq.pdf.

21. Canadian Association of Schools of Nursing. (2015). *Press release: Four in five Canadians believe our nurses should be assessed using a test based on Canadian requirements*. Ottawa: CASN. Retrieved from http://www.casn.ca/2015/10/press-release-four-in-five-canadians-believe-our-nurses-should-be-assessed-using-a-test-based-on-canadian-requirements-2.

22. Ibid.

23. Woodend, K., & Medves, J. (2015, December 14). Kirsten Woodend & Jennifer Medves: We are failing our nurses. *National Post*. Retrieved from http://news.nationalpost.com/full-comment/kirsten-woodend-jennifer-medves-we-are-failing-our-nurses.

24. Barton, A. (2016, May 12). Harmonizing nurse education with U.S. hurts Canada's edge: Association. *Globe and Mail*. Retrieved from http://www.theglobeandmail.com/life/health-and-fitness/health/harmonizing-nurse-education-with-us-puts-canadas-edge-at-risk-association/article29989938.

25. Coghlan, A. (2016, May 19). Letter to the editor. *Globe and Mail*. Retrieved from http://www.ccrnr.ca/assets/2016-05-19-ccrnr-letter-to-the-editor---globe-and-mail.pdf.

26. Canadian Council of Registered Nurse Regulators. (n.d.). *Preparing your nursing students for a successful NCLEX examination experience*. Beaverton, ON: CCRNR. Retrieved from http://www.ccrnr.ca/assets/preparing_your_students_for_a_successful_nclex_experience_final.pdf.

27. Canadian Council of Registered Nurse Regulators. (2016). *NCLEX-RN 2015: Canadian results*. Beaverton, ON: CCRNR. Retrieved from http://www.ccrnr.ca/assets/2015-ccrnr-report-final-for-release-31-mar-2016.pdf.

28. Canadian Federation of Nurses Unions. (2015). *Letter to provincial ministers of health requesting a systemic, comprehensive and transparent review of the process and the exam*. Ottawa: CFNU. Examples are shown at https://www.cna-aiic.ca/en/becoming-an-rn/rn-exam/nclex-rn-communications.

29. Canadian Nurses Association. (2016). *Resolutions at CNA meeting of members 2016: Title of resolution: Support for urgent remediation of NCLEX-RN® issues*. Ottawa: CNA.

30. Peter, E. (2011). Fostering social justice: The possibilities of a socially connected model of moral agency. *Canadian Journal of Nursing Research, 43*(2), 11–17.

31. To learn more about the disaffiliation of Quebec from CNA, see Elliott, J., Rutty, C., & Villeneuve, M. (2013). *The Canadian Nurses Association 1908–2008: One hundred years of service*. Ottawa: CNA, pp. 93–112 (Chapter 6, The Birth of Medicare and a New Era in Canadian Health Care 1967–1990).

32. For detailed information on CNA membership categories, see the *Our Members* page of the CNA website: https://cna-aiic.ca/en/about-cna/our-members.

33. Scarrow, J. (2007). Recommendations from RNAO: After nine months of consultation and discussion, RNAO members vote in favour of six recommendations about RNAO's relations with the Canadian Nurses Association. *Registered Nurse Journal, 19*(1), 22–24, p. 22.

34. Ibid.

35. The resolution was submitted on behalf of the Ottawa region and the Halton, Hamilton, Kawartha-Victoria, Niagara, and South Simcoe chapters, which constituted 25.1 per cent of RNAO's registered nurse and nurse practitioner members as of February 2016. In addition, the resolution was endorsed by the Nursing Leadership Network of Ontario and the Nursing Research Interest Group, whose members fall within and beyond the region/chapters listed.

36. Duncan, S., Thorne, S., & Rodney, P. (2015). Evolving trends in nurse regulation: What are the policy impacts for nursing's social mandate? *Nursing Inquiry, 22*(1), 27–38.

37. Ibid.

38. BC Coalition of Nursing Associations. (2016). *About the coalition*. Vancouver: BCCNA. Retrieved from http://www.bccna.com/about-the-coalition.php.

39. Ibid.

40. Silas, L. (2011). *A message from Linda Silas, President, Canadian Federation of Nurses Unions (CFNU) regarding BCNU's decision to withdraw from CFNU.* Ottawa: Canadian Federation of Nurses Unions. Retrieved from https://nursesunions.ca/news/message-linda-silas-cfnu-president-regarding-bcnu-s-decision-withdraw-cfnu.

41. College of Registered Nurses of British Columbia. (2015). *Information about BCNU lawsuit against CRNBC and ARNBC.* Vancouver: CRNBC. Retrieved from https://www.crnbc.ca/crnbc/Announcements/2015/Pages/info_about_lawsuit.aspx.

42. Ibid.

43. Fraser, J. (2015). *Urgent open letter to all B.C. nurses.* Vancouver: Association of Registered Nurses of British Columbia.

44. Ibid.

45. Supreme Court of Canada. (2015). *Service Employees' International Union, Local no. 333 v. Nipawin District Staff Association et al., [1975] 1 S.C.R. 382.* Ottawa: Supreme Court of Canada. Retrieved from http://scc-csc.lexum.com/scc-csc/scc-csc/en/item/5342/index.do?r=AAAAAQAec2Fza2F0Y-2hld2FuIHJlZZ2lzdGVyZWQgbnVyc2VzAQ.

46. Canadian Federation of Nurses Unions. (2015). *About us.* Ottawa: CFNU. Retrieved from https://nursesunions.ca/about-us.

47. Ontario Nurses' Association. (2015). *What we do.* Toronto: ONA. Retrieved from http://www.onalocal.org/about_us/what_we_do.html.

48. Registered Nurses' Union of Newfoundland and Labrador. (2015). *About us.* St. John's, NL: RNUNL. Retrieved from http://www.rnunl.ca/about.asp.

49. National Nurses United. (2013). *Global nurses united of nurse, healthcare worker unions, born.* Silver Spring, MD: National Nurses United. Retrieved from http://www.nationalnursesunited.org/site/entry/global-nurses-united.

50. International Council of Nurses. (2015). *What we do.* Geneva: ICN. Retrieved from http://www.icn.ch/what-we-do/what-we-do.

51. Liaschenko, J., & Peter, E. (2016). Fostering nurses' moral agency and moral identity: The importance of moral community. *Hastings Center Report, 46*(S1), S18–S21, p. S21.

MODULE II

1. Soroka, S., & Mahon, A. (2012). *An analysis of the impact of current healthcare system funding and financing models and the value of health and healthcare in Canada.*

Ottawa: Canadian Health Services Research Foundation and Canadian Nurses Association.

Chapter 5

1. Parliament of Canada. (n.d.). *Dewar, Marion, C.M., B.Sc.* Ottawa: Parliament of Canada.

2. Statistics Canada. (2012). *Life expectancy at birth, by sex, by province.* Retrieved from http://www.statcan.gc.ca/tables-tableaux/sum-som/l01/cst01/health26-eng.htm; and World Health Organization. (2014). *World health statistics 2014.* Geneva: WHO.

3. Centers for Disease Control and Prevention. (2011). *Achievements in public health, 1900–1999: Control of infectious diseases.* Atlanta, GA: CDC. Retrieved from http://www.cdc.gov/mmwr/preview/mmwrhtml/mm4829a1.htm.

4. Centers for Disease Control and Prevention. (2011). *Ten great public health achievements—United States, 2001–2010.* Atlanta: CDC. Retrieved from http://www.cdc.gov/about/history/tengpha.htm.

5. Brownson, R., Chriqui, J., & Stamatakis, K. (2009). Understanding evidence-based public health policy. *American Journal of Public Health, 99*(9), 1576–1583.

6. Public Health Agency of Canada. (2008). *The Chief Public Health Officer's report on the state of public health in Canada 2008.* Ottawa: PHAC. Retrieved from http://www.phac-aspc.gc.ca/cphorsphc-respcacsp/2008/fr-rc/cphorsphc-respcacsp05b-eng.php.

7. Stern, A., & Markel, H. (2005). The history of vaccines and immunization: Familiar patterns, new challenges. *Health Affairs, 24*(3), 611–621.

8. Centers for Disease Control and Prevention. (2011). *Ten great public health achievements in the 20th century.* Atlanta: CDC. Retrieved from http://www.cdc.gov/about/history/tengpha.htm.

9. Public Health Agency of Canada. (2008). *The Chief Public Health Officer's report on the state of public health in Canada.* Ottawa: PHAC. Retrieved from http://www.phac-aspc.gc.ca/cphorsphc-respcacsp/2008/fr-rc/cphorsphc-respcacsp05b-eng.php.

10. Simpson, J. (2012). *Chronic condition: Why Canada's healthcare system needs to be dragged into the 21st century.* Toronto: Penguin Group Canada, p. 22.

11. Cited in Elliott, J., Rutty, C., & Villeneuve, M. (2013). *The Canadian Nurses Association 1908–2008: One hundred years of service.* Ottawa: CNA, p. 65.

12. Veterans Ombudsman. (2014). *Veterans' long-term care needs: A review of the support provided by Veterans Affairs Canada through its long-term care program.* Ottawa: Government of Canada. Retrieved from

http://www.ombudsman-veterans.gc.ca/eng/reports/reports-reviews/long-term-care-program#d.

13. Statistics Canada. (2014). *Vital statistics and health*. Retrieved from http://www.statcan.gc.ca/pub/11-516-x/sectionb/4147437-eng.htm.

14. Craig. B. (1989–1990). Hospital records and record-keeping, c. 1850-c. 1950. Part 1: The development of records in hospitals. *Archivaria, 29*(Winter), 57–87.

15. Canadian Museum of History. (2015). *Historical overview of immigration to Canada*. Ottawa: Canadian Museum of History. Retrieved from http://www.historymuseum.ca/cmc/exhibitions/hist/medicare/medic-4h03e.shtml.

16. Simpson, J. (2012). *Chronic condition: Why Canada's healthcare system needs to be dragged into the 21st century*. Toronto: Penguin Group Canada, p. 22.

17. McPherson, K. (1996). *Bedside matters: The transformation of Canadian nursing, 1900–1990*. Toronto: Oxford University Press.

18. Lalonde, M. (1974). *A new perspective on the health of Canadians: A working document*. Ottawa: Minister of Supply and Services Canada, p. 11.

19. Lalonde, M. (1974). *A new perspective on the health of Canadians: A working document*. Ottawa: Minister of Supply and Services Canada.

20. Laframboise, H. (1973). Health policy. Breaking it down into more manageable segments. *Journal of the Canadian Medical Association, 108*(3), 388–393.

21. Public Health Agency of Canada. (2008). *The Chief Public Health Officer's report on the state of public health in Canada*. Ottawa: PHAC. Retrieved from http://www.phac-aspc.gc.ca/cphorsphc-respcacsp/2008/fr-rc/cphorsphc-respcacsp05b-eng.php.

22. World Health Organization. (1978). *The declaration of Alma-Ata*. Geneva: WHO. Retrieved from http://www.who.int/hpr/NPH/docs/declaration_almaata.pdf.

23. Health and Welfare Canada. (1986). *Achieving health for all: A framework for health promotion*. Ottawa: Health and Welfare Canada. Retrieved from http://www.hc-sc.gc.ca/hcs-sss/pubs/system-regime/1986-frame-plan-promotion/index-eng.php.

24. World Health Organization. (2015). *Health promotion*. Geneva: WHO. Retrieved from http://www.who.int/healthpromotion/conferences/previous/ottawa.

25. Canadian Public Health Association. (1982). Strong Nursing Leadership and an Inspiration to Nurses Across Canada. *CPHA Health Digest, 6*(2). Retrieved from http://resources.cpha.ca/CPHA/ThisIsPublicHealth/profiles/item.php?l=E&i=329.

26. Health Canada. (2004). *National Forum on Health*. Ottawa: Health Canada. Retrieved from http://www.hc-sc.gc.ca/hcs-sss/ehealth-esante/infostructure/nfoh_nfss-eng.php.

27. National Forum on Health. (1997). *Canada health action: Building on the legacy*, vol. 1, *The final report*. Ottawa: Health Canada. Retrieved from http://www.hc-sc.gc.ca/hcs-sss/pubs/renewal-renouv/1997-nfoh-fnss-v1/index-eng.php.

28. Decter, M. (1994). *Healing medicare: Managing health system change the Canadian way*. Toronto: McGillan Books.

29. Keighley, T., & Villeneuve, M., course leaders. (2013, May 13–14). *Policy and politics: Shaping health policy at the intersection*. 2 Day Workshop, Centre for Professional Development, Lawrence S. Bloomberg Faculty of Nursing, University of Toronto.

30. Goldenberg, E. (2006). *The way it works: Inside Ottawa*. Toronto: McClelland & Stewart, p. 322.

31. Picard, A. (2013). *The path to health care reform: Policy and politics*. Ottawa: Conference Board of Canada, p. 49.

32. Rothwell, R. with revisions by Marshall, T., & Koch, D. (2015). Jean Chrétien. *The Canadian Encyclopedia*. Toronto: Historica Canada. Retrieved from http://www.thecanadianencyclopedia.ca/en/article/joseph-jacques-jean-chretien.

33. Goldenberg, E. (2006). *The way it works: Inside Ottawa*. Toronto: McClelland & Stewart, p. 323.

34. Rothwell, R. with revisions by Marshall, T., & Koch, D. (2015). Jean Chrétien. *The Canadian Encyclopedia*. Toronto: Historica Canada. Retrieved from http://www.thecanadianencyclopedia.ca/en/article/joseph-jacques-jean-chretien.

35. Gray, C. (1999). There's a new sheriff at Tunney's Pasture. *Canadian Medical Association Journal, 161*(4), 426–427.

36. Canadian Intergovernmental Conference Secretariat. (2000). *News release: First ministers' meeting communiqué on health*. Ottawa: CICS. Retrieved from http://www.scics.gc.ca/english/conferences.asp?a=viewdocument&id=1144.

37. Canadian Institutes of Health Research. (2015). *About us*. Ottawa: CIHR. Retrieved from http://www.cihr-irsc.gc.ca/e/37792.html.

38. Canada Health Infoway. (2015). *About Canada Health Infoway*. Toronto: Canada Health Infoway. Retrieved from https://www.infoway-inforoute.ca/en/about-us.

39. Harder, L., & Patten, S. (2006). *The Chrétien legacy: Politics and public policy in Canada.* Montreal: McGill-Queen's University Press.

40. Davies, P. (2005, March 3). *Evidence-based government: How do we make it happen?* Presented at Seventh Annual Workshop of the Canadian Health Services Research Foundation, Montreal, Quebec.

41. Commission on the Future of Health Care in Canada. (2002). *Building on values: The future of health care in Canada.* Ottawa: Commission on the Future of Health Care in Canada, p. xv.

42. Standing Senate Committee on Social Affairs, Science and Technology. (2002). *The health of Canadians—The federal role*, vol. 6, *Recommendations for reform.* Ottawa: Senate of Canada.

43. Government of Canada. (2003). *2003 first ministers' accord on health care renewal.* Ottawa: Government of Canada. Retrieved from http://www.scics.gc.ca/CMFiles/800039004_e1GTC-352011-6102.pdf.

44. Ibid.

45. Health Canada. (2004). *A 10-year plan to strengthen health care.* Ottawa: Health Canada. Retrieved from http://www.hc-sc.gc.ca/hcs-sss/delivery-prestation/fptcollab/2004-fmm-rpm/nr-cp_9_16_2-eng.php.

46. For example, see: House of Commons Standing Committee on Health (2008), *Parliamentary review of "A 10-year plan to strengthen health care"*; and Standing Senate Committee on Social Affairs, Science and Technology (2012), *Time for transformative change: A review of the 2004 health accord.* Both are available online.

47. Standing Senate Committee on Social Affairs, Science and Technology. (2006). *Out of the shadows at last: Transforming mental health, mental illness and addiction services in Canada.* Ottawa: Senate of Canada.

48. Mental Health Commission of Canada. (2012). *Changing directions, changing lives: The mental health strategy for Canada.* Calgary: MHCC.

49. Advisory Panel on Healthcare Innovation. (2015). *Unleashing innovation: Excellent healthcare for Canada.* Executive summary. Ottawa: Health Canada, p. 7. Retrieved from http://www.healthycanadians.gc.ca/publications/health-system-systeme-sante/summary-innovation-sommaire/index-eng.php.

50. Postl, B. (2006). *Final report of the federal advisor on wait times.* Ottawa: Health Canada. Retrieved from http://www.hc-sc.gc.ca/hcs-sss/pubs/system-regime/2006-wait-attente/index-eng.php.

51. Parliament of Canada. (2009). *The wait times issue and the patient wait times guarantee.* Ottawa: Parliament of Canada. Retrieved from http://www.parl.gc.ca/Content/LOP/researchpublications/prb0582-e.htm.

52. Canadian Nurses Association. (2009). *Registered nurses: On the front lines of wait times.* Ottawa: CNA. Retrieved from https://www.cna-aiic.ca/~/media/cna/files/en/wait_times_paper_2011_e.pdf.

53. Adams, O. (2013). Reflection on the health accords: a glass half-full? *Health Council of Canada Guest Blog.* Retrieved from http://healthcouncilcanada.blogspot.ca/2013/09/reflection-on-health-accords-glass-half.html.

54. Advisory Panel on Healthcare Innovation. (2015). *Unleashing innovation: Excellent healthcare for Canada.* Ottawa: Health Canada, p. 2.

55. Advisory Panel on Healthcare Innovation. (2015). *Unleashing innovation: Excellent healthcare for Canada.* Executive summary. Ottawa: Health Canada, p. 7. Retrieved from http://www.healthycanadians.gc.ca/publications/health-system-systeme-sante/summary-innovation-sommaire/index-eng.php.

56. Advisory Panel on Healthcare Innovation. (2015). *Unleashing innovation: excellent healthcare for Canada.* Executive summary. Ottawa: Health Canada, p. xx. Retrieved from http://www.healthycanadians.gc.ca/publications/health-system-systeme-sante/summary-innovation-sommaire/index-eng.php.

57. Lazar, H. (2009). A cross provincial comparison of health care reform in Canada: Building blocks and some preliminary results. *Canadian Political Science Review, 3*(4), 1–14. Retrieved from http://www.queensu.ca/iigr/sites/webpublish.queensu.ca.iigrwww/files/files/Res/crossprov/Lazar--BuildingBlocks.pdf.

58. The Rt. Hon. Justin Trudeau to the Hon. Dr. Jane Philpott (2015, October). *Minister of Health mandate letter.* Retrieved from http://pm.gc.ca/eng/minister-health-mandate-letter.

Chapter 6

1. Nelson, S., & Rafferty, A. (2010). Introduction. In S. Nelson & A. Rafferty (Eds.), *Notes on Nightingale* (pp. 1–8). Ithaca, NY: Cornell University Press.

2. Nursing Task Force. (1999). *Good nursing, good health: An investment for the 21st century.* Toronto: Ontario Ministry of Health and Long-Term Care.

3. Registered Nurses Association of Ontario. (2002). *Tracking the nursing task force (1999): RNs rate their nursing work life.* Toronto: RNAO.

4. Canadian Nursing Advisory Committee. (2002).

Our health our future: Creating quality workplaces for Canadian nurses. Final report of the Canadian Nursing Advisory Committee. Ottawa: Health Canada.

5. Ryten, E. (1997). *A statistical picture of the past, present and future of registered nurses in Canada.* Ottawa: Canadian Nurses Association.

6. Canadian Nurses Association (1998). Nurses take over Ottawa. *CNA Today, 8*(4); see also Rock, A. (1998). *Address to the 1998 biennial convention.* Keynote address presented at the biennial meeting of the Canadian Nurses Association, Ottawa, Ontario.

7. Elliott, J., Rutty, C., & Villeneuve, M. (2013). *The Canadian Nurses Association 1908–2008: One hundred years of service.* Ottawa: CNA, p. 119.

8. Shamian, J., & Villeneuve, M. (2000). Building a national nursing agenda. *Hospital Quarterly, 4*(1), 16–18.

9. Organisation for Economic Co-operation and Development. (2004). *Towards high-performing health systems: Policy studies.* Paris: OECD.

10. Advisory Committee on Health Human Resources. (2000). *The nursing strategy for Canada.* Ottawa: Health Canada, p. 2.

11. Ibid.

12. Advisory Committee on Health Human Resources. (2003). *A report on the nursing strategy for Canada.* Ottawa: Health Canada. Retrieved from http://tools.hhr-rhs.ca/index.php?option=com_mtree&task=att_download&link_id=5921&cf_id=68&lang=en.

13. Ibid.

14. Canadian Canadian Nursing Advisory Committee. (2002). *Our health our future: Creating quality workplaces for Canadian nurses.* Final report of the Canadian Nursing Advisory Committee. Ottawa: Health Canada, p. 1.

15. Nursing Sector Study Corporation. (2006). *Building the future: An integrated strategy for nursing human resources in Canada.* Phase II Final Report. Nursing Sector Study Corporation.

16. Villeneuve, M., & MacDonald, J. (2006). *Toward 2020: Visions for nursing.* Ottawa: Canadian Nurses Association.

17. Canadian Nurse Practitioner Initiative. (2006). *Nurse practitioners: The time is now: A solution to improving access and reducing wait times in Canada.* Ottawa: CNPI.

18. Silas, L. (2012). The research to action project: Applied workplace solutions for nurses. *Nursing Leadership, 25*(March, Special Issue), 9–20.

19. Ibid.

20. Aboriginal Nurses Association of Canada, Canadian Association of Schools of Nursing, & Canadian Nurses Association. (2009). *Cultural competence and cultural safety in First Nations, Inuit and Métis nursing education: An integrated review of the literature.* Ottawa: Aboriginal Nurses Association of Canada, p. 1.

21. Aboriginal Nurses Association of Canada, Canadian Association of Schools of Nursing, & Canadian Nurses Association. (2009). *Cultural competence and cultural safety in nursing education: A framework for First Nations, Inuit and Métis nursing.* Ottawa: Aboriginal Nurses Association of Canada.

22. Canadian Nurses Association. (2016). *National nursing associations sign partnership accord in spirit of authentic Indigenous collaboration.* Retrieved from https://www.cna-aiic.ca/en/news-room/news-releases/2016/national-nursing-associations-sign-partnership-accord-to-improve-indigenous-health.

23. Canadian Medical Association, & Canadian Nurses Association. (2011). *Principles to guide health care transformation in Canada.* Ottawa: CMA & CNA. Retrieved from https://www.cna-aiic.ca/~/media/cna/files/en/guiding_principles_hc_e.pdf.

24. Institute for Healthcare Improvement. (2015). *The IHI triple aim.* Cambridge, MA: Institute for Healthcare Improvement. Retrieved from http://www.ihi.org/Engage/Initiatives/TripleAim/Pages/default.aspx.

25 National Expert Commission. (2012). *A nursing call to action: The health of our nation, the future of our health system.* Ottawa: Canadian Nurses Association.

26. Canadian Nurses Association. (2015). *Framework for registered nurse prescribing in Canada.* Ottawa: CNA. Retrieved from https://www.cna-aiic.ca/~/media/cna/page-content/pdf-en/cna-rn-prescribing-framework_e.pdf.

27. Guardian. (2014, July 4). Good to meet you … Anne Marie Rafferty. *The Guardian.* Retrieved from http://www.theguardian.com/theguardian/2014/jul/04/good-to-meet-you-anne-marie-rafferty.

28. Elliott, J., Rutty, C., & Villeneuve, M. (2013). *The Canadian Nurses Association 1908–2008: One hundred years of service.* Ottawa: CNA, p. 81.

29. Canadian Medical Association. (1926). New business: Training schools for nurses in Canada: Business report of 57th annual meeting of Canadian Medical Association, June 1926, Victoria. *Canadian Medical Association Journal, 16*(September 1926), Supplement, pp. xxxiv–xxxv.

30. Elliott, J., Rutty, C., & Villeneuve, M. (2013).

The Canadian Nurses Association 1908–2008: One hundred years of service. Ottawa: CNA.

31. Pringle, D., Green, L., & Johnson, S. (2004). *Nursing education in Canada: Historical review and current capacity.* Ottawa: Nursing Sector Study Corporation, p. 17.

32. The Canadian Nurse. (1932). Some features of the report of the survey of nursing education in Canada. *The Canadian Nurse, 28*(3), 127–131, p. 127.

33. Mussallem, H.K. (1965). *Nursing education in Canada.* Submission to the Royal Commission on Health Services. Ottawa: Queen's Printer.

34. Ibid.

35. MacMillan, K. (Ed.). (2013). *Proceedings of a think tank on the future of undergraduate nursing education in Canada.* Halifax: Dalhousie University School of Nursing.

36. Registered Nurse Education Review in Nova Scotia. (2015). *Building our future: A new, collaborative model for undergraduate nursing education in Nova Scotia.* Final Report. Halifax: Registered Nurse Education Review in Nova Scotia.

37. Doucette, K. (2015, May 12). N.S. universities to offer new accelerated nursing programs. *CTV News Atlantic.* Retrieved from http://atlantic.ctvnews.ca/n-s-universities-to-offer-new-accelerated-nursing-programs-1.2370399.

38. St. Francis Xavier University. (2016). *StFX is pleased to offer a new pathway for graduates of NSCC's two year LPN diploma program.* Antigonish, NS: St. Francis Xavier University. Retrieved from https://www.stfx.ca/about/news/stfx-pleased-offer-new-pathway-graduates-nsccs-two-year-lpn-diploma-program.

39. CBC News. (2016, April 29). Unhappy nurses vote to turf RN association leaders. *CBC News.* Retrieved from http://www.cbc.ca/news/canada/saskatchewan/unhappy-nurses-vote-to-turf-rn-association-leaders-1.3560021.

40. Lewis, S. (2016, May 9). What's really behind the Saskatchewan RN dispute with LPNs. *Regina Leader Post.* Retrieved from http://leaderpost.com/opinion/columnists/whats-really-behind-the-saskatchewan-rn-dispute-with-lpns.

41. Gkantaras, I., Hahfoud, Z., Foreman, B., Thompson, D., Cannaby, A., Deshpande, D, et al. (2016). The effect of Nurse GraduaTeness on patient mortality: A cross sectional survey (the NuGaT study). *Journal of Advanced Nursing 72*(12), 3034–3044.

42. Registered Nurses' Association of Ontario. (2016). *Mind the safety gap in health system transformation: Reclaiming the role of the RN.* Toronto: RNAO.

43. Ibid., p. 4.

44. Scarrow, J. (2016, May 6). Nursing report calls out to reclaim the role of the RN. *Toronto Star.* Retrieved from https://www.thestar.com/life/nursing/2016/05/06/nursing-report-calls-out-to-reclaim-the-role-of-the-rn.html.

45. Ibid.

46. Registered Practical Nurses Association of Ontario. (2016, June 24). *We're stronger together.* Retrieved from https://www.youtube.com/watch?v=8H4JSdPYkDQ.

47. Martin, D. (2016, July 6). Letter to the editor re: RNAO column. *Hospital News.* Retrieved from http://hospitalnews.com/letter-editor-re-rnao-column.

Chapter 7

1. Birch, S., Tomblin Murphy, G., MacKenzie, A., & Cumming, J. (2015). In place of fear: Aligning health care planning with system objectives to achieve financial sustainability. *Journal of Health Services Research & Policy, 20*(2), 109–114, p. 109.

2. Evans, R. (2011). *Concurrent session presentation.* Address presented at the 8th World Congress on Health Economics, International Health Economics Association, Toronto, Ontario.

3. Merriam-Webster. (2015). *Economics.* Retrieved from http://www.merriam-webster.com/dictionary/economics.

4. Canadian Association for Health Services and Policy Research. (2015). *What is health services and policy research?* Ottawa: CAHSPR. Retrieved from https://www.cahspr.ca/en/community/whatishspr.

5. Palmer, K. (2016, May 15). Why American doctors are calling for Canadian-style medicare. *Toronto Star.* Retrieved from https://www.thestar.com/opinion/commentary/2016/05/15/why-american-doctors-are-calling-for-canadian-style-medicare.html.

6. Canadian Institute for Health Information. (2014). *National health expenditure trends, 1975 to 2014.* Ottawa: CIHI.

7. Ibid.

8. Department of Finance Canada. (2014). *Your tax dollar: 2013–2014 fiscal year.* Ottawa: Department of Finance Canada. Retrieved from http://www.fin.gc.ca/tax-impot/2014/html-eng.asp.

9. Parliament of Canada. (2007). *The federal spending power.* Ottawa: Parliament of Canada. Retrieved

from http://www.parl.gc.ca/content/LOP/Research-Publications/prb0736-e.htm.

10. Canadian Institute for Health Information. (2014). *National health expenditure trends, 1975 to 2014*. Ottawa: CIHI.

11. Parliament of Canada. (2005). *The Canada Health Act: Overview and options*. Ottawa: Parliament of Canada. Retrieved from http://www.parl.gc.ca/content/lop/researchpublications/944-e.htm.

12. Parliament of Canada. (2007). *The federal spending power*. Ottawa: Parliament of Canada. Retrieved from http://www.parl.gc.ca/content/LOP/Research-Publications/prb0736-e.htm.

13. Tholl, W., Bujold, G., & Grimes, K. (2013). *Reframing the federal role in health and health care: A report to the Health Action Lobby*. Ottawa: Health Action Lobby.

14. Commission on the Future of Health Care in Canada. (2002). *Building on values: The future of health care in Canada*. Ottawa: Commission on the Future of Health Care in Canada, p. 37.

15. Health Canada. (2010). *Canada's health care system: Medicare*. Ottawa: Health Canada. Retrieved from http://www.hc-sc.gc.ca/hcs-sss/medi-assur/index-eng.php.

16. Mackenzie, H. (2015). *The Canada health transfer disconnect: An aging population, rising health care costs and a shrinking federal role in funding*. Ottawa: Canadian Federation of Nurses Unions, p. 27.

17. Ibid., p. i.

18. Ibid., p. iv.

19. Advisory Panel on Healthcare Innovation. (2015). *Unleashing innovation: Excellent healthcare for Canada*. Executive summary. Ottawa: Health Canada, p. 121. Retrieved from http://www.healthycanadians.gc.ca/publications/health-system-systeme-sante/report-healthcare-innovation-rapport-soins/alt/report-healthcare-innovation-rapport-soins-eng.pdf.

20. Intergovernmental Affairs. (2010). *Difference between Canadian provinces and territories*. Retrieved from http://www.pco-bcp.gc.ca/aia/index.asp?lang=eng&page=provterr&doc=difference-eng.htm.

21. College of Family Physicians of Canada. (2016). *Physician remuneration in a patient's medical home*. Ottawa: College of Family Physicians of Canada, p. 6; see also Wranik, D., & Durier-Copp, M. (2011). Framework for the design of physician remuneration methods in primary health care. *Social Work in Public Health, 26*(3), 231–259.

22. Canadian Institute for Health Information. (2014). *National health expenditure trends, 1975 to 2014*. Ottawa: CIHI.

23. Porter-O'Grady, T. (1998). A glimpse over the horizon: Choosing our future. *Orthopedic Nursing, 17*(2), 53–60, p. 55.

24. Browne, G., Birch, S., & Thebane, L. (2012). *Better care: An analysis of nursing and healthcare system outcomes*. Ottawa: Canadian Nurses Association and Canadian Health Services Research Foundation.

25. Ontario Association of Community Care Access Centres, Ontario Hospital Association, & Ontario Federation of Community Mental Health and Addiction Programs. (2010). *Ideas and opportunities for bending the health care cost curve: Advice for the government of Ontario*. Toronto: OACCAC, OHA, & Ontario Federation of Community Mental Health and Addiction Programs.

26. Canadian Institute for Health Information. (2016). *Prescribed drug spending in Canada, 2016: A focus on public drug programs*. Ottawa: CIHI.

27. Ontario Ministry of Health and Long-Term Care. (2015). *Transforming Ontario's health care system: Community Health Links provide coordinated, efficient and effective care to patients with complex needs*. Toronto: Ontario Ministry of Health and Long-Term Care. Retrieved from http://www.health.gov.on.ca/en/pro/programs/transformation/community.aspx.

28. Organisation for Economic Co-operation and Development. (2015). *OECD health statistics 2015*. Paris: OECD.

29. Ibid.

30. Peter, E. (2013). Broadening the view of health care ethics/nursing ethics. In J. Storch, P. Rodney, & R. Starzomski (Eds.), *Toward a moral horizon: Nursing ethics for leadership and practice* (2nd ed., pp. 384–397). Toronto: Pearson-Prentice Hall, p. 386.

31. Rodney, P., Buckley, B., Street, A., Serrano, E., & Martin, L.A. (2013). The moral climate of nursing practice: Inquiry and action. In J. Storch, P. Rodney, & R. Starzomski (Eds.), *Toward a moral horizon: Nursing ethics of leadership and practice* (2nd ed., pp. 188–214). Toronto: Pearson-Prentice Hall, p. 188.

Chapter 8

1. Browne, G., Birch, S., & Thebane, L. (2012). *Better care: An analysis of nursing and healthcare system outcomes*. Ottawa: Canadian Nurses Association and Canadian Health Services Research Foundation.

2. Lalonde, M. (1974). *A new perspective on the health of Canadians: A working document.* Ottawa: Minister of Supply and Services Canada, p. 12.

3. World Health Organization. (2007). *Interview on taking office as Director-General.* Geneva: WHO. Retrieved from http://www.who.int/dg/chan/interviews/taking_office.

4. Wald, L. (1902). The nursing settlement of New York. *American Journal of Nursing, 2*(8), 572.

5. Conference Board of Canada. *Life expectancy.* Ottawa: Conference Board of Canada. Retrieved from http://www.conferenceboard.ca/hcp/details/health/life-expectancy.aspx.

6. Conference Board of Canada. *Health: Canada benchmarked against 15 countries.* Ottawa: Conference Board of Canada. Retrieved from http://www.conferenceboard.ca/hcp/details/health.aspx.

7. Statistics Canada. (2013). *Health status.* Ottawa: Statistics Canada. Retrieved from http://www.statcan.gc.ca/pub/82-229-x/2009001/status/int4-eng.htm.

8. Conference Board of Canada. *Health: Canada benchmarked against 15 countries.* Ottawa: Conference Board of Canada. Retrieved from http://www.conferenceboard.ca/hcp/details/health.aspx.

9. Ibid.

10. Baker, G., Norton, P., Flintoft, V., Blais, R., Brown, A., Cox, J., et al. (2004). The Canadian Adverse Events Study: The incidence of adverse events among hospital patients in Canada. *Canadian Medical Association Journal, 170*(11), 1678–1686.

11. Canadian Institute for Health Information. (2011). *Seniors and the health care system: What is the impact of multiple chronic conditions?* Ottawa: CIHI. Retrieved from https://www.cihi.ca/en/info_phc_chronic_seniors_en.pdf.

12. Nasmith, L., Ballem, P., Baxter, R., Bergman, H., Colin-Thomé, D., Herbert, C., et al. (2010). *Transforming care for Canadians with chronic health conditions.* Ottawa: Canadian Academy of Health Sciences. Retrieved from http://www.dfcm.utoronto.ca/Assets/DFCM+Digital+Assets/CAHS+Transforming+Care+for+Canadians+with+Chronic+Health+Conditions.pdf.

13. Public Health Agency of Canada. (2011). *Backgrounder: United Nations NCD summit 2011: Chronic diseases—most significant cause of death globally.* Ottawa: PHAC. Retrieved from http://www.phac-aspc.gc.ca/media/nr-rp/2011/2011_0919-bg-di-eng.php.

14. Alzheimer Society of Canada. (2010). *Rising tide: The impact of dementia on Canadian society.* Toronto: Alzheimer Society of Canada. Retrieved from http://www.alzheimer.ca/en/Get-involved/Raise-your-voice/Rising-Tide.

15. National Expert Commission. (2012). *Non-communicable and chronic diseases.* Ottawa: Canadian Nurses Association. Retrieved from http://www.cna-aiic.ca/~/media/cna/files/en/fact_sheet_14_e.pdf.

16. Public Health Agency of Canada. (2006). *Healthy aging in Canada: A new vision, a vital investment – from evidence to action: A background paper.* Ottawa: PHAC, p. 4.

17. See fact sheets on demographics, determinants of health, and diseases affecting Canadians prepared for the National Expert Commission: http://www.cna-aiic.ca/en/on-the-issues/national-expert-commission/report-and-recommendations#fact_sheets.

18. Canadian Institute for Health Information. (2011). *Seniors and the health care system: What is the impact of multiple chronic conditions?* Ottawa: CIHI. Retrieved from http://secure.cihi.ca/cihiweb/products/air-chronic_disease_aib_en.pdf.

19. Ibid., p. 17.

20. Ramlo, A., & Berlin, R. (2010). *Sustainable: British Columbia's health care system and our aging population.* Retrieved from http://www.urbanfutures.com/sustainable-health.

21. Canadian Institute for Health Information. (2007). *Health care use at the end of life in western Canada.* Ottawa: CIHI.

22. Fowler, R., & Hammer, M. (2013). End-of-life care in Canada. *Clinical & Investigative Medicine, 35*(3), E127–E132.

23. Tanusepturo, P., Wodchis, W., Fowler, R., Walker, P., Bai, Y., Bronskill, S., & Manuel, D. (2015). The health care cost of dying: A population-based retrospective cohort study of the last year of life in Ontario, Canada. *PLoS One, 10*(3). Retrieved from http://www.ncbi.nlm.nih.gov/pmc/articles/PMC4374686.

24. Ibid.

25. Health Council of Canada. (2013). *Progress report 2013: Health care renewal in Canada.* Toronto: Health Council of Canada. Retrieved from http://www.healthcouncilcanada.ca/n3w11n3/ProgressReport2013_EN_2.pdf, p. 1.

26. Canadian Institute for Health Information. (2011). *Health care cost drivers: The facts.* Ottawa: CIHI. Retrieved from https://secure.cihi.ca/free_products/health_care_cost_drivers_the_facts_en.pdf.

27. Canadian Institute for Health Information. (2011). *Health care cost drivers: The facts.* Ottawa: CIHI, p 12.

28. Canadian Institute for Health Information (2011). *CMDB hospital beds staffed and in operation, fiscal year 2009–2010: Quick stats.* Ottawa: CIHI; and Databank of Official Statistics on Quebec. (2011). *Beds, places, internal users and other indicators of service use in public and private facilities, by health region of the reporting institution.* Quebec: Government of Quebec.

29. Canadian Institute for Health Information. (2011). *Health care in Canada, 2011: A focus on seniors and aging.* Ottawa: CIHI.

30. Baker, G.R., Norton, P., Flintoft, V., Blais, R., Brown, A., Cox, J., et al. (2004). The Canadian Adverse Events Study: The incidence of adverse events among hospital patients in Canada. *Canadian Medical Association Journal, 170*(11), 1678–1686.

31. Chan, B., & Cochrane, D. (2016). *Measuring patient harm in Canadian hospitals.* Ottawa: Canadian Institute for Health Information and Canadian Patient Safety Institute, p. 38.

32. Public Health Agency of Canada. (2008). *The chief public health officer's report on the state of public health in Canada 2008.* Ottawa: PHAC. Retrieved from http://www.phac-aspc.gc.ca/cphorsphc-respcacsp/2008/fr-rc/index-eng.php.

33. Browne, G., Birch, S., & Thebane, L. (2012). *Better care: An analysis of nursing and healthcare system outcomes.* Ottawa: Canadian Nurses Association and Canadian Health Services Research Foundation.

34. Keon, J., and Pepin, L. (2009). *A healthy, productive Canada: A determinant of health approach.* Final report of the Subcommittee on Population Health. Ottawa: Senate of Canada, Standing Senate Committee on Social Affairs, Science and Technology, p. 7. Retrieved from http://www.parl.gc.ca/Content/SEN/Committee/402/popu/rep/rephealth1jun09-e.pdf.

35. Rydin, Y., Bleahu, A., Davies, M., Dávila, J., Friel, S., De Grandis, G., et al. (2012). Shaping cities for health: Complexity and the planning of urban environments in the 21st century. *The Lancet, 379,* 2079–2108.

36. Toronto Foundation. (2015). *Toronto's vital signs.* Toronto: Toronto Foundation.

37. Organisation for Economic Co-Operation and Development. (2016). *Resilient cities.* Paris: OECD, p. 13.

38. Ibid., p. 16.

39. Glauser, W., Tepper, J., & Konkin, J. (2016). *8 steps toward addressing Indigenous health inequities.* Retrieved from http://healthydebate.ca/2016/01/topic/8-steps-toward-addressing-indigenous-health-inequities.

40. Muntaner, C., Ng, E., & Chung, H. (2012). *Better health: An analysis of public policy and programming focusing on the determinants of health and health outcomes that are effective in achieving the healthiest populations.* Ottawa: Canadian Health Services Research Foundation and Canadian Nurses Association.

41. National Expert Commission. (2012). *A nursing call to action: The health of our nation, the future of our health system.* Ottawa: Canadian Nurses Association, p. 11.

42. Raza, D., & Goel, R. (2016, May 12). Proper housing is a crucial health issue. *Toronto Star.* Retrieved from https://www.thestar.com/opinion/commentary/2016/05/08/proper-housing-is-a-crucial-a-health-issue.html.

43. Conference Board of Canada. (2012). *Health: Canada benchmarked against 15 countries.* Ottawa: Conference Board of Canada. Retrieved from http://www.conferenceboard.ca/hcp/details/health.aspx.

44. Canadian Institute for Health Information. (2015). *Trends in income-related health inequalities in Canada: Summary report.* Ottawa: CIHI, p. 4.

45. Canadian Health Outcomes for Better Information and Care Project. (n.d.). *About C-HOBIC.* Toronto: C-HOBIC. Retrieved from http://c-hobic.cna-aiic.ca/about/default_e.aspx.

46. Kendall-Gallagher, D., Aiken, L., Sloane, D., & Cimiotti, J. (2011). Nurse specialty certification, inpatient mortality, and failure to rescue. *Journal of Nursing Scholarship, 43*(2), 188–194.

47. Aiken, L., Sloane, D., Bruyneel, L., Van den Heede, K., Griffiths, P., Busse, R., et al. for the RN4CAST consortium. (2014). Nurse staffing and education and hospital mortality in nine European countries: A retrospective observational study. *The Lancet, 383*(9931), 1781–1860.

48. Kendall-Gallagher, D., Aiken, L., Sloane, D., & Cimiotti, J. (2011). Nurse specialty certification, inpatient mortality, and failure to rescue. *Journal of Nursing Scholarship, 43*(2), 188–194.

49. Nelson, A., Powell-Cope, G., Palacios, P., Luther, S.L., Black, T., Hillman, T., et al. (2007). Nursing staffing and patient outcomes in inpatient rehabilitation settings. *Rehabilitation Nursing, 32*(5), 179–202.

50. Dunton, N., Gajewski, B., Klaus, S., & Pierson,

B. (2007). The relationship of nursing workforce characteristics to patient outcomes. *The Online Journal of Issues in Nursing, 12*(3), Manuscript 3. Retrieved from http://www.nursingworld.org/MainMenuCategories/ANAMarketplace/ANAPeriodicals/OJIN/TableofContents/Volume122007/No3Sept07/NursingWorkforceCharacteristics.aspx.

51. Aiken, L., Clarke, S., Sloane, D., Sochalski, J., & Silber, J. (2002). Hospital nurse staffing and patient mortality, nurse burnout, and job dissatisfaction. *Journal of the American Medical Association, 288*, 1987–1993.

52. McGillis Hall, L., Doran, D., & Pink, G. (2004). Nurse staffing models, nursing hours, and patient outcomes. *Journal of Nursing Administration, 34*(1), 41–45.

53. Tourangeau, A., Doran, D., McGillis Hall, L., O'Brien-Pallas, L., Pringle, D., Tu, J., & Cranley, L. (2007). Impact of hospital nursing care on 30-day mortality for acute medical patients. *Journal of Advanced Nursing, 57*(1), 32–44, p. 41.

54. Buhlman, N. (2016). Nurse staffing and patient experience outcomes: A close connection. *American Nurse Today*. Retrieved from https://www.americannursetoday.com/nurse-staffing-and-patient-experience-outcomes.

55. Mitchell, P. (2013). *Nurse staffing—a summary of current research, opinion and policy.* Seattle: Ruckelshaus Center Nurse Staffing Steering Committee, p. 3.

56. Needleman, J. (2015). *Economic and business case for quality and safety.* Presented at the Quality and Safety Summit: Leveraging Nursing Leadership, Toronto, Ontario.

57. McHugh, M., Kelly, L., Smith, H., Wu, E., Vanak, J., & Aiken, L. (2013). Lower mortality in magnet hospitals. *Medical Care, 51*(5), 382–388.

58. Dall, T., Chen, Y., Seifert, R., Maddox, P., & Hogan, P. (2009). The economic value of professional nursing. *Medical Care, 47*(1), 97–104.

59. Wang, L., Vernon-Smiley, M., Gapinski, M., Desisto, M., Maughan, E., & Sheetz, A. (2014). Cost-benefit study of school nursing services. *Journal of the American Medical Association Pediatrics, 168*(7), 642–648. Retrieved from http://www.ncbi.nlm.nih.gov/pubmed/24840710.

60. Royal College of Nursing. (2014). *RCN fact sheet: Nurse prescribing in the UK.* London: Royal College of Nursing.

61. Roots, A., & MacDonald, M. (2014). Outcomes associated with nurse practitioners in collaborative practice with general practitioners in rural settings in Canada: A mixed methods study. *Human Resources for Health, 12*(1), 61.

62. Browne, G., Birch, S., & Thebane, L. (2012). *Better care: An analysis of nursing and healthcare system outcomes.* Ottawa: Canadian Nurses Association and Canadian Health Services Research Foundation.

63. Weiner, J. (2007). Expanding the US medical workforce: Global perspectives and parallels. *British Medical Journal, 335*(7613): 236–238, p. 237.

64. DiCenso, A., & Bryant-Lukosius, D. (2010). *Clinical nurse specialists and nurse practitioners in Canada: A decision support synthesis.* Ottawa: Canadian Health Services Research Foundation.

MODULE III

1. National Expert Commission. (2012). *A nursing call to action: The health of our nation, the future of our health system.* Ottawa: Canadian Nurses Association.

Chapter 9

1. Legislative Assembly of Ontario. (n.d.). *Madeleine Meilleur, MPP.* Toronto: Legislative Assembly of Ontario.

2. Wallace, F. (2016, June 9). Ontario Attorney General Madeleine Meilleur resigning from politics. *Toronto Star.* Retrieved from https://www.thestar.com/news/canada/2016/06/09/ontario-attorney-general-madeleine-meilleur-resigning-from-politics.html.

3. Liberal Arts Instructional Technology Services. (2015). *The public policy process.* Austin: University of Texas at Austin. Retrieved from http://www.laits.utexas.edu/gov310/PEP/policy.

4. Public Health Ontario. (2013). *At a glance: The eight steps to developing a healthy public policy.* Toronto: Public Health Ontario. Retrieved from http://www.publichealthontario.ca/en/eRepository/Eight_steps_to_policy_development_2012.pdf.

5. Office of Nursing Policy. (2003). *Moving forward: Progress report 1999–2003.* Ottawa: Health Canada, p. 3.

6. Kingdon, J. (1995). *Agendas, alternatives, and public policies.* New York: Harper Collins.

7. Milstead, J. (1999). *Health policy and politics: A nurse's guide.* Gaithersburg, MD: Aspen.

8. Mustard, J., Marmot, M., & Tarlov, A. (2000). Opening keynote: Prospects for a healthy future: Comparing Canada with the U.S. and the U.K. In

Proceedings of the 69th annual Couchiching conference: The future of health care in Canada: The art of the possible (pp. 12–26). Willowdale, ON: Couchiching Institute on Public Affairs. Retrieved from https://www.couchichinginstitute.ca/history/2000/CIPA_2000.pdf.

9. Ibid.

10. Tarlov, A. (1999). Public policy frameworks for improving population health. *Annals of the New York Academy of Science, 896*, 281–293.

11. Skelton-Green, J., Shamian, J., & Villeneuve, M. (2013). Policy: The essential link in successful transformations. In M. McIntyre & C. McDonald (Eds.), *Realities of Canadian nursing* (4th ed., pp. 87–113). Philadelphia: Lippincott, Williams & Wilkins; Shamian, J., & Shamian-Ellen, M. (2011). Shaping health policy: The role of nursing research: Three frameworks and their application to policy development. In A. Hinshaw & P. Grady (Eds.), *Shaping health policy through nursing research* (pp. 35–51). New York: Springer; and Shamian, J., & Villeneuve, M. (2011). Two faces, one agenda: Research and policy. In S. Nelson & D. Doran (Eds.), *Mapping the field: Nursing scholarship in health human resources* (pp. 92–104). Toronto: Lawrence S. Bloomberg Faculty of Nursing.

12. Government of Canada. (2017). *Constitution act, 1982*. Ottawa: Department of Justice. Retrieved from http://laws-lois.justice.gc.ca/eng/const/page-15.html.

13. United States of America. (1776). *Declaration of independence*. Washington, DC: National Archives. Retrieved from https://www.archives.gov/founding-docs/declaration-transcript.

14. United Nations. (1948). *The universal declaration of human rights*. New York: United Nations. Retrieved from http://www.un.org/en/documents/udhr.

15. World Health Organization. (2008). *The third ten years of the World Health Organization: 1968–1978*. Geneva: WHO, p. 3. Retrieved from http://www.who.int/global_health_histories/who-3rd10years.pdf.

16. World Health Organization. (1978). *Declaration of Alma-Ata*. International conference on primary health care, 6–12 September. Alma-Ata, USSR: WHO. Retrieved from http://www.who.int/publications/almaata_declaration_en.pdf.

17. Helm, D., & Mayer, C. (2016). Infrastructure: Why it is under provided and badly managed. *Oxford Review of Economic Policy, 32*(3), 343–359, p. 343.

18. Ibid., p. 344.

19. Giacomini, M., Hurley, J., Gold, I., Smith, P., & Ableson, J. (2001). 'Values' in Canadian health policy analysis: *What are we talking about*. Ottawa: Canadian Health Services Research Foundation, p. i.

20. Public Works Department of the Regional Municipality of Peel. (2001). *A case in point: Walkerton's tragedy—water contamination*. Kitchener: Regional Municipality of Waterloo. Retrieved from https://www.peelregion.ca/pw/waterstory/pdf/walkerton-tragedy.pdf.

21. O'Brien-Pallas, L., Tomblin Murphy, G., Shamian, J., Li, X., & Hayes, L. (2010). Impact and determinants of nurse turnover: A pan-Canadian study. *Journal of Nursing Management, 18*, 1073–1086; and O'Brien-Pallas, L., Tomblin Murphy, G., Shamian, J., Li, X., Kephart, G., Laschinger, H., et al. (2016). *Understanding the costs and outcomes of nurses' turnover in Canadian hospitals*. Toronto and Hamilton: Nursing Health Services Research Unit.

22. Akyeampong, E., & Usalcas, J. (1998). *Work absence rates, 1980 to 1997*. Ottawa: Statistics Canada; and Akyeampong, E. (1999). Missing work in 1998—industry differences. *Perspectives on Labour and Income, 11*(3), 30–36.

23. Canadian Nursing Advisory Committee. (2002). *Our health our future: Final report of the Canadian Nursing Advisory Committee*. Ottawa: Health Canada.

24. Dunleavy, J., Shamian, J., & Thomson, D., (2003). Handcuffed by cutbacks. *Canadian Nurse, 99*(3), 23–27, p. 24.

25. Botehlo, J. (2016, July 7). CNE reverses decision to ditch free pass for people with disabilities. *Toronto Star*. Retrieved from https://www.thestar.com/news/gta/2016/07/07/cne-reverses-decision-to-ditch-free-pass-for-people-with-disabilities.html.

26. Crowe, C. (2016, June 28). This is what NIMBY sounds like. *rabble.ca*. Retrieved from http://rabble.ca/blogs/bloggers/cathycrowe/2016/06/this-what-nimby-sounds.

27. Ormsby, M., & Wallace, K. (2016, February 21). Ontario's uncounted homeless dead. *Toronto Star*. Retrieved from https://www.thestar.com/news/insight/2016/02/21/ontarios-uncounted-homeless-dead.html.

28. Rydin, Y., Bleahu, A., Davies, M., Dávila, J., Friel, S., De Grandis, G., et al. (2012). Shaping cities for health: Complexity and the planning of urban environments in the 21st century. *The Lancet, 379*, 2079–2108.

29. CBC News. (2016, January 27). Emergency men's shelter in Leslieville approved by city council. *CBC News*. Retrieved from http://www.cbc.ca/news/canada/toronto/shelter-leslieville-1.3423097.

30. See for example Shamian, J., & Villeneuve, M. (2000). Building a national nursing agenda. *Hospital Quarterly, 4*(1), 16–18. Retrieved from http://www.longwoods.com/content/20521.

31. Ipsos. (2012). *Life-savers, medical professionals top the list of most trusted professionals.* Retrieved from http://www.ipsos-na.com/news-polls/pressrelease.aspx?id=5663.

32. Gray, C. (1999). There's a new sheriff at Tunney's Pasture. *Canadian Medical Association Journal, 161,* 426–427.

33. Longwoods.com. (2005). Judith Shamian: Be true to yourself and your values. *Nursing Leadership, 18*(3), 19–22. Retrieved from https://www.longwoods.com/content/17613/print.

34. Ibid.

35. Canadian Medical Association and Canadian Nurses Association. (2011). *Principles to guide health care transformation in Canada.* Ottawa: CMA & CNA. Retrieved from http://policybase.cma.ca/dbtw-wpd/Policypdf/PD11-13.pdf.

36. Health Action Lobby. (2013). *Welcome to the Health Action Lobby.* Ottawa: Health Action Lobby. Retrieved from http://www.healthactionlobby.ca.

37. Elliott, J., Rutty, C., & Villeneuve, M. (2013). *The Canadian Nurses Association 1908–2008: One hundred years of service.* Ottawa: CNA.

38. See summary file, *Written submissions to the National Expert Commission,* at http://www.cna-aiic.ca/~/media/cna/files/en/commission_submissions_e.pdf.

39. Kingdon, J. (1995). *Agendas, alternatives, and public policies.* New York: Harper Collins.

40. Miljan, L. (2012). *Public policy in Canada: An introduction* (6th ed.). Don Mills, ON: Oxford University Press, p. 88.

41. Change Management Learning Center. (2014). *Change management: The systems and tools for managing change.* Retrieved from http://www.change-management.com/tutorial-change-process-detailed.htm.

42. Ibid.

43. Ibid.

44. The Influencing Public Policy workshop was originally developed by the Canadian Nurses Association in its international affairs department in 2005, and was updated numerous times in the following six years. It was an internal product of the organization that was offered to nurses in Canada and abroad.

45. Office of the Associate Director for Policy. (2014). *Using evaluation to inform CDC's policy process.* Atlanta: Centers for Disease Control and Prevention.

46. National Center for Injury Prevention and Control. (n.d.). *Brief 1: Overview of policy evaluation.* Atlanta: Centers for Disease Control and Prevention. Retrieved from http://www.cdc.gov/injury/pdfs/policy/Brief%201-a.pdf.

Chapter 10

1. UNAIDS. (2016). *About Sheila Dinotshe Tlou, Director, RST for Eastern and Southern Africa, UNAIDS.* Geneva: UNAIDS. Retrieved from http://www.unaids.org/en/aboutunaids/unaidsleadership/bios/rstdirectorforeasternandsouthernafrica.

2. Unknown (Writer), & Bonfiglio, M., Berlinger, J., Marion, A., & Sinofsky, B. (Directors). (2011, February 13). Condoleeza Rice [television series episode]. In O. Winfrey, J. Berlinger, J. Kamen, J. Wilkes, J. Sinclair, & R. Friedman (Producers), *Oprah presents: Master class.* Chicago: Harpo Studios.

3. Cabinet Secretariat in partnership with the Centre for Learning and Development. (n.d.). *Writing briefing notes.* St. John's, NL: Government of Newfoundland and Labrador. Retrieved from http://www.policynl.ca/policydevelopment/documents/Writing-Briefing-Notes.pdf.

4. World Health Organization. (2015). *Evidence briefs for policy.* Geneva: WHO. Retrieved from http://www.who.int/evidence/resources/policy_briefs.

5. McMaster Health Forum. (2015). *Evidence/issue briefs.* Hamilton, ON: McMaster Health Forum. Retrieved from https://www.mcmasterhealthforum.org/stakeholders/evidence-briefs-and-stakeholder-dialogues.

6. Canadian Nursing Students' Association. (2011). *How to write position statement and resolution.* Ottawa: CNSA. Retrieved from http://cnsa.ca/english/publications/resolutions-and-position-statements/how-to-write.

7. Canadian Association of Occupational Therapists. (2015). *CAOT position statements.* Ottawa: CAOT. Retrieved from http://www.caot.ca/default.asp?pageid=4.

8. Simon Fraser University. (n.d.). *Writing a position paper.* Vancouver, BC: Simon Fraser University. Retrieved from http://www.sfu.ca/cmns/130d1/WritingaPositionPaper.htm.

9. Engelli, I., & Allison, C. (2014). *Comparative policy studies: Conceptual and methodological challenges.* London: Palgrave Macmillan.

10. Parliament of Canada. (2009). *Green papers*. Ottawa: Parliament of Canada. Retrieved from http://www.lop.parl.gc.ca/ParlInfo/pages/GreenPapers.aspx.

11. O'Neill, S., & Blackmer, J. (2015). *Assisted reproduction in Canada: An overview of ethical and legal issues and recommendations for the development of national standards*. Ottawa: Canadian Medical Association.

12. Privy Council Office. (2014). *About commissions of inquiry*. Ottawa: Government of Canada. Retrieved from http://www.pco-bcp.gc.ca/index.asp?lang=eng&page=information&sub=commissions&doc=about-sujet-eng.htm.

13. The Lancet. (2014). Editorial. Nursing in the UK: Where next? *The Lancet, 383*(9931), 1781.

14. McGill University. (2017) *Health care in Canada survey*. Montreal: McGill University. Retrieved from http://www.mcgill.ca/hcic-sssc.

15. Office of the Commissioner of Lobbying of Canada. (2012). *Ten things you should know about lobbying: A practical guide for federal public office holders*. Ottawa: Office of the Commissioner of Lobbying of Canada. Retrieved from https://lobbycanada.gc.ca/eic/site/012.nsf/eng/00403.html.

16. Canadian Federation of Nurses Unions. (2014). *The Canada Health Transfer disconnect: An aging population, rising health care costs and a shrinking federal role in funding*. Ottawa: CFNU. Retrieved from https://nursesunions.ca/sites/default/files/page_turner/Canada-Health-Transfer/DD13668CA80CDE-7629C788EC64E79440/CFNU%20Finance%20Book%202015%20final.pdf.

17. Canadian Federation of Nurses Unions. (2015). *Financing interactive map*. Ottawa: CFNU. Retrieved from https://nursesunions.ca/political-action/financing-map.

18. Canadian Federation of Nurses Unions. (2016). *Issue brief*. Ottawa: CFNU. Retrieved from https://nursesunions.ca/sites/default/files/towards_a_health_social_accord_issue_brief.pdf.

19. Canadian Federation of Nurses Unions. (2016). *Towards a health and social accord*. Ottawa: CFNU. Retrieved from https://nursesunions.ca/sites/default/files/1_en_towards_a_health_and_social_accord_0.pdf.

20. Canadian Federation of Nurses Unions. (2016). *National prescription drug plan*. Ottawa: Author. Retrieved from https://nursesunions.ca/sites/default/files/6._handout_4of4_-_national_drug_plan_-_final.pdf.

21. The Canadian Press. (2015). *Press release distribution*. Toronto: The Canadian Press. Retrieved from http://www.thecanadianpress.com/distribution_services.aspx?id=164.

22. International Council of Nurses. (2015). *Position statement: Nurses and social media*. Geneva: ICN. Retrieved from http://www.icn.ch/images/stories/documents/publications/position_statements/E10a_Nurses_Social_Media.pdf.

23. American Nurses Association. (2016). *ANA on social media*. Washington: ANA. Retrieved from http://www.nursingworld.org/FunctionalMenuCategories/AboutANA/Social-Media/default.aspx; and Canadian Nurses Association. (2012). When private becomes public: The ethical challenges and opportunities of social media. *Ethics in Practice for Registered Nurses*. Ottawa: CNA. Retrieved from https://www.cna-aiic.ca/~/media/cna/page-content/pdf-en/ethics_in_practice_feb_2012_e.pdf.

24. Mickoleit, A. (2014). *Social media use by governments*. Paris: OECD. Retrieved from http://www.keepeek.com/Digital-Asset-Management/oecd/governance/social-media-use-by-governments_5jxrcmghmk0s-en#page1.

25. Fraser, R. (2011). *The nurse's social media advantage*. Indianapolis, IN: Sigma Theta Tau International.

Chapter 11

1. Singer, P., & Mapa, J. (1998). Ethics of resource allocation: Dimensions for healthcare executives. *Law & Governance, 2*(2). Retrieved from https://www.longwoods.com/content/16387.

2. Lamarche, P., Pineault, R., Rochon, J., & Sullivan, T. (2011). The policy imperative: Why better evidence in decision making? In T. Sullivan & J.-L. Denis (Eds.), *Building better health care leadership for Canada: Implementing evidence* (pp. 5–22). Montreal & Kingston: McGill-Queen's University Press, p. 10.

3. Van Herck, P., Annemans, L., Sermeus, W., & Ramaekers, D. (2013). Evidence-based health care policy in reimbursement decisions: Lessons from a series of six equivocal case-studies. *PLOS ONE, 8*(10), e78662. Retrieved from http://journals.plos.org/plosone/article?id=10.1371/journal.pone.0078662. See also Davies, P. (2004). *Is evidence based government possible?* Paper presented at the 4th Annual Campbell Collaboration Colloquium, Washington, DC.

4. Hsiao, W., & Heller, P. (2007). *What should macroeconomists know about health care policy?* Washington, DC: International Monetary Fund, p. 4. Retrieved from https://www.imf.org/external/pubs/ft/wp/2007/wp0713.pdf.

5. Frenk, J. (2004). Health and the economy: A vital relationship. *OECD Observer*. Geneva: OECD. Retrieved from http://www.oecdobserver.org/news/archivestory.php/aid/1241/Health_and_the_economy:_A_vital_relationship_.html.

6. Evans, R. (2010). The TSX gives a short course in health economics: It's the prices, stupid! *Healthcare Policy, 6*(2), 13–23.

7. Gibson, J., Martin, D., & Singer, P. (2005). Evidence, economics and ethics: Resource allocation in health services organizations. *Healthcare Quarterly, 8*(2), 50–59.

8. Simoens, S., Villeneuve, M., & Hurst, J. (2005). *Tackling nursing shortages in OECD member countries.* Working Papers No. 19. Paris: OECD.

9. Needleman, J. (2015). *Economic and business case for quality and safety.* Presented at the Quality and Safety Summit: Leveraging Nursing Leadership, Toronto, Ontario.

10. Gibson, J., Martin, D., & Singer, P. (2005). Evidence, economics and ethics: Resource allocation in health services organizations. *Healthcare Quarterly, 8*(2), 50–59.

11. Starzomski, R. (2012, Autumn). Toward a moral horizon: Nursing ethics for leadership and practice. *Communiqué*. Retrieved from http://www.uvic.ca/hsd/nursing/assets/docs/research/communique/2012%20Autumn%20Communique.pdf.

12. Storch, J., & Rodney, P. (n.d.). *Leadership for ethical policy and practice.* Ottawa: Canadian Health Services Research Foundation.

13. Canadian Nurses Association. (2008). *Code of Ethics for Registered Nurses.* Ottawa: CNA, p. 4.

14. Peter, E. (2011). Fostering social justice: The possibilities of a socially connected model of moral agency. *Canadian Journal of Nursing Research, 43*(2), 11–17.

15. Van Herck, P., Annemans, L., Sermeus, W., & Ramaekers, D. (2013). Evidence-based health care policy in reimbursement decisions: Lessons from a series of six equivocal case-studies. *PLOS ONE, 8*(10), e78662. Retrieved from http://journals.plos.org/plosone/article?id=10.1371/journal.pone.0078662.

16. Gibson, J., Martin, D., & Singer, P. (2005). Evidence, economics and ethics: Resource allocation in health services organizations. *Healthcare Quarterly, 8*(2), 50–59.

17. Katikireddi, S., Higgins, M., Bond, L., Bonell, C., & Macintyre, S. (2011). How evidence based is English public health policy? *British Medical Journal, 343*, d7310. Retrieved from doi:10.1136/bmj.d7310.

18. Greenhalgh, T., Howick, J., & Maskrey, N. (2014). Evidence based medicine: A movement in crisis? *British Medical Journal, 348*, g3725. Retrieved from http://dx.doi.org/10.1136/bmj.g3725.

19. Hay, D. (2007). *Developing a Canadian economic case for financing the social determinants of health.* Ottawa: Canadian Policy Research Networks.

20. Brownson, R., Chriqui, J., & Stamatakis, K. (2009). Understanding evidence-based public health policy. *American Journal of Public Health, 99*(9), 1576–1583, p. 1577.

21. Picard, A. (2015, September 27). Life support: Medicare's mid-life crisis [radio broadcast]. *The Sunday Edition with Michael Enright.* Toronto: CBC.

22. Keynes, J. (1937, March 11). Borrowing for defence: Is it inflation? A plea for organised policy. *The Times*, pp. 17–18.

23. Turner, C. (2015, September 16). Stephen Harper's war on experts. *Toronto Star.* Retrieved from https://www.thestar.com/opinion/commentary/2015/09/16/stephen-harpers-war-on-experts.html.

24. Pedwell, T. (2012, July 10). Scientists take aim at Harper cuts with "death of evidence" protest on Parliament Hill. *Globe and Mail.* Retrieved from http://www.theglobeandmail.com/news/politics/scientists-take-aim-at-harper-cuts-with-death-of-evidence-protest-on-parliament-hill/article4403233.

25. Myles, J. (2013). Evidence and decision-making: Bend it like Harper. *The Broadbent Blog.* Toronto: The Broadbent Institute. Retrieved from http://www.broadbentinstitute.ca/evidence_and_decision_making_bend_it_like_harper.

26. Ibid.

27. Walt, G., Shiffman, J., Schneider, H., Murray, S., Brughas, R., & Gilson, L. (2008). "Doing" health policy analysis: Methodological and conceptual reflections and challenges. *Health Policy and Planning, 23*, 308–317, p. 310.

28. Giacomini, M., Hurley, J., Gold, I., Smith, P., & Ableson, J. (2001). *"Values" in Canadian health policy analysis: What are we talking about?* Ottawa: Canadian Health Services Research Foundation, p. 21.

29. Ibid., p. i.

30. Ibid.

31. Greenhalgh, T., Howick, J., & Maskrey, N. (2014). Evidence based medicine: A movement in crisis? *British Medical Journal, 348*, g3725. Retrieved from http://dx.doi.org/10.1136/bmj.g3725.

32. Ibid.

33. Global Policy Forum. (2015). *Globalization*. New York: Global Policy Forum. Retrieved from https://www.globalpolicy.org/globalization.html.

34. World Health Organization. (2015). *Globalization of health*. Geneva: WHO.

35. Schroth, L., & Khawaja, R. (2007). Globalization of healthcare. *Frontiers of Health Services Management, 24*(2), 9–30.

36. Benatar, S., Gill, S., & Bakker, I. (2011). Global health and the global economic crisis. *American Journal of Public Health, 101*(4), 646–653, p. 647.

37. Kickbusch, I. (2011). Global health diplomacy: How foreign policy can influence health. *British Medical Journal, 342*, d3154. Retrieved from http://dx.doi.org/10.1136/bmj.d3154.

38. Ibid.

39. Lenihan, D. (2009). Rethinking the public policy process: A public engagement framework. Ottawa: The Public Policy Forum, p. 7.

40. Libertarian Party of Canada. (2015). *Platform*. Ottawa: Libertarian Party of Canada.

41. Communist Party of Canada. (2010). *Constitution of the Communist Party of Canada*. Toronto: Communist Party of Canada.

42. Wallner, P., & Konski, A. (2008). The impact of technology on health care cost and policy development. *Seminars in Radiation Oncology, 18*(3), 194–200.

43. Merriam-Webster. (2015). *Institution*. Retrieved from http://www.merriam-webster.com/dictionary/politics.

44. Smith, N., Mitton, C., Bryan, S., Davidson, A., Urquhart, B., Gibson, J., et al. (2013). Decision maker perceptions of resource allocation processes in Canadian health care organizations: A national survey. *BMC Health Services Research, 13*, 247. Retrieved from http://www.ncbi.nlm.nih.gov/pmc/articles/PMC3750381.

45. Campaign Life Coalition. (2015). *Ontario's radical sex ed curriculum*. Ottawa: Campaign Life Coalition. Retrieved from http://www.campaignlifecoalition.com/index.php?p=Sex_Ed_Curriculum.

46. Obama, B. (2016). United States health care reform: Progress to date and next steps. *Journal of the American Medical Association, 316*(5), 525–532. Retrieved from http://jama.jamanetwork.com/article.aspx?articleid=2533698.

47. Busby, C., & Blomqvist, Å. (2016). *Challenging vested interests: National priorities for healthcare in 2016. E-Brief.* Toronto: C.D. Howe Institute.

48. Shiffman, J., Quissell, K., Schmitz, H., Pelletier, D., Smith, S., Berlan, D., et al. (2016). A framework on the emergence and effectiveness of global health networks. *Health Policy and Planning, 31*, i3–i16, p. i4.

49. Ibid.

50. Davies, P. (2005, March 3). *Evidence-based government: How do we make it happen?* Keynote address, Seventh Annual Workshop of the Canadian Health Services Research Foundation, Montreal, Quebec.

51. Liberal Party of Canada. (2015). *Carolyn Bennett, MP: Biography*. Ottawa: Liberal Party of Canada. Retrieved from http://carolynbennett.ca/biography.

52. Reich, M. (1995). The politics of health sector reform in developing countries: Three cases of pharmaceutical policy. *Health Policy, 43*(1–3), 47–77.

53. Cerna, L. (2013). *The nature of policy change and implementation: A review of different theoretical approaches*. Paris: OECD.

54. Savoie, D. (2015). *What is government good at? A Canadian answer*. Montreal: McGill-Queen's University Press, p. 179.

55. Glavine, L. (2016). Nurses: Champions for a new health accord. *The Kings County Register/Advertiser*. Retrieved from http://www.kingscountynews.ca/Opinion/Columnists/2016-07-06/article-4578755/GLAVINE-COLUMN%3A-Nurses%3A-champions-for-a-new-health-accord/1.

56. Nelson, S., & Rafferty, A. (2010). Introduction. In S. Nelson & A. Rafferty (Eds.), *Notes on Nightingale* (pp. 1–8). Ithaca, NY: Cornell University Press, p. 6.

57. Emory University Health Sciences Center. (2001, October 11). Global Nursing Partnerships conference addresses international nursing shortage. *EurekAlert*. Retrieved from https://www.eurekalert.org/pub_releases/2001-10/euhs-gnp101101.php.

58. Liaschenko, J., & Peter, E. (2016). Fostering nurses' moral agency and moral identity: The importance of moral community. *Hastings Center Report, 46*, S18–S21.

59. Tronto, J. (1993). *Moral boundaries: A political argument for an ethic of care*. New York: Routledge.

60. Needleman, J. (2015). *Economic and business case for quality and safety*. Presented at the Quality and Safety Summit: Leveraging Nursing Leadership, Toronto, Ontario.

61. Liaschenko, J., & Peter, E. (2016). Fostering

nurses' moral agency and moral identity: The importance of moral community. *Hastings Center Report, 46*, S18–S21, p. S20.

62. Splane, R., & Splane, V. (1994). *Chief nursing officer positions in national ministries of health: Focal points for nursing leadership*. San Francisco: University of California.

63. Harrison, M. (1968). Foot in the door. *The Canadian Nurse, 64*(10), 40–45, p. 41.

64. Ibid.

65. World Health Organization. (2015). *Roles and responsibilities of government chief nursing and midwifery officers: A capacity-building manual*. Geneva: WHO.

66. World Health Organization. (2013). *WHO nursing and midwifery progress report 2008–2012*. Geneva: WHO, p. 9. Retrieved from http://www.who.int/hrh/nursing_midwifery/NursingMidwiferyProgressReport.pdf.

Chapter 12

1. Eliot. T. (1942, September 19). Little Gidding. *New English Weekly*.

2. Picard, A. (2015, September 27). Life support: Medicare's mid-life crisis [radio broadcast]. *The Sunday Edition with Michael Enright*. Toronto: CBC.

3. Greenhalgh, T., Howick, J., & Maskrey, N. (2014). Evidence based medicine: A movement in crisis? *British Medical Journal, 348*, g3725. Retrieved from http://dx.doi.org/10.1136/bmj.g3725.

4. Carthey, J., Walker, S., Deelchand, V., Vincent, C., & Griffiths, W. (2011). Breaking the rules: Understanding non-compliance with policies and guidelines. *British Medical Journal, 343*, d5283. Retrieved from http://dx.doi.org/10.1136/bmj.d5283.

5. Advisory Panel on Healthcare Innovation. (2015). *Unleashing innovation: Excellent healthcare for Canada*. Executive summary. Ottawa: Health Canada. Retrieved from http://www.healthycanadians.gc.ca/publications/health-system-systeme-sante/summary-innovation-sommaire/index-eng.php.

6. Canadian Federation of Nurses Unions. (2016). *United towards a health accord: Issue brief*. Ottawa: CFNU.

7. Goodfellow, C. (2014). The dramatic dehospitalization of health services is a prerequisite for a sustainable and effective health system. *Healthcare Management Forum, 27*, 148–151.

8. National Expert Commission. (2012). *A nursing call to action: The health of our nation, the future of our health system*. Ottawa: Canadian Nurses Association.

9. Truth and Reconciliation Commission of Canada. (2015). *Truth and Reconciliation Commission of Canada: Calls to action*. Winnipeg: TRC, p. 3.

10. Governor General of Canada. (2016). *Making real change happen: Speech from the throne to open the first session of the forty-second Parliament of Canada*. Ottawa: Government of Canada.

11. CBC News. (2016, May 9). Canada removing objector status to UN Declaration on the Rights of Indigenous Peoples. *CBC News*. Retrieved from http://www.cbc.ca/news/aboriginal/canada-position-un-declaration-indigenous-peoples-1.3572777.

12. CBC News. (2016, May 10). Canada officially adopts UN declaration on rights of indigenous peoples. *CBC News*. Retrieved from http://www.cbc.ca/news/aboriginal/canada-adopting-implementing-un-rights-declaration-1.3575272.

13. Advisory Panel on Healthcare Innovation. (2015). *Unleashing innovation: Excellent healthcare for Canada*. Executive summary. Ottawa: Health Canada, p. 120. Retrieved from http://www.healthycanadians.gc.ca/publications/health-system-systeme-sante/summary-innovation-sommaire/index-eng.php.

14. Mark, B., & Harless, D. (2007). Nurse staffing, mortality, and length of stay in for-profit and not-for-profit hospitals. *Inquiry—Excellus Health Plan, 44*(2), 167–182.

15. Devereaux, P., Heels-Ansdell, D., & Lacchetti, C., Haines, T., Burns, K., Cook, D., … Guyatt, G. (2004). Payments for care at private for-profit and private not-for-profit hospitals: A systematic review and meta-analysis. *Canadian Medical Association Journal, 170*, 1817–1824.

16. Hopkins Tanne, J. (2002). Mortality higher at for-profit hospitals. *British Medical Journal, 324*(7350), 1351.

17. Devereaux, P., Schunemann, H., Ravindran, N., Bhandari, M., Garg, A., et al. (2002). Comparison of mortality between private for-profit and private not-for-profit hemodialysis centers: A systematic review and meta-analysis. *Journal of the American Medical Association, 288*, 2449–2457.

18. Comondore, V., Devereaux, P., Zhou, Q., Stone, S., Busse, J., Ravindran, N., et al. (2009). Quality of care in for-profit and not-for-profit nursing homes: Systematic review and meta-analysis. *British Medical Journal, 339*(7717), 381–384. Retrieved from http://dx.doi.org/10.1136/bmj.b2732.

19. llmer, M., Wodchis, W., Gill, S., Anderson, G., & Rochon, P. (2005). Nursing home profit status and

quality of care: Is there any evidence of an association? *Medical Care Research Review, 62,* 139–166.

20. Sutherland, T., & Crump, R.T. (2013). Alternative level of care: Canada's hospital beds, the evidence and options. *Healthcare Policy, 9*(1), 26–34. Retrieved from https://www.longwoods.com/content/23480.

21. Canadian Institute for Health Information. (2009). *Alternate level of care in Canada.* Ottawa: CIHI. Retrieved from https://secure.cihi.ca/free_products/ALC_AIB_FINAL.pdf.

22. Chan, B., & Cochrane, D. (2016). *Measuring patient harm in Canadian hospitals.* Ottawa: Canadian Institute for Health Information and Canadian Patient Safety Institute, p. 38.

23. Prince, M., Wimo, A., Guerchet, M., Ali, G., Wu, Y., Prina, M., & Alzheimer's Disease International. (2015). *World Alzheimer report 2015: The global impact of dementia.* London: Alzheimer's Disease International.

24. Canadian Institute for Health Information. (2012). *Seniors and alternate level of care: Building on our knowledge.* Ottawa: CIHI.

25. Organisation for Economic Co-Operation and Development. (2016). *Health workforce policies in OECD countries: Right jobs, right skills, right places.* Paris: OECD.

26. Obama, B. (2016). United States health care reform: Progress to date and next steps. *Journal of the American Medical Association, 316*(5), 525–532. Retrieved from http://jama.jamanetwork.com/article.aspx?articleid=2533698.

27. Soroka, S., & Mahon, A. (2012). *An analysis of the impact of current health care system funding and financing models and the value of health and health care in Canada.* Ottawa: Canadian Health Services Research Foundation and Canadian Nurses Association.

28. National Expert Commission. (2012). *A nursing call to action: The health of our nation, the future of our health system.* Ottawa: Canadian Nurses Association, p. 16.

29. Browne, G., Birch, S., & Thebane, L. (2012). *Better care: An analysis of nursing and healthcare system outcomes.* Ottawa: Canadian Nurses Association and Canadian Health Services Research Foundation.

30. Canadian Institute for Health Information. (2014). *Sources of potentially avoidable emergency department visits.* Ottawa: CIHI.

31. Fowler, R., & Hammer, M. (2013). End-of-life care in Canada. *Clinical & Investigative Medicine, 35*(3), E127–E132.

32. Duggan, K. (2016, June 27). Civil Liberties Association taking assisted dying law to court. *iPolitics.* Retrieved from https://ipolitics.ca/2016/06/27/b-c-civil-liberties-association-taking-assisted-dying-law-to-court.

33. Canadian Nurses Association. (2015). *Respecting choices in end-of-life care: Challenges and opportunities for RNs.* Ottawa: CNA, p. 32.

34. Baker, G., Norton, P., Flintoft, V., Blais, R., Brown, A., Cox, J., et al. (2004). The Canadian Adverse Events Study: The incidence of adverse events among hospital patients in Canada. *Canadian Medical Association Journal, 170*(11), 1678–1686.

35. Makary, M., & Daniel, M. (2016). Medical error—the third leading cause of death in the US. *British Medical Journal.* Retrieved from http://dx.doi.org/10.1136/bmj.i2139.

36. Chan, B., & Cochrane, D. (2016). Measuring patient harm in Canadian hospitals. Ottawa: Canadian Institute for Health Information and Canadian Patient Safety Institute.

37. Weir, A. (Writer), & Lanning, G. (Director). (2003, October 15). Cutting corners [television series episode]. In A. Barro & B. Vaillot (Executive Producers), *Mayday: Air disasters.* Toronto and Paris: Near-Miss Productions, Inc., Galaxie Production, & Media Production Services, Ltd.

38. Picard, A. (2010, July 14). Universal health care matters, but so does quality. *Globe and Mail.* Retrieved from http://www.theglobeandmail.com/life/health-and-fitness/universal-health-care-matters-but-so-does-quality/article1387165.

39. Shamian, J. (2014). Global perspectives on nursing and its contribution to healthcare and health policy: Thoughts on an emerging policy model. *Canadian Journal of Nursing Leadership, 27*(4), 44–50, p. 44.

40. Quinlan, P. (2014, December 10). Dr. Tim Porter-O'Grady addresses what nurses can expect in the future. *The landscape of nursing's future.* Retrieved from https://www.youtube.com/watch?v=zDCSU3MlWpA.

41. Needleman, J. (2015). *Economic and business case for quality and safety.* Presented at the Quality and Safety Summit: Leveraging Nursing Leadership, Toronto, Ontario.

42. Quinlan, P. (2014, December 10). Dr. Tim Porter-O'Grady addresses what nurses can expect in the future. *Nursing Success TV.* Retrieved from https://www.youtube.com/watch?v=zDCSU3MlWpA.

43. Snowdon, A., Schnarr, K., Hussein, A., & Alessi,

C. (2012). *Measuring what matters: The cost vs. values of health care*. London, ON: Ivey International Centre for Health Innovation, Western University.

44. Harris, A., & McGillis Hall, L. (2012). *Evidence to inform staff mix decision-making: A focused literature review*. Ottawa: Canadian Nurses Association. Retrieved from https://www.cna-aiic.ca/~/media/cna/page-content/pdf-en/staff_mix_literature_review_e.pdf.

45. Unknown (Writer), & Bonfiglio, M., Berlinger, J., Marion, A., & Sinofsky, B. (Directors). (2011, January 16). Maya Angelou [television series episode]. In O. Winfrey, J. Berlinger, J. Kamen, J. Wilkes, J. Sinclair, & R. Friedman (Producers), *Oprah presents: Master class*. Chicago: Harpo Studios.

46. Davis, Sister E. (2005, March 3). *Dory, rainbow and inuksuk*. Keynote address, Seventh Annual Workshop of the Canadian Health Services Research Foundation, Montreal, Quebec.

47. Nelson, S., Turnbull, J., Bainbridge, L., Caulfield, T., Hudon, G., Kendel, D., Mowat, D., Nasmith, L., Postl, B., Shamian, J., & Sketris, I. (2014). *Optimizing scopes of practice: New models for a new health care system*. Ottawa: Canadian Academy of Health Sciences.

48. Ipsos Reid. (2015, June). *Expectations of the health care system*. Presented at HealthCareCAN, Ottawa, Ontario.

49. Nelson, S., Turnbull, J., Bainbridge, L., Caulfield, T., Hudon, G., Kendel, D., Mowat, D., Nasmith, L., Postl, B., Shamian, J., & Sketris, I. (2014). *Optimizing scopes of practice: New models for a new health care system*. Ottawa: Canadian Academy of Health Sciences.

50. Canadian Nurses Association. (2015). *Framework for registered nurse prescribing in Canada*. Ottawa: CNA. Retrieved from https://www.cna-aiic.ca/~/media/cna/page-content/pdf-en/cna-rn-prescribing-framework_e.pdf.

51. Needleman, J., Buerhaus, P., Stewart, M., Zelevinsky, K., & Mattke, S. (2006). Nurse staffing in hospitals: Is there a business case for quality? *Health Affairs, 25*(1), 204–211.

52. Canadian Federation of Nurses Unions. (2015). *Trends in own illness- or disability-related absenteeism and overtime among publicly-employed registered nurses: Quick facts 2015*. Ottawa: CFNU. Retrieved from https://nursesunions.ca/sites/default/files/2015-05-05_absenteeism_and_overtime_quick_facts_en.pdf.

53. Advisory Panel on Healthcare Innovation. (2015).

Unleashing innovation: Excellent healthcare for Canada. Executive summary. Ottawa: Health Canada, p. 120. Retrieved from http://www.healthycanadians.gc.ca/publications/health-system-systeme-sante/summary-innovation-sommaire/index-eng.php.

54. Nagle, L. (2015). Editorial: The ties that bind us. *Nursing Leadership, 28*(2), 1–4.

55. Duncan, S., Thorne, S., & Rodney, P. (2015). Evolving trends in nurse regulation: What are the policy impacts for nursing's social mandate? *Nursing Inquiry, 22*(1), 27–38.

56. Osman, F. (2002). Public policy making: Theories and their implications in developing countries. *Asian Affairs, 24*(3), 37–52. Retrieved from http://www.cdrb.org/journal/2002/3/3.pdf.

57. Lenihan, D. (2009). Rethinking the public policy process: A public engagement framework. Ottawa: The Public Policy Forum, p. 26.

58. Duncan, S., Thorne, S., & Rodney, P. (2015). Evolving trends in nurse regulation: What are the policy impacts for nursing's social mandate? *Nursing Inquiry, 22*(1), 27–38, p. 35.

59. Diamandis, P. (2013, February 19). Blog: Why billion-dollar, 100-year-old companies die. *Huffington Post*. Retrieved from http://www.huffingtonpost.com/peter-diamandis/why-billion-dollar-100-ye_b_2718262.html.

60. World Health Organization. (2015). *Roles and responsibilities of government chief nursing and midwifery officers: A capacity-building manual*. Geneva: WHO.

61. Health Canada. (2013). *World Health Organization*. Ottawa: Health Canada. Retrieved from http://www.hc-sc.gc.ca/ahc-asc/intactiv/orgs/organi-eng.php.

62. World Health Organization. (2013). *Health workforce: Networks*. Retrieved from http://www.who.int/hrh/nursing_midwifery/networks.

63. World Health Organization. (2013). *WHO nursing and midwifery progress report 2008–2012*. Geneva: WHO, p. 9. Retrieved from http://www.who.int/hrh/nursing_midwifery/NursingMidwiferyProgressReport.pdf.

64. World Health Organization. (2015). *Options analysis report on strategic directions for nursing and midwifery (2016–2020)*. Geneva: WHO.

65. World Health Organization. (2015). *Global strategy on human resources for health: Workforce 2030*. Geneva: WHO, p. 8.

66. Harrison, M. (1968). Foot in the door. *The Canadian Nurse, 64*(10), 40–45, p. 41.

67. Shamian, J. (2014). Global perspectives on nursing and its contribution to healthcare and health policy: Thoughts on an emerging policy model. *Canadian Journal of Nursing Leadership, 27*(4), 44–50.

68. Ibid., p. 48.

69 United Nations Development Programme. (2017). *Millennium development goals.* New York: United Nations. Retrieved from http://www.undp.org/content/undp/en/home/sdgoverview/mdg_goals.html.

70. United Nations. (2016). *Transforming our world: The 2030 agenda for sustainable development.* Retrieved from https://sustainabledevelopment.un.org/post2015/transformingourworld.

71. High-Level Commission on Health Employment and Economic Growth. (2016). *Working for health and growth: Investing in the health workforce.* Geneva: WHO, pp. 11–12.

72. Decter, M. (1994). *Healing medicare: Managing health system change the Canadian way.* Toronto: McGillan Books.

73. Sandberg, S. (2013.) *Lean in.* New York: Knopf.

74. Obama, B. (2016). United States health care reform: Progress to date and next steps. *Journal of the American Medical Association, 16*(5), 525–532. Retrieved from http://jama.jamanetwork.com/article.aspx?articleid=2533698.

75. Ipsos Reid. (2015, June). *Expectations of the health care system.* Presented at HealthCareCAN, Ottawa, Ontario.

76. Rodney, P., Buckley, B., Street, A., Serrano, E., & Martin, L.A. (2013). The moral climate of nursing practice: Inquiry and action. In J. Storch, P. Rodney, & R. Starzomski (Eds.), *Toward a moral horizon: Nursing ethics of leadership and practice.* 2nd ed. Toronto: Pearson-Prentice Hall, p. 190.

77. Watson, J. (n.d.). *Overview: The Watson Caring Science Institute.* Retrieved from http://www.watsoncaringscience.org/images/features/library/WCSI_Overview_Mission_Statement_2_08.pdf.

COPYRIGHT ACKNOWLEDGEMENTS

Figure 3.2: © All rights reserved. *A Partner in Health for all Canadians*. Health Canada, 2014. Adapted and reproduced with permission from the Minister of Health, 2016.

Figure 6.1: © All rights reserved. *The Nursing Strategy for Canada – October 2000*. Health Canada, 2000. Adapted and reproduced with permission from the Minister of Health, 2016.

Figures 7.7, 7.9, 7.12, and 12.1: Canadian Institute for Health Information. (2015). *National Health Expenditure Trends, 1975 to 2015*. Ottawa: CIHI. Available at: https://www.cihi.ca/sites/default/files/document/nhex_trends_narrative_report_2015_en.pdf. Used by permission of the Canadian Institute for Health Information.

Figure 8.3: Davis, K., Stremikis, K., Squires, D., and Schoen, C. (2014, June). *Mirror, Mirror on the Wall: How the Performance of the U.S. Health Care System Compares Internationally*. New York: The Commonwealth Fund. Available at: http://www.commonwealthfund.org/publications/fund-reports/2014/jun/mirror-mirror. Used by permission of The Commonwealth Fund.

Figure 12.6: Sustainable development goals, United Nations, 2016. Image used by permission of the United Nations. Available at: http://www.globalgoals.org/.

INDEX